THE OCCUPATIONAL THERAPY EXAMINATION REVIEW GUIDE

Debra N. Anderson, OTR
Administrative Director of Occupational Therapy
Frye Regional Medical Center
Hickory, North Carolina

and

Adjunct Instructor
Department of Occupational Therapy
Lenoir-Rhyne College
Hickory, North Carolina

Jolene Marie Jacobson, OTR
Occupational Therapist
Health South
Northern Kentucky Rehabilitation Hospital
Edgewood, Kentucky

Mary Kathryn Cowan, MA, OTR, FAOTA
Professor
Department of Occupational Therapy
Eastern Kentucky University
Richmond, Kentucky

Jean Steffan Smith, MS, OTR
Associate Professor
Department of Occupational Therapy
Eastern Kentucky University
Richmond, Kentucky

F. A. DAVIS COMPANY • Philadelphia

F. A. Davis Company
1915 Arch Street
Philadelphia, PA 19103

Printed in the United States of America

Last digit indicates print number: 10 9 8 7 6 5 4 3

Publisher: Jean-François Vilain
Editor: Lynn Borders Caldwell
Production Editor: Glenn L. Fechner
Cover Designer: Steven R. Morrone

As new scientific information becomes available through basic and clinical research, recommended treatments and drug therapies undergo changes. The authors and publisher have done everything possible to make this book accurate, up to date, and in accord with accepted standards at the time of publication. The authors, editors, and publisher are not responsible for errors or omissions or for consequences from application of the book, and make no warranty, expressed or implied, in regard to the contents of the book. Any practice described in this book should be applied by the reader in accordance with professional standards of care used in regard to the unique circumstances that may apply in each situation. The reader is advised always to check product information (package inserts) for changes and new information regarding dose and contraindications before administering any drug. Caution is especially urged when using new or infrequently ordered drugs.

Library of Congress Cataloging-in-Publication Data

The occupational therapy examination review guide / Debra N. Anderson
. . . [et al.].
    p.   cm.
    Includes bibliographical references.
    ISBN 0-8036-0029-1
    1. Occupational therapy--Examinations, questions, etc.
I. Anderson, Debra N., 1961–
RM735.32.024   1996
616.8′515′076--dc20   95-46117

To Jean Steffan Smith, friend and colleague
1952–1996

FOREWORD

The purpose of this book is to support preparation for the National Board for Certification in Occupational Therapy (NBCOT) regulatory examination, "the certification exam." It accomplishes that purpose admirably! *The Occupational Therapy Examination Review Guide* prepares the reader for the test and provides five simulated examinations that cover occupational therapy curriculum content according to the major subject areas of the certification examination.

Introductory information describes the certification examination and its regulations, instructions for how to use the book, and test taking tips. These data suggest how best to structure the process of applying for the test, establishing study schedules, and reviewing curriculum content in preparation for the examination.

Following the introduction, five simulated examinations, each 200 questions in length, are presented. The simulations match the content outline of the certification examination: pediatrics, physical disabilities, psychosocial dysfunctions, and management and administration. Each examination is followed by answers to the questions. A major strength of this text is that not only are the answers given, but the clinical reasoning used to arrive at the correct answer is explained. Answers are referenced to current literature. The questions are well constructed and challenge the reader to use critical thinking skills to arrive at the correct responses. Similar questions appear in dif-ferent modes from one examination to another, which is an excellent way for the reader to test his or her knowledge. A comprehensive bibliography is provided for easy reference. These unique features make this text useful for instruction, as well as for review in preparation for the certification examination.

For most candidates, anticipating the required certification examination is the occasion of excitement at nearing professional status, but it also evokes some anxiety about taking and passing the examination. This book provides an approach to exam preparation and study that can significantly reduce test anxiety.

The Occupational Therapy Examination Review Guide is written in a style that is clear and easy to understand. It will be most welcome by students or foreign-trained therapists preparing for the certification examination, therapists changing practice areas or reentering practice who wish to update their knowledge, and occupational therapy educators responsible for preparing students for the examination. The authors have created a significant contribution to occupational therapy education and literature with this work.

Lorraine Williams Pedretti, MS, OTR
Professor Emeritus
San José State University
San José, California

PREFACE

This workbook has been written to provide occupational therapy students with a general review of the profession and to give them study tools to use while preparing to take the certification examination. It will also serve as an excellent review for occupational therapists who may be reentering the field or changing areas of practice.

The textbooks used as references for the questions are those most commonly required for purchase by students in occupational therapy educational programs across the United States. Realizing that original sources may not be available to students, the authors chose to cite materials to which students have easy access. In this way, *The Occupational Therapy Examination Guide* has been designed to complement occupational therapy curricula; encouraging individuals to synthesize knowledge and become comfortable with the format of the National Board for Certification in Occupational Therapy (NBCOT) certification examination.

Please keep in mind that this workbook will not:

- be a comprehensive guide to the practice of occupational therapy as represented in textbooks available to students,
- replicate the exam or any of the questions on the exam, or
- offer the student a guarantee of passing the exam.

This workbook will:

- provide a general review of the practice of occupatonal therapy,
- assist the student in identifying strengths and weaknesses in knowledge of occupational therapy,
- acquaint the student with the format of questions used on the exam,
- help the student organize and set priorities for study time, and
- provide the student with a reference list from which further study may be pursued.

ACKNOWLEDGMENTS

There are many individuals who have been helpful in the development of this book. Our deepest appreciation goes to our families and friends for their moral support and encouragement throughout the project. In addition, we would like to thank the students of Pi Theta Epsilon at Eastern Kentucky University for providing us with a forum to "test" many of the questions and tips in this book.

For their time and ideas in the review process, we thank

Barbara Borg, MA, OTR
Lecturer
Department of Occupational Therapy
Colorado State University
Ft. Collins, Colorado

Brent H. Braveman, MEd, OTR
Director, Clinical Services
Department of Occupational Therapy
University of Illinois at Chicago
Chicago, Illinois

Jane Case-Smith, EdD, OTR
Assistant Professor
Department of Occupational Therapy
Ohio State University
Columbus, Ohio

Linda Duncombe, MS, OTR
Clinical Associate Professor
Department of Occupational Therapy
Boston University
Boston, Massachusetts

Jim Hinojosa, PhD, OTR, FAOTA
Associate Professor
Department of Occupational Therapy
New York University
New York, New York

Caryn Johnson, MS, OTR
Assistant Academic Fieldwork Coordinator
Department of Occupational Therapy
Thomas Jefferson University
Philadelphia, Pennsylvania

Elizabeth M. Kanny, MA, OTR, FAOTA
Lecturer and Head
Division of Occupational Therapy
Department of Rehabilitation Medicine
University of Washington
Seattle, Washington

Judith G. Kimball, PhD, OTR, FAOTA
Chair
Department of Occupational Therapy
University of New England
Biddeford, Maine

Paula Kramer, PhD, OTR
Professor and Chair
Department of Occupational Therapy
Kean College of New Jersey
Union, New Jersey

Shelly J. Lane, PhD, OTR, FAOTA
Assistant Professor
Department of Occupational Therapy
State University of New York
Buffalo, New York

Lela A. Llorens, PhD, OTR, FAOTA
Associate Vice President/Faculty Affairs
San Jose State University
San Jose, California

Gladys N. Masagatani, MEd, OTR, FAOTA
Professor
Department of Occupational Therapy
Eastern Kentucky University
Richmond, Kentucky

Jaime Phillip Muñoz, MS, OTR
Clinical Instructor
Department of Occupational Therapy
Duquesne University
Pittsburgh, Pennsylvania

Lorraine Williams Pedretti, MS, OTR
Professor Emeritus
Department of Occupational Therapy
San Jose State University
San Jose, California

Nancy Jane Powell, PhD, OTR, FAOTA
Associate Professor
Department of Occupational Therapy
Wayne State University
College of Pharmacy and Allied Health Professions
Detroit, Michigan

Patricia Nuse Pratt, MOT, OTR, FAOTA
Private Practice
Cleveland, Georgia

Linda Kohlman Thomson, MOT, OTR, OT(C), FAOTA
Manager
Occupational Therapy
St. Joseph Hospital
Bellingham, Washington

We would especially like to thank Lynn Borders Caldwell for her vision and guidance throughout the project.

CONTENTS

PREPARING FOR THE EXAMINATION

WHAT IS THE NBCOT EXAMINATION?

Successful completion of the certification examination is required for any individual who wishes to practice as a registered occupational therapist (OTR). The culmination of academic and fieldwork study rests on passing the National Board for Certification in Occupational Therapy (NBCOT) regulatory examination. The examination tests the student's *depth* of knowledge. The questions require that the student apply knowledge of occupational therapy or synthesize bits of knowledge to select the correct answer. The purpose of the examination is to identify those candidates that exhibit entry-level competence for the practice of occupational therapy. Once a candidate has successfully completed the examination, he or she is certified as an occupational therapist. Certification exams are given on the third Saturdays in March and September. Examinations are given for both certified occupational therapy assistant (COTA) and registered occupational therapy (OTR) candidates. Approximately 66,500 occupational therapy practitioners have been certified in the past 65 years.

WHO CAN TAKE THE CERTIFICATION EXAMINATION?

The NBCOT oversees the certification examination and eligibility of candidates. Candidates must have graduated from an accredited or approved occupational therapy program and successfully completed fieldwork assignments in order to take the certification examination. Beginning in 1997, candidates are required to submit course transcripts from accredited occupational therapy programs. In addition, program directors from the educational settings provide the NBCOT with a list of students who have met the educational criteria to sit for the examination. The NBCOT then sends the candidate handbook to those students who are eligible. It is important that your program director have your correct mailing address to give to the NBCOT.

WHAT IS THE FORMAT OF THE EXAMINATION?

The certification examination is composed of 200 multiple choice questions that use the four-option format. Candidates are given 4 hours in which to complete the examination.

The actual questions for the examination have been developed by the Certification Examination Development Committee. The committee consists of a group of content experts, occupational therapists, and occupational therapy assistants from all over the United States and from a variety of treatment settings. A content outline for the certification examination was developed from the 1991 AOTCB (now the NBCOT) "National Study of the Profession of Occupational Therapy" (American Occupational Therapy Certification Board 1995). This approach provides a comprehensive overview of the service areas and issues pertaining to the practice of occupational therapy.

For each administration of the examination, a new set of questions is drawn from a "pool" or "item bank." Separate item banks exist for the OTR and COTA examinations. The questions on each examination correspond to the content outline for either OTR or COTA candidates. The content outline identifies how many items should be asked for each major practice area. Each item has the same weight in scoring, and every question on the examination has only one correct answer. There is not a penalty for guessing. The raw scores of correct answers are statistically converted to a "scaled score," which ranges from 300 to 600 points. A scaled score of 450 or higher is required to pass the examination.

WHAT HAPPENS AFTER THE EXAMINATION?

Test results are mailed approximately 1 month after the certification examination. The rate of students who pass the examination is usually in the 94th percentile range or higher. As previously stated, a score of 450 or higher is required to pass the certification examination.

Candidates may request that results be sent to the licensing agency of the state in which they will choose to practice. Candidates will have three opportunities to pass the exam. A fourth attempt may be allowed after filing an approved remedial plan. The three opportunities are counted consecutively from the time that the candidate is eligible to take the exam. Each time the exam is offered, the score is counted in the attempt total, whether the candidate actually takes the exam or not.

It is recommended that the candidate complete an application for state licensure before taking the examination. Often, these applications require a notarized copy of transcripts from an accredited occupational therapy program, letters of reference, a picture identification, and so forth.

Depending on the state licensure laws and facility requirements, therapists may or may not be able to work on a temporary permit until examination results are received. Contact the licensing agency as soon as you know in which state you will be practicing (if the state requires licensure for occupational therapy). **Candidates should learn as early as possible what information will be necessary for licensure and when applications should be submitted.**

HOW DO I APPLY FOR THE EXAMINATION?

A candidate handbook is sent to eligible candidates by the NBCOT approximately 4 months before the examination. Within this handbook is an application for the examination, a few study questions, and general information regarding the examination. The basic fee for taking the examination is $250. (Additional fees may be incurred for requesting a special test site, reporting of scores to state regulatory agencies, or processing of a late application.) Late applications may be processed for an additional fee.

Individuals from outside the United States have different deadline dates and should verify these dates with the NBCOT. Information specific to these candidates can be found in the "Foreign Graduate Packet," which may be requested from the NBCOT. Foreign candidates are required to successfully complete three English proficiency tests prior to taking the NBCOT exam. If a candidate does not receive his or her handbook, which outlines all of this information, he or she may call the NBCOT at (301) 990-7979. Once the NBCOT has received the application, the candidate will be mailed a confirmation; however, individuals may choose to send the application by certified mail to receive a returned receipt from the post office.

There are more than 50 testing sites within the United States and approximately 8 other sites located in foreign countries, including Canada, China, England, India, and Israel.[1]

HOW DO I USE THIS BOOK?

This book has five complete sample tests of 200 questions that simulate the actual examination by asking questions in a four-option multiple-choice format. At the end of this chapter, there is also a section that offers test taking "tips." The tips provide the reader with tools to identify his or her strengths and weaknesses as well as to organize and to set priorities for study time. The test taking tips are followed by the five practice examinations. The first four examinations provide questions that are divided by the general topics that reflect practice areas. For example, all of the questions are grouped for pediatrics, physical disabilities, psychosocial dysfunctions, or administration and management. Within the first three topic areas (pediatrics, physical disabilities, and psychosocial dysfunctions), a specific percentage of questions are asked pertaining to the following items:

15%—Assessment of occupational performance
23%—Development of the treatment plan
19%—Implementation of the treatment plan
10%—Evaluation of the treatment plan
 9%—Discharge planning

The topic area of Administration and Management is divided into two item categories:

12%—Organize and manage services
12%—Promote professional practice

These areas are the same as those used by the NBCOT (formerly the AOTCB) in the content outline (American Occupational Therapy Certification Board 1995). The content outline identifies the percentage of questions to be asked for each major area of practice and is printed in the candidate handbook.

By dividing each of the first four simulation examinations into the above categories, the reader is able to focus on one topic per item at a time. The final examination, Simulation Examination 5, mixes the topic areas, as is done in the actual examination. This format is a bit more difficult in that it requires the reader to change clinical focus frequently. This final examination also allows the reader to evaluate how well he or she has retained and been able to implement the techniques recommended in this book.

The mix of questions in each test covers the range of occupational therapy interventions from referral through discharge, thus providing a general review of the profession. A complete set of answers follows each examination. The format of the answers provides additional benefit to the reader because they explain why wrong answers are wrong and why right answers are right. In addition, each answer provides the reader with a reference from which further information may be obtained.

A complete bibliography, including primary textbooks that the reader is likely to own, is located at the end of this book. These texts were selected based on results of a survey of educators, which assisted the authors in identifying which textbooks are most frequently used in occupational therapy curricula.

WHERE DO I BEGIN?

Preparing to take the examination can be overwhelming when you look at the "big picture." By breaking the process into smaller parts, it is easier to manage. The first step to work through is to identify your areas of strength as well as your weaknesses. A personal study plan (Tables 1 and 2) will help you through this process. Once this has been completed, the second step is to invest time into completing the study plan. The final step is to pull all of the information together to take the practice examinations. It may be helpful to review the test taking tips frequently and to integrate these techniques into working through the practice examinations.

TEST TAKING TIPS

Test Taking Tip 1

Create a personal study plan. The question most frequently asked by occupational therapy students preparing for the examination is "How do I start?" This guide will assist you in pulling the process of educational preparation together, organizing your study time, and helping you to become comfortable with answering multiple-choice questions. Whether or not they use this book, students preparing for the examination first need to have their course work at their fingertips. This material includes books, notes, handouts, and so forth.

Once the student is settled with the stacks of information that have taken years to accumulate, the question arises, "Where do I start?" See the following examples:

1. Complete Table 2 by first defining your areas of strength as well as those that may be weaker. An example is provided in Table 1. This is done by choosing a main practice area and then working down the page through all the component parts for that category.
2. Classify areas from the weakest area with an "A" to the strongest area with a "D." Those areas that are neither a strength nor a weakness will be a "B" or "C," with "B" being weaker than "C."
3. Within each letter grouping, identify the weakest subject with a number 1 and sequentially number through to the strongest subject.

Once this step has been completed, *your* individualized studying needs have been organized and priorities have been set for accomplishment. The lower the number, the higher it is on the priority list for study.

Now that priorities have been set for studying, the next activity is to write target dates for review for each area and subject. For instance, one individual may choose to work on the area of pediatrics during the month of March. Another individual may choose to review pediatric assessments the first week of March, developmental stages the second week of March, and so forth. Design *your* study plan to meet *your* needs. Set target dates that are realistic and attainable.

Now that the planning is complete, it is time for the study to begin. Start with the area listed as "A1" (high priority and need) and work your way through to the last "A" item. Once this is finished, continue with the "B", and "C", and "D" items. When all areas have been reviewed, you may choose to begin again at item A1 or to reset priorities for your studying needs.

The easiest part of this task is defining the time frames in which to study specific topics. The toughest challenge is implementing the examination review plan!

Test Taking Tip 2

Be prepared. The more prepared you are to take the examination, the more comfortable the examination will be. Preparation includes studying the knowledge base of occupational therapy, getting a good night's sleep, and bringing the right tools to the examination. Once the studying is complete, the majority of the preparation is complete; however, when asked to identify the one most important thing in preparing for the examination, a graduating class of students all agreed that the answer was getting a good night's sleep. Plan to arrive at the test site 20 to 30 minutes before the examination. Doing so will allow time for registration and for becoming acclimated to the environment. In addition, it is recommended that each examinee bring three to four sharpened no. 2 pencils and an eraser.

Test Taking Tip 3

Prepare your body as well as your mind! Eating a well-balanced breakfast can actually affect your performance on the examination. A breakfast high in carbohydrates and low in fat will increase your energy and not produce a sluggish feeling. Avoid caffeine because its ultimate effect will leave you tired and drowsy in the midst of the examination. Finally, wear comfortable clothes in layers to allow you to adjust as necessary to the temperature of the room.

Test Taking Tip 4

Review the test packet briefly before starting the test. As you review the test booklet to verify that all of the test materials needed are provided, you will have a basic idea of the length of the test. If something is missing from the booklet, the error can be quickly corrected at the beginning of the examination and need not break your concentration later on.

Test Taking Tip 5

Pace yourself. The test is to be completed within 4 hours. Within this time frame, 200 multiple-choice questions are to be completed. One technique for pacing the examination is to divide the test booklet into four equivalent sections by bending the corner of the page in the top right-hand corner. The goal should be to complete each of the four sections within 50 minutes to 1 hour. By understanding the format of the test and budgeting your time, you may work more efficiently through the questions in the allotted time. The second technique is to use a watch to help pace yourself. This may be done in one of two ways. The first is to synchronize a watch with the clock being used by the individual administering the examination. At the end of every few pages of questions, briefly glance at your watch to keep an eye on your pace. If questions remain incomplete within the last 10 minutes of the examination, use discretion to select one letter and fill in all of the remaining answers with that letter. *Remember, there is no penalty for guessing—only for leaving questions unanswered!* The second option is to wear a watch that signals on the hour. Set the watch for 12:00 when the examination begins. In doing this, you will know that when it is 4:00, the time will have expired for taking the examination. Between 12:00 and 4:00, the watch will signal each hour and you may check your pace without having to "clock-watch." The goal is to complete at least 25 percent of the examination, or 50 questions, within each hour. Avoid wasting time by looking frequently at your watch.

Test Taking Tip 6

Write as needed in the test booklet. It is permissible and often helpful to write in the test booklet, underlining key words in questions, crossing off answers as they are eliminated, or circling logical answers. The key here is to mark the correct answer on the answer sheet after completing each question. Those who attempt to save time by writing the answers in the book and later transferring them to the answer sheet run the risk of making errors. These errors ultimately affect their scores or their constructive use of time. In so doing, a candidate may color in the correct answer, but in the wrong number on the answer sheet. The item is then scored as a wrong answer. One technique to prevent this problem is to avoid skipping any questions and answers in the test booklet or on the answer sheet. If you are uncertain of an answer, make the best logical guess, and fill it in on the answer sheet. In general, you will be able to eliminate one or two of the incorrect answers. As an answer is eliminated, cross off the letter of the answer in the booklet. Again, there is no penalty for guessing, only for leaving questions unanswered!

Test Taking Tip 7

When you use the same letter for more than three answers in a row, double check the questions to verify each answer. Test writers usually break up strings of four or more of the same letter or answer. The multiple-choice format is usually set so that three of the same letters in a row are the maximum run of correct answers. If there are four or more of the same letters in a row, and if time allows, it may be beneficial to recheck the answers. *Save this task for the end of the examination*!

Test Taking Tip 8

Mark your answers clearly on the score sheet. Stray marks may invalidate answers. If the answer is too light, it may not be scanned appropriately by the scoring machine.

If the answer is too big, it may be interpreted incorrectly as one of the adjacent letters. If you anticipate problems of this type, you can have the answer sheet hand scored. There is an extra charge for this service, but it may make the difference between passing and failing the examination. Look at the following examples of correct and incorrect marking of answers.

22. Ⓐ Ⓑ Ⓒ ⬤   Overmarking an answer.

23. Ⓐ ⬤ Ⓒ Ⓓ   Stray mark on answer sheet.

24. ⬤ Ⓑ Ⓒ Ⓓ   Incomplete marking of an answer.

25. Ⓐ Ⓑ ⬤ Ⓓ   Correct marking of an answer.

Test Taking Tip 9

Use key techniques to help select the correct answer.

1. **Follow your instincts when answering questions.** The first answer chosen is usually the correct one. Only change an answer if you later realize that it is absolutely incorrect.

2. **Ask, "What is this question about?"** One technique used by a colleague is to try to decipher what the question is testing. This is done by selecting the key terms in the question and not being distracted by peripheral information. By sorting through the information provided to identify what the question is testing, you may be more likely to select the correct answer.

3. **Anticipate the answer.** Many times, you may anticipate an answer while reading a question. Once this is done, you may look for the anticipated answer among the options. It is important to read and consider all of the options to verify that the anticipated answer is the correct answer.

4. **Use logical reasoning.** A commonly used technique is the process of reasonable deduction by eliminating answers that are incorrect. Once this is done, time is spent working with the options that remain. (It is permissible to cross off answers in the test booklet as they are eliminated.) As you complete the questions in this book, remember these techniques and practice using them when you have difficulty in answering a question.

Test Taking Tip 10

Read the questions before reading a case history. Reading the questions first prepares your mind to seek out the answers while you read the selection. A small percentage of questions on the examination are grouped with a case history. In such instances, approximately three questions correspond to the case history. Try your skills in the following case history and three questions:

Case History

The patient is a 49-year-old white woman who was referred to an occupational therapist for evaluation. In the initial assessment, the individual is unable to move her shoulder, wrist, and hand voluntarily, but wrist extension

Table 1. EXAMPLE OF COMPLETED CERTIFICATION EXAMINATION STUDY PLAN

	PEDIATRICS	PHYSICAL DISABILITIES	PSYCHOSOCIAL DYSFUNCTIONS
Referral sources and acknowledgment of referrals	D/3	D/1	D/4
Documentation of an individual's history and/or interview	D/2	D/2	C/5
Implications of values/beliefs	A/2	D/4	B/1
Observation of individual skills and behavior	B/3	D/3	C/4
Documentation formats and information sharing	B/2	D/5	C/3
Written and verbal communication standards	C/1	D/10	C/2
Licensing regulating agency requirements	A/1	A/1	A/1
Medical terminology	B/1	D/9	C/1
Standardized assessment tools	D/1	D/7	D/1
Nonstandardized assessment tools	D/4	D/6	D/3
Establishing goals and objectives	D/5	D/8	D/2
Frames of reference	A/3	A/2	A/2
Population norms	D/8	D/12	D/5
Normal/abnormal development	C/4	C/1	C/6
Procedures	C/5	B/2	A/5
Indications for use of activities	C/3	C/2	A/4
Common treatment activities	D/6	B/1	A/3
Grading of treatment activities	B/4	B/3	B/2
Group formats and group development	D/7	D/11	A/6
Group activities and group process	D/9	D/13	D/7
Roles of team members	C/6	D/14	D/6
Assessment for adaptive equipment	C/2	A/3	C/7

Table 1. *(continued)*

	PEDIATRICS	PHYSICAL DISABILITIES	PSYCHOSOCIAL DYSFUNCTIONS
Fabrication of adaptive equipment	A/4	B/4	D/11
Advanced technology	B/7	A/4	C/9
COTA Roles	B/6	B/5	B/4
OTR Roles	B/5	B/4	B/3
Community Resources	C/8	C/4	C/10
Development of home programs	C/7	C/3	C/8
ADL training	D/11	D/15	D/9
Discharge planning and recommendations	D/10	D/17	D/8
Patient/family education	D/12	D/16	D/10

	ADMINISTRATION & MANAGEMENT
Standards of practice	C/4
Code of ethics	C/2
Uniform terminology	C/3
Roles of AOTA	B/1
Roles of NBCOT	B/2
Student supervision	A/4
COTA supervision	A/2
Reimbursement	C/1
Disciplinary processes	A/3
Marketing occupational therapy services	A/1
Patient rights	D/2
Liability and malpractice issues	D/1
Program evaluation	B/3
Quality improvement	B/4

Table 2. CERTIFICATION EXAMINATION STUDY PLAN

	PEDIATRICS	PHYSICAL DISABILITIES	PSYCHOSOCIAL DYSFUNCTIONS
Referral sources and acknowledgment of referrals			
Documentation of an individual's history and/or interview			
Implications of values/ beliefs			
Observation of individual skills and behavior			
Documentation formats and information sharing			
Written and verbal communication standards			
Licensing regulating agency requirements			
Medical terminology			
Standardized assessment tools			
Nonstandardized assessment tools			
Establishing goals and objectives			
Frames of reference			
Population norms			
Normal/abnormal development			
Procedures			
Indications for use of activities			
Common treatment activities			
Grading of treatment activities			
Group formats and group development			
Group activities and group process			
Roles of team members			
Assessment for adaptive equipment			

Table 2. *(continued)*

	PEDIATRICS	PHYSICAL DISABILITIES	PSYCHOSOCIAL DYSFUNCTION
Fabrication of adaptive equipment			
Advanced technology			
COTA Roles			
OTR Roles			
Community Resources			
Development of home programs			
ADL training			
Discharge planning and recommendations			
Patient/family education			

	ADMINISTRATION & MANAGEMENT
Standards of practice	
Code of ethics	
Uniform terminology	
Roles of AOTA	
Roles of NBCOT	
Student supervision	
COTA supervision	
Reimbursement	
Disciplinary processes	
Marketing occupational therapy services	
Patient rights	
Liability and malpractice issues	
Program evaluation	
Quality improvement	

is facilitated with tapping and vibration. Passive range of motion is within normal limits for the elbow and hand, but the shoulder is limited to 90 degrees of pain-free shoulder flexion. The therapist notes a 1½ finger width of subluxation in the shoulder. The individual has intact sensations for hot/cold, light touch/localization, and sharp/dull.

Based on this information, answer the following questions:

1. **What systems did the occupational therapist assess in the above scenario?**
   A. Visual-perceptual.
   B. Cognitive.
   C. Psychosocial.
   D. Sensorimotor.

2. **What type of positioning technique would most likely be recommended based on an neurodevelopmental treatment (NDT) approach?**
   A. A lap tray for support of the affected extremity.
   B. A sling for support of the extremity.
   C. A Bobath hand splint.
   D. Placement of the affected arm in the patient's lap.

3. **The likelihood of muscle return is good based on:**
   A. the within-normal-limits range of the elbow and hand.
   B. intact sensory perception of hot/cold, light touch/localization, and sharp/dull.
   C. subluxation of the shoulder.
   D. facilitation of movement by tapping and vibration.

The answers are as follows:

1. (D) Sensorimotor. Because both active and passive movements were assessed as well as sensation, the correct answer is "sensorimotor." Based on the information given, the areas involving memory, problem solving, concentration, and visual perception were not assessed. Thus, answers A and C are incorrect. Answer B is also incorrect because information regarding the individual's living situation and interests were not documented, as would be seen in a psychosocial assessment.

2. (A) Lap tray to support the affected extremity. Based on the case study, the affected arm is flaccid but beginning to exhibit characteristics of Brunnstrom's recovery stage II. For this reason, the safest position for the arm would involve providing support and avoiding positioning that would increase tone or patterns of synergy. Answer B is incorrect because a therapist would not want to position the patient in a synergistic pattern of elbow flexion and shoulder adduction that would be accomplished with a sling. Answer C is incorrect because there is no device referred to as the Bobath splint for the hand. Finally, an unsupported flaccid arm resting in the lap can lead to increased pain, subluxation, and deformity; therefore, answer D is incorrect.

3. (B) Intact sensory perception of hot/cold, light touch/localization, and sharp/dull. This answer is correct because it indicates that the pathways that carry sensory and motor messages are intact; however, the amount of return may not be predicted. Individuals with normal passive range of motion do not always regain muscle tone in the arm; therefore, answer A is incorrect. Answer D is incorrect because a subluxation will be more likely to hinder return instead of enhancing return of muscle function.

Answers to questions provide the student with an explanation for the correct selection. In addition, references are listed so that the students may obtain further information for study. References are listed by the author of the book; followed by the chapter author and chapter title of the work referenced. Simply cross reference the book author with the bibliography of *The Occupational Therapy Examination Review Guide* to find the title of the work referenced.

The tips provided here are not an exhaustive list of what individuals have found to be useful in preparing for examinations. You may have developed some of your own techniques that have been proven successful. Select only the tips that feel comfortable to you, and practice using these techniques as you work through this book.

REFERENCES

American Occupational Therapy Certification Board: *Certification Examination for Occupational Therapist, Registered and Certified Occupational Therapy Assistant, Candidate Handbook*, 1995. The American Occupational Therapy Certification Board, Rockville, MD, 1994.

American Occupational Therapy Certification Board: *Questions Most Frequently Asked by Students About Certification.* The American Occupational Therapy Certification Board, Rockville, MD, 1922.

AOTCB Information Exchange. The American Occupational Therapy Certification Board, Rockville, MD, Winter 1994.

Gronlund, N: *How to Construct Achievement Tests.* Prentice-Hall, Englewood Cliffs, NJ, 1987.

Martinson, T: *SuperCourse for the GMAT*, ed 3. Prentice-Hall, New York, 1991.

Millman, J, and Pauk, P: *How to Take Tests.* McGraw-Hill, New York, 1969.

Robinson, A, and Katzman, J: *The Princeton Review: Cracking the GRE 1995.* Villard Books, New York, 1992.

McFadden, S, and Wooldridge, E: *Certification. OT Week's Today's Student.* The American Occupational Therapy Association, Rockville, MD, Spring 1995.

SIMULATION EXAMINATION 1

Directions: Circle the correct answer to the following questions. When you have completed this examination, check your answers against the answer key that follows. As you will see, an explanation is given for each answer along with a reference for further study. The book author is listed as well as the chapter author. See the bibliography for complete references. Study the areas in which your comprehension was low, then test yourself again by taking Simulation Examination 2.

PEDIATRIC QUESTIONS

Assessment of Occupational Performance

1. The therapist has designed a checklist for evaluating a child's eating performance skills. The term that best describes this type of evaluation tool is:
   A. norm-referenced.
   B. criterion-referenced.
   C. clinical observation.
   D. valid and reliable.

2. A standardized test is called "valid" when it:
   A. measures the skill or function it claims to measure.
   B. provides similar scores on serial test administrations.
   C. provides similar scores when administered by two different examiners.
   D. is based on a normative population.

3. "Norm referencing" of a test for children means the test:
   A. measures normal behavior.
   B. compares performance to a normal standard.
   C. is valid and reliable.
   D. should be used with a normal population.

4. Standardization of a test for children means that the test:
   A. is valid.
   B. has normative data.
   C. has a standard format.
   D. is reliable.

5. The following procedure should be followed when administering standardized tests to young children:
   A. Test in a stimulating environment.
   B. Follow test manual directions.
   C. Remove all test materials before presenting the next item.
   D. Carry on a conversation with the child.

6. The Milani-Comparetti Motor Development Screening Test measures the following in children:
   A. Primitive reflexes and postural reactions.
   B. Developmental prehension skills.
   C. Cognitive skills.
   D. Language skills.

7. Assessment of a child indicates a normally developing infant. The occupational therapist documents presence of a postural reaction associated with development of the extensor tone needed for sitting and standing. This reaction would be:
   A. tonic labyrinthine in prone.
   B. asymmetric tonic neck.
   C. neck righting.
   D. Landau reaction.

8. Chart review of a newly referred child indicates that the child has dyslexia. This term is applied to an:
   A. inability to print or write.
   B. inability to read.
   C. inability to calculate mathematics.
   D. inability to plan motor actions.

9. The parents of a child report that the child has been diagnosed with autism. This information indicates to the therapist that the child has a condition classified as a(n):
   A. anxiety disorder of childhood.
   B. childhood conduct disorder.
   C. affective disorder.
   D. pervasive developmental disorder of childhood.

10. In assessing a child diagnosed with cerebral palsy resulting in spastic diplegia, the occupational therapist would anticipate involvement in the following extremities:
    A. Both upper limbs.
    B. Both legs.
    C. Lower extremity, trunk, and mild upper extremity.
    D. All extremities.

Development of the Treatment Plan

11. If a 9-year-old child with sensory integration problems has not developed a preferred hand for printing or writing, the best option for the occupational therapist would be to:
    A. develop right-hand skills, as most children are right-handed.
    B. wait a few more years until the child decides for herself or himself which hand is preferred.
    C. let the teacher decide on a preferred hand.
    D. consider and treat underlying sensory integration problems as a possible cause.

12. At a team planning meeting for a 2-year-old child with multiple handicaps, it is decided that the occupational therapist will fulfill the roles of other therapies needed as well. This decision requires a "role release" from the teacher, physical therapist, and speech therapist. Which of the following team approaches for young children does this method describe?
    A. Unidisciplinary.
    B. Multidisciplinary.
    C. Interdisciplinary.
    D. Transdisciplinary.

13. When planning treatment for a child with high tone or spasticity, the occupational therapist would MOST likely use the neurodevelopmental treatment (NDT) principle of:
    A. weight bearing and compression with movement.
    B. small movements with stability.
    C. stability, reduction of movements, and development of midline orientation.
    D. passive movement followed by slow, rhythmic movement.

14. A child with spina bifida needs a chair adapted to provide stability while sitting and working at school. The following seating principle of hip/knee/ankle position should be used to begin planning the adaptation process:
    A. 45/45/45 degrees at hip/knee/ankle joints.
    B. 90/90/90 degrees at hip/knee/ankle joints.
    C. 90/45/45 degrees at hip/knee/ankle joints.
    D. 125/125/125 degrees at hip/knee/ankle joints.

15. On completion of an evaluation of a child with cerebral palsy, the occupational therapist has identified the primary objective of inhibition of flexor spasticity in the hand. The activity that would be MOST appropriate in meeting this objective would be:
    A. building a block tower.
    B. active release of blocks into a container.
    C. traction on the finger flexors.
    D. weight bearing over a small bolster in prone.

16. An occupational therapist is working with a 7-year-old child with mild, spastic cerebral palsy. The evaluation has shown the therapist that the child has poor "in-hand manipulation" skills. What type of activity would develop this ability?
    A. Grasping blocks to build a building.
    B. Placing pegs from one pegboard to another.
    C. Carrying a bag of Lego blocks with a handle.
    D. Removing a nut from a bolt.

17. Following an assessment, the occupational therapist develops the following objective: "Mary will feed herself solid foods using a spoon without spilling in a 20-minute period." The underlined portion of this objective is called:
    A. the learner.
    B. the behavioral statement.
    C. the performance criterion.
    D. the conditions statement.

18. Development of a treatment plan for a child with an underreactive vestibular system would most likely provide specific activities to address:
    A. poor postural responses.
    B. discomfort with motion activities.
    C. anxiety when feet are off the ground.
    D. gravitational insecurity.

19. The occupational therapist is writing a "problem list" based on a child's performance. This list is usually developed at which point in the occupational therapy process?
    A. After the observation or screening.
    B. After the interview.
    C. After the evaluation.
    D. After the writing of the goals and objectives.

20. When writing a program plan for a child, the occupational therapist includes in the documentation:
    A. long-term goals written to the anticipated period of rehabilitation.
    B. long-term goals written in specific terms.
    C. short-term objectives written to the anticipated period of rehabilitation.
    D. short-term objectives written in general terms.

21. In writing the goals and objectives for a child's occupational therapy program, the therapist should include:
    A. the child's priorities.
    B. the priorities of the parents or caregivers.

C. the problems identified in the occupational therapy evaluation.

D. the priorities of the child, caregiver, and therapist.

22. **The occupational therapist is developing a treatment plan for a child with praxis, or motor planning deficits. "Praxis" refers to a problem performing an unfamiliar motor task using primarily the function of:**
    A. automatic movement.
    B. reflexes.
    C. coordination.
    D. cognition.

23. **The caregiver, child, and occupational therapist are working toward a goal of developing the child's oral skills. Which of the following, in terms of developmental sequence, would be the highest achievement?**
    A. Munching.
    B. Rotary chewing.
    C. Vertical chewing.
    D. Sucking and swallowing.

24. **The occupational therapist is developing the treatment plan after an assessment. The first step in the general problem analysis of a child's occupational therapy evaluation is to:**
    A. define and describe the child's problem.
    B. describe precautions associated with the problem.
    C. identify the critical elements of development and role performance for the age of the child.
    D. consider the effects of the problem on developmental tasks and performance.

25. **Treatment planning for a child with the quadriplegic athetoid type of cerebral palsy would take into consideration the involvement of:**
    A. one upper limb.
    B. one side of the body.
    C. both legs.
    D. all extremities.

Implementation of the Treatment Plan

26. **As a part of the treatment plan, the occupational therapist sets up an unstructured obstacle course for the child. Which type of play does this exemplify?**
    A. Exploratory.
    B. Symbolic.
    C. Creative.
    D. Recreational.

27. **When treating a child with "tactile defensiveness," the occupational therapist handles the child as if the child were:**
    A. underreactive to being touched.
    B. overreactive to being touched.

C. craving touch.
D. unaffected by light touch.

28. **While in occupational therapy, a child has a seizure that barely interrupts activity performance. This would be reported as what type of a seizure?**
    A. Grand mal.
    B. Psychomotor.
    C. Petit mal.
    D. Akinetic.

29. **During treatment, the occupational therapist is providing activities that assist the child in integrating rotary motion. Sensory receptors for this type of vestibular processing are located in the:**
    A. semicircular canals.
    B. utricle.
    C. saccule.
    D. cochlea.

30. **A child diagnosed with mental retardation is also categorized in the moderate or trainable range of intellectual ability. The child probably functions in the following manner:**
    A. Requires nursing care for basic survival skills.
    B. Can usually handle routine daily functions.
    C. Requires supervision to accomplish most tasks.
    D. Is able to learn academic skills at the third- to seventh-grade level.

31. **The occupational therapist observes that a child moves from a completely prone position to a prone-on-elbow position. As a result, the child is gaining control in the midline position through the development of:**
    A. primitive reflexes.
    B. prehensile reactions.
    C. righting reactions.
    D. equilibrium reactions.

32. **After 6 months of treatment, the occupational therapist observes that a child has begun to integrate the postural reflex that brings her into a four-point kneeling position. This reflex is:**
    A. crossed extension.
    B. asymmetric tonic neck.
    C. symmetrical tonic neck.
    D. tonic labyrinthine.

33. **The Early Intervention Developmental Profile (EIDP) was designed specifically to guide the interdisciplinary teams in program planning for young children with disabilities. Which one of the following terms best describes this type of test?**
    A. Therapist-made checklist.
    B. Clinical observations.
    C. Criterion-referenced test.
    D. Norm-referenced test.

34. The occupational therapist is documenting the muscle tone of a child with athetoid cerebral palsy. This muscle tone would be described as:
    A. fluctuating.
    B. spastic.
    C. flaccid.
    D. rigid.

35. An occupational therapist is working with an infant and observes and documents the presence of the first stage of voluntary grasp. This type of grasp would be noted as:
    A. radial palmar.
    B. pincer.
    C. ulnar palmar.
    D. palmar.

36. The occupational therapist documents that a child has "tactile defensiveness." Which part of the central nervous system is thought to be involved with this disturbance?
    A. Discriminative tactile system.
    B. Protective tactile system.
    C. Vestibular system.
    D. Olfactory system.

37. The occupational therapist is using a pediatric occupational therapy frame of reference that is based on facilitation of growth and development. This frame of reference was established by:
    A. Lela Llorens.
    B. Gilfoyle and Grady.
    C. A. Jean Ayres.
    D. Mary Reilly.

38. The occupational therapist is using a pediatric occupational therapy frame of reference that is defined as "the organization of sensory input in the brain for the emitting of adaptive responses." This frame of reference was established by:
    A. Lela Llorens.
    B. Gilfoyle and Grady.
    C. A. Jean Ayres.
    D. Mary Reilly.

39. The occupational therapist is using a pediatric occupational therapy frame of reference that describes normal maturation of the nervous system in terms of "spatiotemporal" adaptation. This frame of reference was established by:
    A. Lela Llorens.
    B. Eleanor Gilfoyle and Ann Grady.
    C. A. Jean Ayres.
    D. Mary Reilly.

40. In discussions with a child's caregiver, the occupational therapist explains that the normal developmental pattern of infants is to sit without support:
    A. before they lift their heads in prone.
    B. after back extension in prone develops.
    C. before primitive reflexes disappear.
    D. after they are able to walk alone.

41. A child's caregiver asks the occupational therapist at what age a normal child begins to "cruise," or walk sideways while holding onto furniture. The therapist reports that this behavior usually occurs between the ages of:
    A. 3 and 5 months.
    B. 6 and 8 months.
    C. 9 and 12 months.
    D. 13 and 15 months.

Evaluation of the Treatment Plan

42. The occupational therapist has set up an unstructured play setting to reassess a child. This method of evaluation is MOST effective for a(n):
    A. observation.
    B. interview.
    C. performance-based screening test.
    D. standardized test.

43. The occupational therapist observes that through treatment, the child is now developing a reflex or reaction that allows rotation of the trunk. This reflex or reaction is:
    A. neonatal neck righting.
    B. asymmetric tonic neck.
    C. body righting.
    D. tonic labyrinthine.

44. A 6-month-old child with a visual impairment is being seen for reevaluation. Tactile defensive behavior has decreased as seen in less crying when handled by family members. Given that tactile defensiveness continues to be observed, which of the following activities would best meet this child's tactile needs at this time?
    A. Using a vibrator on the child's stomach.
    B. Brushing the child with various brushes.
    C. Swaddling the child before handling.
    D. Touching the child lightly while she wears a blindfold, and asking "Where did I touch you?"

45. A 24-month-old child with Down syndrome is being evaluated after a sensorimotor program. She has made gains in mobility and motor skills. Her parents are concerned about continued temper outbursts that often occur during physical handling, as well as difficulty "being still." The most appropriate adjustment in this child's program would be to:
    A. coach the parents in skills needed for decreasing apparent tactile defensiveness.
    B. increase therapy time per week.
    C. suggest that the parents visit a child psychologist.
    D. suggest that the child be enrolled in a preschool program.

Discharge Planning

46. **Parents are more motivated to carry out treatment programs when the:**
    A. occupational therapy program works for the child.
    B. parents are constantly challenged by the difficulty of the occupational therapy program.
    C. therapist has set the goals.
    D. home program is separate from daily family routines.

47. **The therapist is working with a child with an autosomal recessive inherited condition in which the exocrine glands produce abnormal mucus. This child has a condition referred to as:**
    A. cystic fibrosis.
    B. Duchenne's disease.
    C. pediatric acquired immunodeficiency syndrome (AIDS).
    D. Down syndrome.

48. **Occupational therapists working in the area of early intervention have frequent contact with a child's parent. Which of the following statements BEST describe how parents should be involved in the occupational therapy program?**
    A. Parents should not be present during occupational therapy sessions.
    B. Parents should be trained as substitute therapists.
    C. Parents' needs and wishes should be included in program planning.
    D. Only one parent needs to be present when the occupational therapy program is discussed.

49. **A 6-year-old child will be discharged from an outpatient occupational therapy program, and the therapist will be meeting with the classroom teacher and parents. Which of the following activities would best treat the child's visual perception problem of "position in space"?**
    A. Identifying letters on a distracting page.
    B. Finding geometric shapes scattered in a box.
    C. Following directions about objects located in front, in back, and to the side.
    D. Making judgments about moving through space.

50. **An 18-year-old student with mental retardation is being discharged from an occupational therapy program in a large metropolitan school to a community-sheltered workshop. What information from the occupational therapist's standard evaluation is most necessary in discharge planning?**
    A. Leisure interests.
    B. Ability to follow rules and instructions.
    C. Gross motor skills.
    D. Reflex integration.

PHYSICAL DISABILITY QUESTIONS

Assessment of Occupational Performance

51. **A therapist is evaluating an individual with a peripheral nerve injury for strength, range of motion, and endurance. The occupational therapist is MOST likely using which theory?**
    A. Rehabilitative.
    B. Neurodevelopmental.
    C. Biomechanical.
    D. Psychoanalytic.

52. **A therapist is evaluating the posture and movement of an individual who had a stroke. The therapist is MOST likely using which theory?**
    A. Rehabilitative.
    B. Neurodevelopmental.
    C. Psychoanalytic.
    D. Maturational.

53. **A sensory-perceptual evaluation is MOST likely to:**
    A. ascertain the need for facilitation of sensation.
    B. determine the need for corrective lenses.
    C. assess the need for training in compensatory techniques.
    D. determine visual deficits.

54. **The occupational therapist is assessing an individual whose diagnosis is cerebrovascular accident. The most appropriate technique to be used in assessing sensory awareness is to:**
    A. test the individual's affected extremity before the unaffected extremity.
    B. demonstrate the procedure on the unaffected extremity, then occlude the individual's vision.
    C. demonstrate the procedure on the affected extremity then establish rapport with the individual.
    D. interview the individual and assess only the areas that he or she reports are impaired.

55. **The occupational therapist is preparing to complete an evaluation for an individual whose diagnosis is cerebrovascular accident. The sensory portion of the test would be invalid for an individual with which one of the following impairments?**
    A. Expressive aphasia.
    B. Receptive aphasia.
    C. Agnosia.
    D. Ataxia.

56. **An individual with a head injury has been referred for occupational therapy services. Assessment of her affected extremity indicates that she is capable of performing gross movement combinations with minimal evidence of synergy. However, flexion synergy is evident when she attempts activities that are strenuous for her. This patient is in what stage of return?**

A. Stage 3.
B. Stage 4.
C. Stage 5.
D. Stage 6.

57. **The occupational therapist is performing an initial bedside consultation with an individual who had a stroke. The individual presents with a flaccid left upper extremity and demonstrates impaired sensation throughout the arm. The therapist also notes marked pitting edema of the affected hand. Based on prioritization of the individual's needs, the initial recommendations would include:**
    A. positioning, compression glove, and edema massage followed by passive range-of-motion exercises.
    B. splinting, elevation of the arm, and active range-of-motion exercises.
    C. no action until the edema subsides.
    D. having the individual attempt to squeeze a ball.

58. **A paper-and-pencil test that can be used with an individual to determine unilateral neglect is:**
    A. six-block assembly.
    B. line bisection.
    C. proverb interpretation.
    D. identification of the square in four overlapping figures.

59. **An individual who had a myocardial infarction (MI) had been transferred from the acute care unit to a rehabilitation unit. During the initial interview, he displays good memory of information processed before the MI but poor recall of the period spent in the acute care facility. He is able to recall information since the transfer. This individual has difficulty with:**
    A. orientation.
    B. long-term memory.
    C. anterograde amnesia.
    D. retrograde amnesia.

60. **The instrument used to measure range of motion of the hand is called:**
    A. a goniometer.
    B. a dynamometer.
    C. a pinch meter.
    D. an aesthesiometer.

Development of the Treatment Plan

61. **The SOAP note method of documentation is used in an acute care hospital setting to record information regarding an individual with dementia. Which statement is an example of subjective information?**
    A. The therapist will establish a daily self-feeding routine using verbal and physical cues to encourage the individual to open containers on the lunch tray.

B. The individual has been able to identify closed liquid-beverage containers on the meal tray for four of six presentations.
    C. The individual is able to identify and drink liquids presented in cups without lids but leaves beverages in closed containers untouched.
    D. The individual asks for more beverages during meals, but appears surprised when the therapist indicates beverages in closed containers are on the meal tray.

62. **An individual who had a cerebrovascular accident, is dependent with self-care, and transfers with the assistance of two people has expressed the goal of returning home with a transfer status of needing the assistance of only one person. A long-term goal would be that:**
    A. the individual will complete upper-extremity sponge bathing with setup of equipment and verbal cues.
    B. the individual will perform lower-extremity dressing with the maximal assistance of one person.
    C. the individual will complete upper-extremity self-care using appropriate adaptive equipment with the supervision of a family member.
    D. the individual will complete a modified sit-pivot transfer to the commode with the moderate assistance of two people.

63. **After evaluation, the goal for an individual who had a total hip replacement was minimal assistance with verbal cues for memory. After 2 weeks of treatment, the individual is able to dress with standby assistance. What skills does this person need to demonstrate before changing the goal?**
    A. Less time needed to perform dressing.
    B. Improved concentration.
    C. Ability to remember two of three hip precautions.
    D. Consistent and appropriate use of adaptive equipment.

64. **In establishing long-term goals for an individual with T-3 paraplegia, the occupational therapist would MOST likely predict that the patient will attain what level of independence with self-care bathing and dressing and activities of daily living (ADL) transfers?**
    A. Complete independence with self-care and transfers.
    B. Independence with self-care and minimal assistance with transfers.
    C. Minimal assistance with self-care and moderate assistance with ADL transfers.
    D. Dependence with both self-care and transfers.

65. **An individual with right unilateral neglect is able to track from the left side to the midline of the body on paper-and-pencil tasks. What treatment activity could be used with this person to work on crossing the midline to improve writing?**

A. Have the individual practice wheeling a wheelchair following a taped line on the floor.

B. Place commonly used self-care items on the left side.

C. Have the individual trace lines across the page with the right index finger from the left to the right side.

D. Place playing cards in a horizontal row from right to left in sequence.

66. **A prerequisite for an individual to use a mobile arm support would be:**

A. incoordination.

B. lateral trunk stability.

C. fair + elbow flexion.

D. poor head control.

67. **Which of the following are among the methods used for sensory desensitization?**

A. Textured material, rubbing, tapping, and prolonged contact.

B. Massage, facilitory electrical stimulation, and a progressive desensitization program.

C. Pressure, percussion, vibration, icing, and edema massage.

D. Visual compensation and functional use of the extremity.

68. **An individual referred for occupational therapy has a diagnosis of ulnar nerve injury. Which splint would be MOST appropriate?**

A. A wrist cock-up.

B. An anticlaw.

C. A resting hand splint.

D. A cone.

69. **The therapist is planning the sequence of activities in the treatment plan for a patient who has had a cerebrovascular accident. In planning active range-of-motion exercises, the therapist must also be aware of what may limit range of motion so that those issues may be addressed before the activity is performed. Those issues that the therapist needs to consider are:**

A. muscle tone, edema, sensation, and diadokinesis.

B. edema, proprioception, and muscle tone.

C. edema, contracture, muscle tone, and pain.

D. contracture, stereognosis, and sensation.

70. **An individual has a diagnosis of shoulder encapsulitis or frozen shoulder. The treatment plan would include:**

A. pendulum exercises, icing, and active and passive range-of-motion exercises.

B. resistive exercise and active and passive range-of-motion exercises.

C. active range-of-motion exercises, functional activities, weight lifting, and heat treatments.

D. overhead pulley exercises, manipulation, resistive exercise, and passive range-of-motion exercises.

71. **The best method of compensation for both unilateral neglect and absence of sensation in an upper extremity is:**

A. to avoid the use of sharp tools or scissors and to avoid extreme water temperatures.

B. to wear noisy bracelets on the wrist or ankle as a reminder to visually scan toward the affected side.

C. to use an electric shaver.

D. to wear elbow pads on the affected side.

72. **An example of limiting the amount of work needed for a task when educating an individual in energy-conservation techniques would be to use:**

A. a side-loading washer.

B. permanent-press clothing.

C. an extended-handle dustpan.

D. good body mechanics.

73. **Stabilizing the forearm on the table when writing is necessary for someone with:**

A. decreased vision.

B. poor endurance.

C. limited fine movement.

D. incoordination.

74. **An individual who has difficulty finding white socks on a bed with white sheets has a deficit in:**

A. figure-ground discrimination.

B. unilateral neglect.

C. position in space.

D. cognitive mapping.

75. **Drawing a map of a familiar place such as a route to work or a floor plan of a home requires:**

A. position in space.

B. figure-ground discrimination.

C. topographic orientation.

D. visual closure.

Implementation of the Treatment Plan

76. **Rood inhibition techniques include:**

A. joint approximation and slow stroking.

B. slow rolling and light touch.

C. neutral warmth and fast brushing.

D. slow icing and fast brushing.

77. **Neurophysiologic and developmental treatment approaches include:**

A. Rood, Bobath, Ayres, and proprioceptive neuromuscular facilitation (PNF).

B. Rood, Bobath, Mosey, and PNF.

C. Rood, Bobath, Brunnstrom, and PNF.

D. Bobath, Brunnstrom, Mosey, and Ayres.

78. **Treatment for unilateral neglect includes:**

A. stimulating the uninvolved limbs with ice.

B. exercises using the uninvolved arm to move the involved arm across the midline.

C. participation in tasks that do not cross the midline.

D. participation in tasks placed on the uninvolved side.

79. **According to Brunnstrom, a head-injured individual in stage 2 of muscle return would be most likely to demonstrate the following movement in treatment:**
    A. Isolated joint movement.
    B. Voluntary gross motor movements 25% of range.
    C. Flexor synergy and voluntary or associated reactions.
    D. Gross motor movements such as reaching arm forward to 90 degrees and pronating or supinating the forearm.

80. **Sensory retraining is:**
    A. successful for hypersensitivity.
    B. successful for hyposensitivity.
    C. successful for both hypersensitivity and hyposensitivity.
    D. unsuccessful for both hypersensitivity and hyposensitivity.

81. **Scapulohumeral rhythm is defined as:**
    A. a ratio of movement of 2:1 as the humerus moves on the scapula.
    B. a ratio of movement of 2:1 as the scapula moves on the humerus.
    C. a ratio of movement of 5:1 as the scapula moves on the humerus.
    D. a ratio of movement of 1:5 as the humerus moves on the scapula.

82. **Constructional apraxia, body scheme disturbances, and unilateral neglect all contribute to self-care difficulties called:**
    A. spatial relations.
    B. dressing apraxia.
    C. anosognosia.
    D. figure-ground discrimination.

83. **Which one of the following senses does the somatosensory system include?**
    A. Taste.
    B. Smell.
    C. Vision.
    D. Touch.

84. **A common criterion for splints that are made or issued by an occupational therapist is that the:**
    A. fingers should be flexed in a functional position.
    B. thumb is opposed and abducted.
    C. splint should be worn at all times.
    D. pressure marks or redness should disappear after 20 minutes.

85. **When selecting an area in the clinic to perform Rood inhibition techniques on an individual, the therapist would most likely choose:**

A. a mat table facing the individual toward a busy clinic.
B. a private treatment room with a bright light.
C. a mat table in a cool room.
D. a private treatment room with a dimmer light.

86. **An individual with a cerebrovascular accident and his or her family members would most likely be taught to perform transfers:**
    A. only to the unaffected side of the body.
    B. only to the affected side of the body.
    C. to both sides of the body.
    D. only to the side from which the commode will be approached.

87. **An individual with a short above knee amputation is taught to wrap the stump with the end of the ace wrap:**
    A. running horizontally with the end on the good side between the waist and the iliac crest.
    B. running vertically between the waist and the iliac crest on the amputated side.
    C. on the front of the leg running diagonally from below the crease of the hip on the amputated side.
    D. on the front of the leg running horizontally below the crease of the hip on the amputated side.

88. **A safety function which should be incorporated into a power wheelchair in addition to mobility is:**
    A. a portable ventilator.
    B. arm troughs.
    C. adaptations for pressure relief.
    D. adjustable speed.

Evaluation of the Treatment Plan

89. **An individual with a left hemisphere cerebrovascular accident is given a paper typed with letters of the alphabet randomly dispersed. The individual is instructed to cross out all the M's. After completing the task, the missed letters are in a random pattern throughout the page. This person demonstrates:**
    A. a left visual field cut.
    B. a right visual field cut.
    C. functional illiteracy.
    D. decreased attention.

90. **In assessment of an individual with rheumatoid arthritis, the occupational therapist has her raise her left arm. Range of motion is limited to 85 degrees of shoulder flexion. While in this position, the patient is able to tolerate moderate resistance. The therapist observes passive range of motion to be the same as active range of motion. The patient's manual muscle test score would be:**

A. normal (5).
B. good (4).
C. fair (3).
D. fair minus (3-).

91. **What approximate Celsius temperature range is recommended for testing of hot and cold sensation?**
    A. Hot is 40 to 45°C; cold is 5 to 10°C.
    B. Hot is 45 to 50°C; cold is 10 to 15°C.
    C. Hot is 30 to 35°C; cold is 0 to 5°C.
    D. Hot is 25 to 30°C; cold is -5 to 0°C.

92. **When performing sensation testing on an individual, the occupational therapist should do the following:**
    A. Apply the stimuli distally to proximally.
    B. Test the involved area first, then the uninvolved area.
    C. Present test stimuli in an organized pattern to improve reliability during retesting.
    D. Occlude the vision of the therapist during testing.

93. **During manual muscle testing of shoulder flexion, the individual can move the arm through the full range of motion, but can tolerate only minimal resistance against gravity to the arm. The strength according to the manual muscle test (MMT) is:**
    A. fair minus (3-).
    B. fair (3).
    C. fair plus (3+).
    D. good minus (4-).

94. **What is the position used to measure tip pinch?**
    A. Thumb against the tip of the index finger.
    B. Thumb against the side of the index finger.
    C. Thumb against the tips of the index and middle fingers.
    D. Thumb against the tips of all the fingers.

95. **The name of the instrument used to test two point discrimination is:**
    A. a goniometer.
    B. a dynamometer.
    C. a pinch meter.
    D. an aesthesiometer.

Discharge Planning

96. **In what manner must an individual with burns perform a home program of positioning or splinting, or both, to prevent deformity?**
    A. A home program would not be necessary.
    B. Continue the same positioning and splinting program as was indicated before discharge.
    C. Have the individual follow through with splinting only during the day.
    D. Have the individual follow through with positioning and splinting only during the night.

97. **An individual with left-side weakness and balance problems wishes to vacuum the floors on returning home. Which type of vacuum cleaner would the therapist recommend?**
    A. A canister vacuum cleaner.
    B. An upright vacuum cleaner.
    C. A self-propelled vacuum cleaner.
    D. A hand-held cordless vacuum cleaner.

98. **An individual begins therapy with a blood-thinning medication after surgery for an endarterectomy. Which grooming tool will be recommended by his therapist to use in the hospital as well as after discharge?**
    A. An electric razor.
    B. A single-blade safety razor.
    C. A straight razor.
    D. A double-blade safety razor.

99. **An individual who is able to ambulate with a quadripod cane has been discharged. What recommendations should be made on the home evaluation regarding safety?**
    A. Remove all throw or scatter rugs.
    B. Place lever handles on faucets.
    C. Install a ramp if steps exist.
    D. Install a hand-held shower.

100. **An individual with chronic obstructive pulmonary disease is taught to modify his bathing techniques for carryover after discharge. What method should be used?**
    A. A tub bath using hot water.
    B. A hot shower using a bath chair.
    C. A lukewarm shower using a bath chair.
    D. A tub bath using lukewarm water.

PSYCHOSOCIAL QUESTIONS

Assessment of Occupational Performance

101. **The therapist is interested in objectively assessing an individual's general behaviors, such as appearance; interpersonal behaviors, such as self-assertion; and task behaviors, such as following directions. The psychosocial assessment instrument that provides this information is the:**
    A. Milwaukee Evaluation of Daily Living Skills (MEDLS).
    B. Kohlman Evaluation of Living Skills (KELS).
    C. Comprehensive Occupational Therapy Evaluation (COTE) Scale.
    D. Allen Cognitive Level (ACL).

102. **The projective assessment that is recommended for administration by an occupational therapist is:**
    A. the magazine picture collage.
    B. the Rorschach inkblot test.
    C. proverb interpretation.
    D. the House-Tree-Person (H-T-P) Test.

103. In the assessment of individuals in whom the early and middle stages of most dementias are diagnosed, the functional ability that will MOST likely remain intact for the longest duration is:
    A. the ability to read written information.
    B. the ability to write basic information.
    C. the ability to engage in superficial social conversation.
    D. the ability to dress and undress oneself.

104. The assessment instrument designed for use as a screening of self-care, physical, and social behaviors through the observations of caregivers familiar with the individual's daily care is the:
    A. Bay Area Functional Performance Evaluation (BaFPE).
    B. Comprehensive Occupational Therapy Evaluation (COTE).
    C. Role Checklist.
    D. Parachek Geriatric Rating scale.

105. The occupational therapy frame of reference that is consistent with psychoanalytic perspectives used by other members of the health care team is:
    A. occupational behavior.
    B. human occupation.
    C. object relations.
    D. role acquisition.

106. The most appropriate ADL assessment instrument for an adult in an acute care psychosocial setting is the:
    A. Kohlman Evaluation of Living Skills (KELS).
    B. Milwaukee Evaluation of Daily Living Skills (MEDLS).
    C. Functional Independence Measures (FIM).
    D. Katz Index of ADL.

107. This assessment provides the occupational therapist with a computer-generated summary of an individual's overall occupational performance functioning:
    A. Occupational Case Analysis and Interview Rating Scale (OCAIRS).
    B. OT FACT.
    C. Assessment of Occupational Functioning (AOF).
    D. Leisure Diagnostic Battery (LDB).

108. The occupational therapist reviews an individual's chart after receiving a referral for evaluation and treatment. The psychiatrist's admission report includes an Axis II diagnosis in addition to the Axis I diagnosis of major depression. Axis II reveals:
    A. that there is a complicating medical condition.
    B. that there is a personality disorder or a prominent maladaptive personality feature.
    C. the severity of the Axis I diagnosis.
    D. the existence of a dual diagnosis of substance abuse.

109. The occupational therapist reviews the available records as part of the screening assessment. The individual's demographic information reveals that the referral is for a grade-school-aged male child. The available social history indicates that this child's relationships with peers is characterized by grabbing their toys and disrupting group games. In addition, several descriptions by adults indicate that he displays annoying behaviors in the company of others. In general, these behaviors are most often linked to individuals with a diagnosis of:
    A. autism.
    B. attention-deficit hyperactivity disorder.
    C. personality disorder.
    D. anxiety disorder.

110. The assessment instrument that evaluates orientation is:
    A. the Lower Cognitive Level (LCL).
    B. the Allen Cognitive Level (ACL).
    C. The Kitchen Task.
    D. the Mini Mental Status Examination.

Development of the Treatment Plan

111. The occupational therapist selects activities appropriate for young adults who are taking tricyclic antidepressant medications. The activity that is contraindicated is:
    A. counted cross-stitch needlework projects.
    B. cooking foods that include aged cheese or coffee.
    C. a gross motor activity that can be graded between moderate to heavy metabolic equivalents (METS).
    D. an outdoor activity that involves being in direct sunlight.

112. The occupational therapist is planning treatment for individuals with a variety of personality disorders who have inaccurate perceptions of others and unrealistic perceptions of themselves. The treatment method that best addresses these problem areas is a:
    A. small group that provides a wide range of craft activities from which the members are encouraged to select.
    B. session focused on understanding and changing the individual's way of relating with the therapist.
    C. social skills training program completed in small groups.
    D. cooperative group activity that both provides and elicits consistent and accurate feedback about interactions within the group.

113. Comprehensive psychiatric rehabilitation services often include recreational therapy. The primary role that is expected of recreational therapy is to:

A. provide a variety of therapeutic sports, arts, crafts, music, and recreation activities to develop and reinforce healthy interest patterns.
B. provide specially designed learning experiences that stimulate awareness of social skills and behaviors.
C. provide acting-doing experiences that enable the individual to acquire leisure, work, and self-care skills at a maximum level of independence and to gain a sense of self-satisfaction and personal worth.
D. support the work-related behaviors and habits of time management, organization, and dependability through a variety of activities.

114. **If drawing is the treatment activity selected for adolescent females being treated for eating disorders, the most appropriate activity consists of the following:**
A. The occupational therapist asks a group member to lean against a wall where a large piece of paper has been posted. The therapist then draws around the individual's body shape. Other group members are then asked to draw in where clothes and accessories would be placed on this drawing.
B. Each member of a small group is asked to draw a picture of himself or herself on a piece of paper. The occupational therapist then leads a discussion about body-image concerns and links the discussion to the group's drawings.
C. All group participants are asked to draw pictures of their family. The occupational therapist leads a discussion that focuses on the underlying family dynamics that are symbolized in the drawings.
D. The individual is seen privately and is asked to draw a picture of a person performing an activity. After the picture is drawn, the occupational therapist asks the person to describe the action that the person in the drawing is doing and asks what skills the individual used while drawing this picture.

115. **Identify the goal that BEST reflects the cognitive-disabilities frame of reference.**
A. The individual will initiate and complete laundry activities in his or her own laundry area while the caregiver provides verbal cues about matching colors and shapes and monitors the individual's performance for unanticipated problems.
B. Within the next 2 weeks, the individual will choose and participate in two activities that relate to his or her current and future community roles.
C. The individual will demonstrate improved ability to maintain standing balance as evidenced by his or her use of weight shifting during a variety of throwing and catching games.
D. The individual will increase interactions with others by contacting two peers and asking them to join him or her in attending a movie within the next 2 months.

116. **The clinical-reasoning strategy that can lead to therapist bias during the problem-solving phase is demonstrated by the following:**
A. The therapist attributes an individual's problems to internal causes versus problems within the situation or environment.
B. The therapist appreciates that similarities and differences can occur between the therapist and his or her clients.
C. The therapist looks at reasons to support and disprove his or her proposed solutions to a problem.
D. The therapist considers the person's perceptions of the severity of the problem.

117. **The performance components that are particularly important to consider when analyzing activities for use with adults with psychosocial problems are:**
A. the amount of self-control demands, time-management demands, self-expression opportunities, and interest in the activity.
B. age appropriateness, prehension patterns required, and the presence of small pieces that could be mistakenly swallowed.
C. tactile, kinesthetic, visual, and olfactory properties.
D. space requirements, equipment and supply needs, cost, and safety considerations.

118. **Limit setting concerning impulsivity would be most important with these diagnoses in an inpatient setting:**
A. Depression and anxiety.
B. Alcoholism and anorexia nervosa.
C. Mania and borderline personality disorder.
D. Delirium and dementia.

119. **The following example of limit setting by the therapist enhances most therapeutic relationships:**
A. Reassuring the individual that you are his or her friend.
B. Telling the individual "I know how you feel."
C. Encouraging the individual to focus on positive feelings to open up communication.
D. Encouraging the individual to reconnect with his or her current and future personal life.

120. **The occupational therapist plans to use several parachute activities, involving cooperative demands and only limited competition demands, for a 30-minute meeting of young adults in a psychosocial treatment setting. This stage of group development is a(n):**
A. project group.
B. egocentric-cooperative group.
C. cooperative group.
D. mature group.

121. **The occupational therapist is training an adult developmentally disabled worker to put the**

pencil in the box before the score pad for a game packaging task in a sheltered workshop assembly line. The employee has not done this task before. The type of reinforcement schedule that will BEST achieve the goal of learning this task sequence is:

A. intermittent reinforcement with correct responses.
B. reinforcement every 10 minutes.
C. reinforcement for every fourth correct response.
D. continuous reinforcement of correct responses.

122. The BEST reinforcer for learning the task sequence described in question 121 is:

A. social reinforcers.
B. consumable reinforcers.
C. punishment.
D. activity reinforcers.

123. The occupational therapist realizes that the worker is having difficulty learning the game assembly sequence for question 121. The therapist decides to use backward chaining. Backward chaining would be:

A. encouraging the individual to reverse the packaging sequence.
B. having the worker put only the last piece into the game package.
C. putting only the pencil or the pad into the game box.
D. that the therapist demonstrates and repeats the correct sequence before each of the worker's attempts.

124. The occupational therapy treatment approach that will meet the overall needs experienced by individuals identified with alcohol abuse problems is to:

A. monitor and encourage the use of fine motor, tactile, figure-ground, and visuospatial functions; involve individual in expressive arts to focus on verbalization of feelings; and provide leisure-time education.
B. educate the family members about making safety modifications to the kitchen area.
C. encourage Alcoholics Anonymous (AA) involvement; provide retraining of neglected ADLs; explore work-related values.
D. make aftercare arrangements for vocational counseling and AA; provide time-management education for self-care activities.

125. The occupational therapist uses a remediation of functional performance deficits approach in addressing individuals treated in a psychosocial setting. The activity that is consistent with this approach is:

A. an expressive group magazine collage.
B. a class about job-seeking strategies.
C. the modification of the environment to provide familiar visual cues.
D. a review of the individual's balance of time among ADLs, work, and leisure activities.

126. When planning a meal preparation activity with an individual who is receiving a MAO inhibitor for depression, the safest food item to include would be:

A. aged cheddar cheese.
B. smoked turkey.
C. chocolate chips.
D. rice.

127. The best description of stressors is:

A. the process by which individuals adjust to daily stressful events within their environments.
B. the body's reactions to threat, often described as 'fight or flight.'
C. the precipitating conditions and events that elicit stress reactions.
D. the process of "fit" between the individual and his or her environment.

128. The therapist has determined that an individual's main problem is increased neck and shoulder tension that leads to headaches. The tension occurs primarily while the individual is at work as a word processor in a recently restructured corporation. The BEST stress management approach for this situation is:

A. assertiveness training focusing on increasing the individual's assertiveness with his or her boss.
B. Electromyography (EMG) biofeedback training combined with relaxation training.
C. training in cognitive reappraisal to decrease the frequency of the individual's tendency to generalize and exaggerate the negative side of work events.
D. teaching the individual more effective problem-solving strategies.

129. The activity feature that is most consistent with a behavioral frame of reference is:

A. the level of skill required is appropriate for the generally expected skills for that age.
B. the symbolic potential of the activity.
C. the combined activity demands of sensations, perceptions, and motor skills.
D. the measurability of activity performance.

130. Overall, what percentage of occupational therapists report the use of a group format to achieve individual goals?

A. 10 to 20 percent
B. 30 to 40 percent
C. 50 to 60 percent
D. 80 to 90 percent

Implementation of the Treatment Plan

131. The group format that is used most often by occupational therapists is:

A. cooking groups.
B. activity-of-daily-living groups.
C. arts-and-crafts groups.
D. exercise groups.

132. **Asking a middle-aged individual about the grade school he or she attended is one way of obtaining data about this individual's:**
    A. retention.
    B. remote memory.
    C. orientation.
    D. recent memory.

133. **The occupational therapist selects a "pie of life" activity to use with a group of individuals in a stress-management group. The therapist states, "I see that at least half of you have drawn your pie of life with too little time for rest and relaxation. Why don't we spend some group time exploring some ways to add more relaxation and rest into our days? Why don't we each give one suggestion?" The phase of group development this therapist's interaction describes is:**
    A. opening the group.
    B. processing the group.
    C. developing the group.
    D. group closure.

134. **The scenario described in question 133 is an example of an activity and therapist-group interaction that is consistent with the following developmental groups:**
    A. Project groups.
    B. Egocentric-cooperative groups.
    C. Cooperative groups.
    D. Mature groups.

135. **Personality disorders, in general, are marked by impaired functioning in:**
    A. activities of daily living (ADLs).
    B. instrumental activities of daily living.
    C. relationships with others.
    D. sensorimotor skills.

136. **The most common feature of occupational therapy task groups is that:**
    A. the group provides opportunities to evaluate areas of function that have been specified by a frame of reference.
    B. the focus of the group is a topic that is in common to all of the members and can be discussed by the members.
    C. the focus of the group is to encourage here-and-now explorations of member behaviors and issues while promoting learning through "doing."
    D. the focus of the group is to encourage the members to develop sequentially organized social interaction skills with the other members.

137. **The condition classified as an anxiety disorder is:**
    A. cyclothymic disorder.
    B. dysthymia.
    C. schizophrenia.
    D. posttraumatic stress disorder.

Evaluation of the Treatment Plan

138. **Which dressing ability is consistent with an individual assessed as functioning within Allen's cognitive level 3?**
    A. When reminded to dress and when clothing has been selected by another individual, the individual is able to put on his or her clothing.
    B. The individual moves spontaneously to assist a caregiver in dressing him or her.
    C. The individual does most of the dressing tasks independently with occasional minor errors.
    D. The individual is unable to perform any dressing task.

139. **The group composition that is most likely to result in an increased focus on the group leader and decreased interaction among the group members is a:**
    A. group size of less than 5 members.
    B. group made up of members of differing ages.
    C. group size between 7 and 10 members.
    D. group with members who have similar goals and abilities.

140. **According to group-development principles, when group members engage in increased conflict or fighting with the other members or the leaders, the most likely reason is that:**
    A. the members acting this way feel that the group topic or activity is not important to them.
    B. the members had little input into making group decisions.
    C. there have been several recent changes in the group membership.
    D. the members are frustrated with an inability to successfully meet the demands of the group or activity.

141. **An adult female experienced repeated sexual abuse by her father as a child and now describes her father's abusive actions as being caused by his stress of being fired from a job because of new management. The defense mechanism she is using is:**
    A. identification.
    B. projection.
    C. denial.
    D. rationalization.

142. **The extrapyramidal side-effect syndrome experienced by individuals receiving antipsychotic medications that impairs swallowing and leads to involuntary jerky arm and leg movements is:**
    A. parkinsonian syndrome.
    B. antipsychotic medication overdose.
    C. tardive dyskinesia.
    D. lithium toxicity.

143. **The BEST word to describe an individual's pervasive and sustained emotion that influences his or her perception of situations is:**

A. affect.
B. anxiety.
C. ideas of reference.
D. mood.

Discharge Planning

144. The following list of items can be considered gradations of caregiver assistance with housekeeping tasks according to the cognitive-disabilities frame of reference. The item that indicates an individual needing the MOST caregiver assistance according to this theoretic perspective is:
    A. the caregiver provides the individual with familiar tools such as a broom and dustpan and provides verbal cues about sequencing a sweeping task.
    B. the caregiver hands the individual a dust cloth and points to the location to dust. The caregiver redirects the individual to continue dusting if the individual stops before finishing.
    C. the caregiver provides the individual with verbal cues about the direction to spray and the necessary ventilation when using a general household cleanser in a spray container.
    D. the caregiver provides suggestions about methods of improving the appearance of objects being cleaned or arranged after cleaning.

145. The therapist is considering possible topics for a discharge planning group for individuals on an inpatient psychiatric unit. Which of the following topics would be important to cover because it is significantly related to rehospitalization?
    A. Managing family conflicts.
    B. Living skills needed for keeping aftercare appointments.
    C. Coping strategies for continuing medication compliance.
    D. Education about problems with alcohol and substance use.

146. Adults with mental retardation can be offered a variety of work alternatives. Which alternative usually involves simple assembly or sorting and packaging tasks with supervision and subcontracted piecework?
    A. Adult activity center.
    B. Supervised employment.
    C. Job coaching.
    D. Sheltered workshop.

147. The individual tells the therapist, "I don't know about going home tomorrow. I wanted to be discharged yesterday and the doctor suggested I stay in the hospital another day." You respond by saying, "It sounds as if you're not sure whether you're ready to be discharged." Your response is an example of:
    A. paraphrasing.
    B. social chitchat.

C. proposing a solution.
D. confrontation.

148. The BEST work program for individuals who experience difficulty accepting supervision, difficulty relating to co-workers, and difficulty accepting the value of punctuality is:
    A. competitive job placement.
    B. a job coach.
    C. supported employment.
    D. work adjustment.

149. The therapist is a member of a treatment team reviewing the treatment options for an individual who is experiencing acute psychiatric symptoms but who is not suicidal. This individual has been living with family members. The BEST treatment environment for this individual to receive occupational therapy services is:
    A. Partial hospitalization.
    B. Daycare.
    C. Day treatment.
    D. A community mental health center.

150. The therapist is working in a long-term psychiatric inpatient setting for adults. The therapist is asked by the treatment team to assess the individual's ability to maintain clothing, get dressed, eat a meal, and bathe because these are required skills for discharge to a group home. The MOST appropriate assessment to obtain this information is the:
    A. Milwaukee Evaluation of Daily Living Skills (MEDLS).
    B. Allen Cognitive Level (ACL).
    C. Kohlman Evaluation of Living Skills (KELS).
    D. Barthel Self-Care Index.

ADMINISTRATION AND MANAGEMENT QUESTIONS

Organize and Manage Services

151. Health care for disabled individuals, people with end-stage renal disease, or those older than 65 years of age is most likely paid for by:
    A. Medicare.
    B. Medicaid.
    C. Third-party payors.
    D. Private pay.

152. Quality-of-care components that are defined by a set of predetermined measures and are developed by professionals based on their expertise are called:
    A. thresholds.
    B. criterion.
    C. norms.
    D. monitors.

153. Outcome measures demonstrate the effectiveness and efficiency of a therapeutic program. What is the format generally used to collect, analyze, and report results of therapy in a rehabilitative program in relationship to costs?
    A. Quality improvement.
    B. Peer review.
    C. Cost accounting.
    D. Program evaluation.

154. Quality improvement is:
    A. patient-care monitoring.
    B. a method of cost accounting.
    C. one form of peer review.
    D. health accounting.

155. An occupational therapy job description will most likely contain:
    A. the title of the job, past experience, and job requirements.
    B. a summary of primary job functions, references, and job requirements.
    C. the organizational relationships, personality characteristics desired in a job candidate, and accomplishments of the candidate.
    D. the title of the job, organizational relationships, essential job functions, and the job requirements.

156. A technique frequently used by occupational therapy managers to prioritize patients to receive occupational therapy (OT) services during a personnel shortage is:
    A. status of reimbursement.
    B. triage.
    C. attrition.
    D. date of referral.

157. The manager of occupational therapy is planning for re-allocation of space that the department occupies. He or she studies and identifies the flow of staff and patients through the clinic, offices, and ADL apartment. In so doing, the manager has:
    A. identified elements critical for selecting a new location for the department.
    B. determined equipment needs.
    C. analyzed the work flow.
    D. determined functional areas.

158. The theory of cost containment is exemplified in the:
    A. Medicare Diagnosis-Related Groups (DRG) system.
    B. departmental charge structure.
    C. fee for service structure.
    D. per diem rates.

159. While completing the assessment and treatment planning process, the occupational therapist confers with the individual to establish program goals. As the therapist writes these goals, they should be:

A. specific measurable statements with time frames.
B. time frames for what will be accomplished.
C. specific measurements of the individual's skill and performance.
D. activities to be completed that correspond with the goals and objectives.

160. Objectives are:
    A. specific measurable statements with time frames.
    B. time frames for what will be accomplished.
    C. specific measurements of the individual's skill and performance.
    D. statements of how the goals will be achieved.

161. Medical documentation should include:
    A. concise objective information.
    B. speculative and judgmental information.
    C. objective and speculative information.
    D. subjective information and personal opinions.

162. A treatment plan or "plan of care":
    A. specifies directions for the therapist.
    B. measures the progress toward an individual's goal.
    C. organizes the individual's priorities.
    D. summarizes the approach of management of an individual.

163. An individual educational plan is completed for:
    A. occupational therapists as a part of the continuing education plan.
    B. adults who have sustained a head injury.
    C. all children with disabilities before they receive special education services.
    D. families before discharge of a significant other from occupational therapy services.

164. The subjective section of the SOAP format includes:
    A. measurement results.
    B. analysis of measurements recorded.
    C. speculative information.
    D. quotes from the individual.

165. The objective section of the SOAP format includes:
    A. functional performance levels.
    B. subjective and objective findings.
    C. conclusions and assumptions of performance measures.
    D. quotes from the individual and the family.

166. The supervising occupational therapist asks an experienced COTA to complete a portion of the assessment. The portion most appropriate for the COTA to complete independently would be:
    A. collecting chart review information.
    B. analyzing and interpreting assessment information.
    C. establishing the treatment goals.
    D. establishing the treatment plan.

167. **A budget format in which the occupational therapy manager is to justify all anticipated expense activities is referred to as:**
    A. incremental.
    B. programmatic.
    C. cost accounting.
    D. zero-based.

168. **The order in which the budgeting process MOST frequently occurs is:**
    A. budgeting, planning, controlling, and monitoring.
    B. monitoring, planning, controlling, and budgeting.
    C. planning, budgeting, monitoring, and controlling.
    D. controlling, monitoring, planning, and budgeting.

169. **A student has successfully fabricated a resting hand splint. The supervisor then assigns the student to fabricate an antispasticity splint. This process is based on which educational foundation?**
    A. Meet the learner at his or her current level.
    B. Generalization of learning.
    C. Use spaced learning intervals.
    D. Proceed from the complex to simple but unfamiliar.

170. **A standard formula for identifying space needs for an inpatient occupational therapy department is:**
    A. 1 to 4 square feet per bed.
    B. 4 to 8 square feet per bed.
    C. 8 to 12 square feet per bed.
    D. 12 to 14 square feet per bed.

171. **The theory of a hospital increasing its prices charged to all payors to make up for shortfalls in reimbursement by some payors is called:**
    A. prospective payment.
    B. cost shifting.
    C. account billing.
    D. cost accounting.

172. **A system of uniform terminology that is used to code health care services provided and that is used nationally for billing purposes is the:**
    A. UB-82.
    B. HCFA 1450.
    C. CPT.
    D. DRG.

173. **Benefits paid under Medicare Part A would include:**
    A. inpatient hospitalization.
    B. in-home occupational therapy services (psychiatric).
    C. outpatient occupational therapy.
    D. comprehensive outpatient rehabilitation facility.

174. **The therapist is treating an adult whose medical coverage is provided by a state payment system. The system MOST likely to be involved would be:**
    A. Medicaid or Medicare.
    B. Medicaid, the Education for All Handicapped Children Act, or workers' compensation.
    C. workers' compensation or Medicaid.
    D. the Education for All Handicapped Children Act or workers' compensation.

175. **The therapist is treating a middle-aged woman who has carpal tunnel syndrome. The employer's industrial nurse indicated that the condition was a result of repetitious fine motor skill execution required as an essential job function. The payment program MOST likely to provide payment of occupational therapy services is:**
    A. Medicare.
    B. Medicaid.
    C. workers' compensation.
    D. the Education for All Handicapped Children Act.

Promote Professional Practice

176. **Performance appraisals are for the PRIMARY purpose of:**
    A. objectively assessing worker performance.
    B. documenting employee disciplinary issues.
    C. awarding a merit increase.
    D. writing yearly professional goals and objectives.

177. **Agencies that provide services to the developmentally disabled population are accredited by:**
    A. JCAHO.
    B. CARF.
    C. AC MRDD.
    D. NLN/APHA.

178. **Agencies that provide health care services in nursing homes and are not part of a hospital system are accredited by:**
    A. JCAHO.
    B. CARF.
    C. AC MRDD.
    D. NLN/APHA.

179. **An academic fieldwork educator is responsible for:**
    A. administrative and day-to-day supervision of the student program.
    B. direct day-to-day supervision of students.
    C. acting as a liaison between the academic setting, facility, and students.
    D. establishing objectives for the fieldwork site.

180. **A productivity percentage that is frequently used as a standard in establishing workloads for staff occupational therapists is:**
    A. 45 percent.
    B. 60 percent.
    C. 75 percent.
    D. 90 percent.

181. **A target market is:**
    A. a broad-based marketing approach to services.
    B. segmentation of the market into distinct groups with a focus on a specified area.
    C. assessment of the consumer's social class, lifestyle, and personality characteristics.
    D. analysis of the economic and financial environment of the market base.

182. **An accrediting agency that surveys inpatient and comprehensive outpatient rehabilitation programs is the:**
    A. AOTA.
    B. JCAHO.
    C. CARF.
    D. NBCOT.

183. **Advertising may include:**
    A. direct mailings.
    B. holding an open house.
    C. lecturing.
    D. developing a free speakers bureau.

184. **A document that encompasses the underlying values and basic moral beliefs to be used by occupational therapists is the:**
    A. Standards of Practice.
    B. Uniform Terminology System for Reporting Occupational Therapy Services, third edition.
    C. licensure guidelines.
    D. Occupational Therapy *Code of Ethics.*

185. **Informed consent is:**
    A. the process of providing sufficient information so that an individual can make an informed decision about his or her own health care.
    B. a clinical judgment by the therapist to implement a particular treatment for the individual.
    C. a verbal agreement made by the prospective employee to accept a job offer.
    D. written acknowledgment of ability to complete a job with or without accommodation.

186. **An occupational therapist is required to have graduated from an accredited occupational therapy program, successfully completed fieldwork experience, and passed the National Board for Certification in Occupational Therapy (NBCOT) certification examination to obtain:**
    A. malpractice insurance.
    B. mandatory certification.
    C. employment.
    D. membership in the state association.

187. **An occupational therapist has engaged in a dereliction of duty causing actual damage to the plaintiff secondary to substandard care. The therapist may be found guilty, and the plaintiff awarded monetary rewards, through the:**
    A. local ordinances.
    B. "tort" law.
    C. NBCOT.
    D. state licensing board.

188. **An increase in public awareness of occupational therapy and the promotion of functional independence for individuals with disabilities have:**
    A. reduced the supply of therapists and reduced the demand.
    B. increased the supply of occupational therapists to meet the demand.
    C. created an increase in demand resulting in an inadequate supply of therapists.
    D. not affected the supply or demand of occupational therapists.

189. **A private-practice occupational therapist is preparing to act as a consultant to a community agency. The first step should be to:**
    A. negotiate the contract.
    B. establish trust.
    C. assess the environment.
    D. identify problems.

190. **Medical care, dental coverage, sick leave, disability insurance, and tuition reimbursement are all a part of:**
    A. a vacation package.
    B. a recruitment package.
    C. a benefits package.
    D. orientation.

191. **A manager may financially reward employees through:**
    A. disciplinary actions.
    B. performance reviews.
    C. clinical education.
    D. merit increases.

192. **Marketing and promotion of occupational therapy are most frequently done by personal selling. This would include:**
    A. consumer analysis.
    B. a presentation to physicians.
    C. a self-audit.
    D. an environmental assessment.

193. **The Americans with Disabilities Act (ADA) of 1990 was landmark legislation on behalf of individuals with disabilities. A key term used in the ADA is "essential functions." Essential functions are:**
    A. accommodations provided for the disabled.
    B. any modifications to a job that allow a disabled worker to perform the job tasks.
    C. job tasks that are fundamental to the position.
    D. modified work tasks.

194. **The document that provides the following occupational therapy guidelines for screening, referral, evaluation, treatment planning, implementation, discontinuation of services, quality assurance, indirect services, and legal and ethical issues is called the:**

A. Uniform Terminology System for Reporting Occupational Therapy Services, third edition.
B. Standards of Practice.
C. licensure regulations.
D. AOTA Policies and Procedures.

195. **A research design that tests a hypothesis by measuring the differences of two or more variables and "looking" at their relationship is:**
A. experimental design.
B. quasi-experimental design.
C. factorial design.
D. correlation design.

196. **After identifying a potential research question, the next step in the process is:**
A. stating the purpose.
B. designing the research.
C. completing a review of the literature.
D. establishing boundaries for the study.

197. **State organizations that were established to assure appropriate cost-effective care and protect the consumer are:**
A. JCAHOs.
B. CARFs.
C. PROs.
D. ARAs.

198. **JCAHO is an acronym for:**
A. Justified Care of Adolescent Hospital Organizations.
B. Juvenile Council of Adolescent Health Organizations.
C. Joint Council on Accessibility of Health Organizations.
D. Joint Commission on Accreditation of Hospital Organizations.

199. **The manager of occupational therapy is writing a report to justify additional staff. The information that would provide the STRONGEST support for additional staff would be:**
A. a cost-accounting report.
B. a definition of Relative Value Units (RVUs) report.
C. a productivity report.
D. a market analysis.

200. **A program that ensures that disabled children receive educational services in the least restrictive environment is:**
A. the Americans with Disabilities Act.
B. the Education for All Handicapped Children Act.
C. Children's Protective Services.
D. Medicare.

ANSWERS FOR SIMULATION EXAMINATION 1

1. (C) Clinical observation. Checklists are simple lists of factors or behaviors that a therapist thinks are important to observe as a support for referral or screening of a child. Although checklists may appear in a standard format, they are not well developed enough to include establishment of normative data and other attributes of tests, such as validity and reliability. If a checklist is researched, it may become criterion-referenced. See reference: Case-Smith, Allen, and Pratt (eds): Stewart, KB: Occupational therapy assessment in pediatrics: Purposes, process, and methods of evaluation.

2. (A) Measures the skill or function it claims to measure. There are several kinds of validity, including logical, content, and construct validity; however, they all indicate whether the test measures what it claims to measure. Answers B and C describe reliability, which indicates the strength of the test's consistency. A test based on a normative population (answer D) is not necessarily valid, because it has collected statistics on only that group. Scores obtained by the sample population are usually compared with scores on tests measuring similar functions in order to establish validity. See reference: Case-Smith, Allen, and Pratt (eds): Richardson, PK: Use of standardized tests in pediatric practice.

3. (B) Compares performance to a normal standard. "Norm referencing" is a term applied to standardized or formal tests that have been given to a specific population

called the "normative sample." It does not guarantee that the test is valid and reliable unless evidence for these characteristics is provided. See reference: Dunn, W: Cook, DG: The assessment process.

4. (C) Has a standard format. Standardization of a test means that the test is administered in a prescribed manner, and that scoring and interpretation of scores are also completed in a prescribed way. The presence of data from giving the test to a normal population, and the establishment of reliability and validity, are often included with standardized tests but are not stated as a required part of the definition. See reference: Case-Smith, Allen, and Pratt (eds): Richardson, PK: Use of standardized tests in pediatric practice.

5. (B) Follow test manual directions. As a standardized test, directions from the test manual should be followed closely to ensure the reliability of test results. Test environments should be nonstimulating so that the child can concentrate on the test items. Test items with young children are best presented with the last item on the table so that the child can make the transition more easily. Although the overall success of an evaluation can depend on the therapist's ability to establish rapport with the child and the family, too much conversation with the child may be distracting and may detract from optimal performance. See reference: Dunn, W: Cook, DG: The assessment process.

6. (A) Primitive reflexes and postural reactions. The Milani-Comparetti Motor Development Screening Test measures the disappearance of primitive reflexes and the emergence of postural reactions. These reactions are linked to locomotor patterns. Neither cognitive nor language skills are included on this test. See reference: Case-Smith, Allen, and Pratt (eds): Nichols, DS: The development of postural control.

7. (D) Landau reaction. The Landau reaction is stimulated by the lifting of the head when the child is suspended horizontally. Extensor tone is created throughout the body and is needed for sitting and standing. The tonic labyrinthine reflex in prone involves body flexion. The asymmetrical tonic neck reflex is characterized by extension on the face side and flexion on the skull side with head turning. The neck righting reaction is characterized by head and body alignment on the rotational axis. None of these other reactions develop extensor tone. See reference: Case-Smith, Allen, and Pratt (eds): Nichols, DS: The development of postural control.

8. (B) Inability to read. The term "dyslexia" literally means dysfunction in reading. Answer A is technically called dysgraphia. Answer C is dyscalculia, and answer D is dyspraxia. See reference: Case-Smith, Allen, and Pratt (eds): Gordon, CY, Schanzenbacher, KE, Case-Smith, J, and Carrasco, R: Diagnostic problems in pediatrics.

9. (D) Pervasive developmental disorder of childhood. This disorder includes extreme social isolation, difficulty or inability in communication, and unusual responses to the environment. Anxiety disorders of childhood are usually reactions to real or perceived stress (therefore, answer A is incorrect). An example of a childhood conduct disorder is repetitive and persistent antisocial behavior (therefore, answer B is incorrect). An example of an affective disorder is childhood depression (therefore, answer C is incorrect). See reference: Case-Smith, Allen, and Pratt (eds): Gordon, CY, Schanzenbacher, KE, Case-Smith, J, and Carrasco, R: Diagnostic problems in pediatrics.

10. (C) Lower extremity, trunk, and mild upper extremity. The correct answer is C because diplegia refers to these specific areas of the body. Involvement of both legs is called paraplegia (answer B), and all extremities and neck involvement describes quadriplegia (answer D). Answer A is also incorrect because there is no specific classification or name for involvement of both upper limbs when describing cerebral palsy. See reference: Case-Smith, Allen, and Pratt (eds): Gordon, CY, Schanzenbacher, KE, Case-Smith, J, and Carrasco, R: Diagnostic problems in pediatrics.

11. (D) Consider and treat underlying sensory integration problems as a possible cause. Often, children's sensory integration problems interfere with the development of hand dominance. The cause could be decreased ability to cross the body midline, poor sensory perception in the arms and hands, delayed integration of reflex patterns, and so forth. Answers A, B, and C are incorrect because they do not address possible underlying causes for poorly established hand dominance. See reference: Case-Smith, Allen, and Pratt (eds): Parham, LD, and Mailloux, Z: Sensory integration.

12. (D) Transdisciplinary. The concept of "role release" or of one team member fulfilling the roles of others to ease communication with the family is called the transdisciplinary method of teamwork. Answer A is incorrect because a unidisciplinary team is not really a team; as the term implies, there is only one member. Answer B is not correct because the multidisciplinary team uses several disciplines, but they may not work in a collaborative manner. Answer C is also incorrect because in the interdisciplinary team, although it has group consensus regarding program planning, the members carry out their programs in their own environments. See reference: Case-Smith, Allen, and Pratt (eds): Allen, AS: Relationships with other service providers.

13. (D) Passive movement followed by slow, rhythmic movement. According to Erhardt, therapy for the child with spasticity should include the neurodevelopmental treatment principle of passive movement to reduce tone. This type of movement is important because, initially, it will elongate the muscles and prepare the child for gentle movement, such as rocking on a therapy ball in prone, to further reduce tone. Answer A is wrong because it is the treatment principle for children with low muscle tone, who need the additional tactile and proprioceptive input of weight bearing and compression with movement. Answer B is wrong because it is the principle underlying treatment of low-to-normal muscle tone or ataxia, where the child needs to move to develop righting and balance reactions without losing stability. Answer C is wrong because it applies to the treatment of children with athetosis, who move too much in very asymmetric patterns. See reference: Hopkins and Smith (eds): Erhardt, RP: Cerebral palsy.

14. (B) 90/90/90 degrees at hip/knee/ankle joints. A 90-degree position at each joint places the body in a neutral position without too much flexion or extension, which might cause deformity and interfere with function in sitting. Answer A is incorrect because 45 degrees at each of these joints places the body in extreme flexion. Answer C is incorrect because 45 degrees at any joint is excessive flexion. Answer D is incorrect because 125 degrees places each joint in excessive extension. See reference: Hopkins and Smith (eds): Erhardt, RP: Cerebral palsy.

15. (D) Weight bearing over a small bolster in prone. Basic hand skills are developed through weight bearing on the arms. Inhibition of flexor spasticity occurs through slow joint compression from weight bearing, as well as facilitation of ulnar to radial function in the hand. Answers A and B are incorrect because they require voluntary control of release of objects without inhibition. Answer C is incorrect because traction on the finger flexors would increase spasticity in the flexor muscles and make opening of the hand more difficult. See reference: Case-Smith, Allen, and Pratt (eds): Exner, CE: Development of hand skills.

16. (D) Removing a nut from a bolt. Answer D describes one type of "in-hand manipulation" called "rotation." Rotation is the movement of an object around one or more of its axes, where objects may be turned horizontally or end over end with the pads of the fingers. Answers A, B, and C are incorrect because they describe hand activities that essentially keep the object in a certain position as it is grasped, released, or carried. See reference: Case-Smith, Allen, and Pratt (eds): Exner, CE: Development of hand skills.

17. (D) The conditions statement. This is the "conditions statement" because it defines the circumstances under which the child will feed herself. "Self-feeding" is the behavioral component of this statement. The performance criterion is "without spilling in a 20-minute period" because it defines how acceptable performance is measured. The child is called "the learner." See reference: Case-Smith, Allen, and Pratt (eds): Case-Smith, J: Planning and implementing services.

18. (A) Poor postural responses. Poor postural responses, such as poor balance and postural control against gravity, are often symptoms of an underreactive vestibular system. Possible symptoms of an overreactive vestibular system are answers B, C, and D, which are problems of intolerance for motion and gravitational insecurity. See reference: Ayres: Disorders involving the vestibular system.

19. (C) After the evaluation. The information received from observation, interview, and evaluation gives the therapist a comprehensive picture of the child's performance dysfunctions; therefore, the problem list is constructed after the evaluation (answer C). See reference: Case-Smith, Allen, and Pratt (eds): Case-Smith, J: Planning and implementing services.

20. (A) Long-term goals written to the anticipated period of rehabilitation. Long-term goals are usually written with a possible discharge date in mind or, in the case of a school program, toward the end of the school year (answer A). They are written in general terms. Conversely, the short-term objectives are written toward shorter periods and indicate that a child is making progress toward the long-term goal. Short-term objectives are written in specific terms to measure specific areas of progress. See reference: Case-Smith, Allen, and Pratt (eds): Case-Smith, J: Planning and implementing services.

21. (D) The priorities of the child, caregiver, and therapist. The problems established in the occupational therapy (OT) evaluation are not the only basis for writing OT goals and objectives. The child's priorities as well as the caregiver's needs and concerns must be addressed so that immediate needs are met and so that everyone is committed to the success of the program. See reference: Case-Smith, Allen, and Pratt (eds): Case-Smith, J: Planning and implementing services.

22. (D) Cognition. "Praxis" or "motor planning" refers to the ability to attend to and plan a motor act cognitively, based on adequate sensory input (answer D). Dr. Ayres referred to this function as the highest, most complex, of children's motor functions, involving conscious attention that is closely linked to mental and intellectual functions. Automatic and reflex motor activity, as well as coordination of the motor act, do not require attention or volition—it is enough to have a general goal in mind. Therefore, answers A, B, and C are incorrect. See reference: Ayres: Developmental dyspraxia: A motor planning problem.

23. (B) Rotary chewing. Rotary chewing is the highest level of oral motor development among these choices (answer B). In order of developmental appearance, sucking and swallowing appear first, followed by munching of food (an early form of chewing), then vertical chewing, and last, rotary chewing. See reference: Case-Smith, Allen, and Pratt (eds): Case-Smith, J, and Humphry, R: Feeding and oral motor skills.

24. (C) Identify the critical elements of development and role performance for the age of the child. Answer C is correct because it is the necessary step to understanding delays in development and the needs of the child. Next, the therapist defines and describes the child's problem, which includes course and outcome. Finally, in general problem analysis, the effects of the problem on tasks and performance (including the components of performance) are considered. This process can begin with referral of a child and continue through evaluation to the planning of intervention. See reference: Case-Smith, Allen, and Pratt (eds): Case-Smith, J: Planning and implementing services.

25. (D) All extremities. The word "quadriplegia" refers to involvement of all four extremities and in cerebral palsy describes trunk, neck, and often oral motor involvement as well. One-limb involvement is called monoplegia and is very rare. The involvement of one side of the body is called hemiplegia, so this term is an incorrect answer. Answer C, the involvement of both legs, is called paraplegia. See reference: Case-Smith, Allen, and Pratt (eds): Gordon, CY, Schanzenbacher, KE, Case-Smith, J, and Carrasco, RC: Diagnostic problems in pediatrics.

26. (A) Exploratory. Exploratory play provides the child with experiences that develop body scheme, sensory integrative and motor skills, and concepts of sensory characteristics and actions on objects. Therefore, the obstacle course is an example of exploratory play. Symbolic play is associated with the development of language and concepts (the use of "dress up" materials would be an example of this type of play). Creative play and interests are characterized by refinement of skills in activities that allow construction, social relationships, and dramatic play (finger painting is an example of creative play). Recreational play consists of play-leisure experiences that allow exploration of interests and roles, such as sports or arts and crafts. See reference: Case-Smith, Allen, and Pratt (eds): Stewart, KB: Occupational therapy assessment in pediatrics: Purposes, process, and methods of evaluation.

27. (B) Overreactive to being touched. "Touch defensiveness" or "tactile defensiveness," as described by A.

Jean Ayres, is an overreaction or negative reaction to sensations of touch. These sensations may be overwhelming probably because of a lack of central nervous system inhibitory influences. Answer A is not correct, because an underreactivity to touch is thought to indicate touch sensations are not being adequately received or perceived by the central nervous system. Although children with tactile defensiveness may touch objects and people excessively, they usually do not crave being touched by others, therefore, answer C is not correct. Light touch is particularly uncomfortable to the child with touch defensiveness; therefore, answer D is also incorrect. See reference: Ayres: Tactile defensiveness.

28. (C) Petit mal. Petit mal is the correct name for a seizure that barely interrupts a child's performance (answer C is correct). Answer A, grand mal seizure, usually involves loss of consciousness. Answer B, psychomotor or tonic-clonic seizure affects automatic movements and therefore is incorrect. Answer D, akinetic seizure, involves loss of muscle tone, and therefore this answer is also incorrect. See reference: Case-Smith, Allen, and Pratt (eds): Gordon, CY, Schanzenbacher, KE, Case-Smith, J, and Carrasco, RC: Diagnostic problems in pediatrics.

29. (A) Semicircular canals. Although the vestibular system functions are not completely understood, it is generally believed that the semicircular canals receive sensory information about motion. The utricle and saccule receive sensory information about gravity, and the cochlea receives auditory sensory information. See reference: Ayres: The nervous system within.

30. (B) Can usually handle routine daily functions. Answer B is correct because it describes the skills of an individual with moderate or trainable-level mental retardation. This child can usually complete activities of daily living, live in a group home setting, and do unskilled work in a sheltered workshop situation. Answer A describes a child with profound mental retardation. Answer C describes a child with severe mental retardation. And answer D describes a child who is mildly mentally retarded, or educable. See reference: Case-Smith, Allen, and Pratt (eds): Gordon, CY, Schanzenbacher, KE, Case-Smith, J, and Carrasco, RC: Diagnostic problems in pediatrics.

31. (C) Righting reactions. Righting reactions develop after the integration of primitive reflex patterns, which are thought to be necessary for survival in the normal newborn. Righting reactions allow children to right their heads against gravity and to realign their bodies around the movement of the head in that process. Prehensile reactions refer to grasping patterns and reach, which differentiate humans from other primates. Equilibrium reactions develop after righting reactions and allow the child to maintain a standing and walking posture. See reference: Hopkins and Smith (eds): Simon, CJ, and Daub, MM: Human development across the life span.

32. (C) Symmetrical tonic neck. The symmetrical tonic neck reflex is elicited by neck dorsiflexion, and the re-

sponse consists of flexion of hips and knees and extension of the arms. This pattern of movement brings the child into four-point position for the first time, but eventually it must be integrated for creeping to occur. The asymmetrical tonic neck response (extension on the face side of the body and flexion on the skull side) interferes with the achievement of four-point position. A crossed extension reflex causes extension of legs on stimulation of the foot. The tonic labyrinthine reflex involves total flexion or extension patterns in response to placement in prone or supine positions. None of the latter patterns bring the child into a quadruped position. See reference: Hopkins and Smith (eds): Simon, CJ, and Daub, MM: Human development across the life span.

33. (C) Criterion-referenced test. A test that guides program planning (such as the EIDP) is usually called a "criterion-referenced test," according to Pratt and colleagues. The normative data may be based on other tests or studies. Answers A and B are not correct because therapist-made checklists and clinical observations are informal observations that a therapist finds useful with certain client groups. They are often written in different formats from one program to another. A norm-referenced test has a higher level of normative standardization than the criterion-referenced tests; therefore, answer D is not correct. See reference: Case-Smith, Allen, and Pratt (eds): Richardson, PK: Use of standardized tests in pediatric practice.

34. (A) Fluctuating. Children with athetoid cerebral palsy have fluctuating muscle tone (answer A), which usually fluctuates from low to normal. Spastic muscle tone is characteristic of children with spastic cerebral palsy (answer B). Flaccid muscle tone (answer C) or low muscle tone is usually seen in young children with cerebral palsy and usually is later classified as spastic, athetoid, or ataxic. Rigid muscle tone is characterized by tonic muscle activity that does not fluctuate; therefore, answer D is incorrect. See reference: Case-Smith, Allen, and Pratt (eds): Gordon, CY, Schanzenbacher, KE, Case-Smith, J, and Carrasco, RC: Diagnostic problems in pediatrics.

35. (C) Ulnar palmar. Ulnar palmar grasp precedes the other types of grasp. The infant first grasps on the ulnar side of the hand against the palm, then with all four fingers against the palm (palmar grasp), and finally the grasp moves to the radial side of the hand (radial grasp). The highest level of grasp is pincer grasp, in which the pad of the index finger meets the opposed thumb. See reference: Case-Smith, Allen, and Pratt (eds): Exner, CE: Development of hand skills.

36. (B) Protective tactile system. The protective tactile system is not being modulated properly when touch-defensive responses are seen in a child; therefore, answer B is correct. Children who have difficulty identifying where they are touched or difficulty identifying shapes of objects have a disorder of the discriminative tactile system. Touch or tactile sensations are not carried via vestibular or olfactory pathways, and therefore these answers are also incorrect. See reference: Ayres: Developmental dyspraxia: A motor planning problem.

37. (A) Lela Llorens. Lela Llorens was broadly influenced by developmental theorists, and her frame of reference addresses the individual's functions and their integration during specific periods of life (horizontal developmental) and over the course of time (longitudinal development). See reference: Case-Smith, Allen, and Pratt (eds): Hinojosa, J, Kramer, P, and Pratt, PN: Foundations of practice: Developmental principles, theories, and frames of reference.

38. (C) A. Jean Ayres. A. Jean Ayres formulated sensory integration theory, which describes how the brain organizes sensory input for use in adaptive responses. See reference: Case-Smith, Allen, and Pratt (eds): Hinojosa, J, Kramer, P, and Pratt, PN: Foundations of practice: Developmental principles, theories, and frames of reference.

39. (B) Eleanor Gilfoyle and Ann Grady. Gilfoyle and Grady have used the term "spatiotemporal" to describe a process of interactions between the child and his or her environment of time and space. Their frame of reference is differentiated from that of the other theorists. If the adaptation process is interrupted or not completed, the results are spatiotemporal distress and dysfunction. See reference: Case-Smith, Allen, and Pratt (eds): Hinojosa, J, Kramer, P, and Pratt, PN: Foundations of practice: Developmental principles, theories, and frames of reference.

40. (B) After back extension in prone develops. Answer B is correct because back extension developed in prone is a basic requirement for trunk control in sitting. Answer A is incorrect because lifting the head in prone is only the beginning of back extension, and the child has little trunk control. Answer C is not correct because primitive reflexes interfere with the development of back control. Answer D is incorrect because walking alone requires further development of trunk and leg control than sitting alone. See reference: Case-Smith, Allen, and Pratt (eds): Nichols, DS: The development of postural control.

41. (C) 9 and 12 months. Children usually begin to "cruise" (walk sideways holding on to a rail) between 9 and 12 months. See reference: Case-Smith, Allen, and Pratt (eds): Case-Smith, J, and Shortridge, SD: The developmental process: Prenatal to adolescence.

42. (A) Observation. The "uncontrived" activity setting allows the therapist to observe the child's natural use of functional abilities and social and play skills without structure or adult influence. In this way, the therapist can compare interview and test findings with information from observation notes to formulate recommendations. See reference: Case-Smith, Allen, and Pratt (eds): Stewart, KB: Occupational therapy assessment in pediatrics: Purposes, process, and methods of evaluation.

43. (C) Body righting. The body righting reaction replaces the neonatal neck righting reflex (log rolling) and provides the infant with the ability to rotate the trunk on the vertebral axis. The asymmetric tonic neck reflex interferes with development of rotation because of arm extension on the face side and shoulder retraction on the skull side. The tonic labyrinthine reflex interferes with development of rotation also because it acts on the body in flexion and extension patterns only. See reference: Hopkins and Smith (eds): Simon, CJ, and Daub, MM: Human development across the life span.

44. (C) Swaddling the child before handling. Swaddling provides a child who is still very tactilely defensive some deep pressure before being handled. Deep pressure "breaks through" the light-touch receptors on the skin, which are thought to be lacking modulation as they are processed to the central nervous system. Answers B and D, besides stimulating light-touch receptors, also are being applied by an adult. These activities, if controlled by the child, would be more acceptable. Answer A is incorrect and involves an improper use of vibration. Vibrators should not be applied on the stomach, where there can be possible ill effects to various organs of the body located in that area. See reference: Hopkins and Smith (eds): Kinnealey, M, and Miller, L: Sensory integration/learning disabilities.

45. (A) Coach the parents in skills needed for decreasing apparent tactile defensiveness. Training the parents meets the need of spreading more therapeutic intervention into the daily activities and addresses the problem of behavior that may be related to touch defensiveness. Answer B is not the most appropriate choice but would be correct if the parents were unable to work on home programming. Answers C and D are incorrect because they do not address a problem that may be improved through occupational therapy or sensorimotor intervention. See reference: Hopkins and Smith (eds): Kinnealey, M, and Miller, L: Sensory integration/learning disabilities.

46. (A) Occupational therapy program works for the child. Answer A is correct because parents need to see the success of the occupational therapy program in order to continue. A program that is too challenging (answer B) may be frustrating for the child and parent alike. Answer C is incorrect because parents are more invested in the program if they have participated in goal setting. Incorporating a home program into the family's daily routine makes it easier in terms of time schedules and makes the program more meaningful to both parent and child (answer D is incorrect). See reference: Case-Smith, Allen, and Pratt (eds): Humphry, R, and Case-Smith, J: Working with families.

47. (A) Cystic fibrosis. Cystic fibrosis (answer A) is the only correct answer. Duchenne's disease is a neuromuscular condition; therefore, Answer B is incorrect. Pediatric AIDS is an acquired immune deficiency syndrome, so that answer C is incorrect. Down syndrome is a birth defect characterized by an additional chromosome 21 and is also incorrect. See reference: Case-Smith, Allen, and Pratt (eds): Gordon, CY, Schanzenbacher, KE, Case-Smith, J, and Carrasco, RC: Diagnostic problems in pediatrics.

48. (C) Parents' needs and wishes should be included in program planning. An individual parent's needs and wishes should be considered when decisions about parent involvement in the occupational therapy program are discussed (answer C is correct). Parents should be encouraged to observe their child in therapy so that they may better understand the program and their child's problems; therefore answer A is incorrect. Although some parents may carry out therapy programs at home, many therapists and parents feel that too much responsibility for the program may detract from normal family life and socialization. It is also recommended that both parents be present when an occupational therapy program is discussed (answer D is incorrect), so that one does not become dependent on the other for information and communication. See reference: Case-Smith, Allen, and Pratt (eds): Humphry, R, and Case-Smith, J: Working with families.

49. (C) Following directions about objects located in front, in back, and to the side. Answer C is correct because a visual perceptual problem of position in space refers to difficulty perceiving the relationship of an object to the self. Answer A, identifying letters on a distracting page, is not correct because it refers to a problem of size and shape (form) constancy. Answer D, making judgments about moving through space, is incorrect because it refers to a problem in perceiving spatial relationships. See reference: Case-Smith, Allen, and Pratt (eds): Schneck, CM: Visual perception.

50. (B) Ability to follow rules and instructions. Answer B is correct because it gives information about the student's basic ability to learn and adapt in a work situation. Answer A, leisure interests, is not correct because although important to the student's life, leisure interest knowledge is not essential to work. Answers C and D are not correct because, although they describe the student's motor control function, which can affect which type of job he or she performs, adaptation can be made to either of these areas of need. See reference: Case-Smith, Allen, and Pratt (eds): Gordon, CY, Schanzenbacher, KE, Case-Smith, J, and Carrasco, RC: Diagnostic problems in pediatrics.

51. (C) Biomechanical. The biomechanical approach is based on enhancing strength, range of motion and endurance. The biomechanical approach is typically used when impairment does not affect the intact central nervous system. This approach is primarily used for individuals who have had a traumatic injury or illness that has affected the musculoskeletal system. The rehabilitative approach (answer A) emphasizes making an individual as independent as possible and compensating for limitations. The neurodevelopmental approach (answer B) is used for individuals who are born with a central nervous system dysfunction, have experienced an illness, or have had an injury to the neural system. The neurodevelopmental approach is based on using sensory input and developmental sequences to promote function. The psychoanalytic approach (answer D) is based in working with an individual's internal conflicts and past experiences. It is most frequently used in mental health environments. See reference: Trombly: Theoretical foundations for practice.

52. (B) Neurodevelopmental. The neurodevelopmental approach is a theory of practice that was developed for individuals who were either born with a central nervous system dysfunction or have experienced a trauma or injury to the central nervous system. The principles of treatment are based on the integration of primitive reflexes, development of voluntary movement, normalization of tone, positioning, controlled sensory input, and learning. The rehabilitative approach (answer A) emphasizes making an individual as independent as possible and compensating for limitations. The psychoanalytic approach (answer C) is based on working with an individual's internal conflicts and past experiences. It is most frequently used in mental health environments. The maturational approach (answer D) is based on a child's skill development occurring as the central nervous system matures. See reference: Trombly: Theoretical foundations of occupational therapy.

53. (C) Assess the need for training in compensatory techniques. Sensory-perceptual evaluations include assessment of proprioception, stereognosis, motor planning, visual form and space, and visual-field deficits. Treatment of sensory impairment includes reeducation of sensation as well as instruction in compensatory techniques. Training in compensatory techniques includes the use of vision to guide an extremity during movement. Also, caretakers may need to be trained in protective precautions for those individuals who demonstrate impaired cognition. See reference: Trombly, CA (ed): Bentzel, K: Remediating sensory impairment.

54. (B) Demonstrate the procedure on the unaffected extremity, then occlude the individual's vision. The presentation of stimuli in sensory evaluation is extremely important. Because of the compensation that may occur with vision, it is necessary to occlude the individual's vision. Also, the unaffected extremity should be assessed before the affected extremity, the opposite of answer A, to reduce anxiety in the individual. Stimuli should be presented in a random proximal-to-distal pattern. A rapport (answer C) should be established before beginning any of the evaluation procedures, also to reduce anxiety. An individual may not be aware of any deficit areas (answer D), so the whole extremity should be assessed to ensure accuracy. Picture cards are helpful in assessing individuals with expressive aphasia. See reference: Trombly, CA (ed): Bentzel, K: Evaluation of sensation.

55. (B) Receptive aphasia. Individuals with receptive aphasia are unable to comprehend spoken or written words and symbols; therefore, they cannot accurately understand verbal directions or consistently respond to stimuli. Individuals with receptive aphasia may be able to imitate or follow demonstration. However, these techniques may not be used with a sensory evaluation. Expressive aphasia interferes with an individual's verbal or written expression, but not comprehension of verbal or written information. An individual with expressive aphasia would be able to indicate the response by pointing to the stimulus used or a card that has been marked with the correct response. An individual who has agnosia or ataxia would be able to understand directions, but unable to indicate an area accurately because of impaired recognition of the body part or impaired coordination. The method of response may be adapted by using verbal description of an area or cue cards. See reference: Trombly, CA (ed): Woodson, AM: Stroke.

56. (B) Stage 4. Brunnstrom defined the recovery of muscle function in six stages: (1) flaccidity, (2) development of synergies, (3) voluntary movement within synergy, (4) gross motor movement within synergy, (5) movement outside of synergies, and (6) near normal movement with isolated joint movement. Brunnstrom also defined three movements to represent stage 4. These are (1) placing the hand behind the back, (2) flexing the shoulder at 90 degrees with the elbow fully extended, and (3) pronating and supinating the forearm. See reference: Trombly· Movement therapy of Brunnstrom.

57. (A) Positioning, compression glove, and edema massage followed by passive range-of-motion exercises. These four measures can be effective in the reduction of edema and prevention of further edema. The goal is to promote the movement of fluid back into normal circulation rather than allowing it to collect in one area or body part. Gentle passive range of motion is necessary to help maintain joint structure and provide nutrients to the joint. The actual movement of the extremity may serve as a "pump" to assist in moving excess fluid back into the body. These techniques are contraindicated for individuals who have deep vein thrombosis. In addition, edema is partially a result of the loss of movement in an extremity, which does not allow the contraction of muscles to pump the fluid to the heart. A person who performs active or active-assisted range-of-motion exercise would be able to use that exercise to reduce the edema, and the muscle tone in the individual's arm world be considered low tone, but not flaccid. See reference: Trombly, CA (ed): Woodson, AM: Stroke.

58. (B) Line bisection. Line bisection is used as a method of determining unilateral neglect. The block assembly (used for constructional apraxia) is not a paper-and-pencil task, and the other test may be performed with or without the individual writing. Proverb interpretation (abstraction) may be performed verbally, and overlapping figures (figure-ground discrimination) testing may be performed by pointing. See reference: Trombly, CA (ed): Quintana, LA: Evaluation of perception and cognition.

59. (C) Anterograde amnesia. Anterograde amnesia is the inability to recall events after a trauma. Retrograde amnesia is the inability to recall events before a trauma. Long-term memory is the storage of information for recall at a later time. Orientation is the awareness of person, place, and time. See reference: Trombly, CA (ed): Quintana, LA: Evaluation of perception and cognition.

60. (A) A goniometer. A goniometer measures available joint movement. A pinch meter is used to measure available thumb-to-finger pinch strength in all available positions. A dynamometer measures grip strength in the

hand. An aesthesiometer measures two-point discriminations. See reference: Trombly, CA: Evaluation of biomechanical and physiological aspects of motor performance.

61. (D) The individual asks for more beverages during meals, but appears surprised when the therapist indicates beverages in closed containers are on the meal tray. The subjective portion of the SOAP note should contain information that is gained through a chart review, or communication with the patient, his or her family, or staff. This information is not measurable and therefore is considered subjective. Answer A would be in the program plan. Answers B and C would be in the objective portion because they are either measurable or based on specific observations. See reference: Trombly: Planning, guiding, and documenting therapy.

62. (C) The individual will complete upper-extremity self-care using appropriate adaptive equipment with the supervision of a family member. A long-term goal is written in conjunction with the individual and family to specify the end result of a longer period of treatment. A short-term goal breaks the long-term goal into manageable steps to be accomplished by the individual within a certain time frame or number of treatment sessions. Performing upper-extremity bathing, lower-extremity dressing, or a commode transfer with clothing adjustment were all short increments toward the stated goal of the individual returning home with the assistance of one person. The goal that encompassed the long-range plan was to complete upper-extremity self-care with the supervision of a family member. See reference: Trombly: Planning, guiding, and documenting therapy.

63. (D) Consistent and appropriate use of adaptive equipment and hip precautions. Many factors are considered when a long-term goal is reset. These factors may include items such as consistency, cognitive or perceptual impairments, the amount of time required, and any change in attention or concentration. For the long-term goal to be changed, the individual needs to be able to demonstrate consistency of performance, because improved memory and increased performance have already been demonstrated. The amount of time needed or concentration have not been problems or they would have been as part of the goal originally. The ability to remember two of three hip precautions does not demonstrate improved memory, so the long-term goal would not change. See reference: Trombly: Planning, guiding, and documenting therapy.

64. (A) Complete independence with self-care and transfers. An individual with T-3 paraplegia will have the trunk balance and upper extremity strength and coordination to complete self-care and work activities independently. See reference: Wilson, DJ, McKenzie, M, Barber, L, and Watson, KL: Goals and treatment planning.

65. (C) Have the individual trace lines across the page with the right index finger from the left to the right side. A person who follows a line when wheeling a wheelchair is focusing on midline positioning, not crossing the midline. Placing objects commonly used on the unaffected side is a compensatory technique that does not involve crossing the midline. The individual with midline problems would need cueing to avoid starting at the midline when attempting to lay cards out from the right to left side. Also, the person would have difficulty accurately completing a sequencing task on the neglected side, making it difficult to complete the midline crossing successfully. However, when tracing a line across the page, the individual receives the same proprioceptive input from the movement, and uses the same amount of space in the visual field, as when writing on paper. This task makes the transfer of skills easier when performing writing. See reference: Zoltan, B, Siev, E, and Freishtat, B: Body image and body scheme disorders.

66. (B) Lateral trunk stability. An individual who is uncoordinated or has poor head control would not be able to control the mobile arm support to bring the hand safely to the mouth without hitting the face or some other area. Also, poor head control would mean that the individual's head would be out of alignment for the hand to reach, or the person would be unable to see properly to control the mobile arm support. An individual with fair plus (3+) elbow flexion would be able to stabilize the elbow on the table to bring the hand to the mouth and would have enough strength to move the arm without the mobile arm support. For the mobile arm support to perform properly, the individual's trunk needs to be stabilized laterally by his or her own control or with positioning devices to provide a stable base from which the arm may move. See reference: Trombly (ed): Linden, CA, and Trombly, CA: Orthoses: Kinds and purposes.

67. (A) Textured material, rubbing, tapping, and prolonged contact. Sensory desensitization helps the individual recalibrate altered sensory perceptions and improve sensibility. This type of program is initiated when light-touch sensation is intact. The above listed modalities are used as graded tactile stimuli. Treatment is most successful when carried out and controlled by the individual. With a severe injury such as a burn, it is also necessary to train the individual in protective precautions. Any techniques that provide an ungraded or nonspecific level of touch, such as massage, pressure, percussion, or electrical stimulation, would be tolerated with difficulty by a person with hypersensitivity, because much of the input is facilitory and would be interpreted as painful. Visual compensation and functional use of the extremity are techniques used with individuals who have impaired sensation. See reference: Trombly (ed): Bentzel, K: Remediating sensory impairment.

68. (B) An anticlaw. An ulnar nerve injury influences the flexion of the ring and small fingers that occurs during grasp as well as wrist flexion and ulnar deviation. This injury may cause hyperextension of the metacarpophalangeal joint, resulting in a claw hand. See reference: Kisner and Colby: The elbow and shoulder complex.

69. (C) Edema, contracture, muscle tone, and pain. Edema or swelling limit range of motion because of the increase of fluid in the extremity. A contracture can result

when joint motion is limited by a prolonged spasticity or change in the tissues, causing resistance to passive stretch. Muscle tone may also be a limiting factor in one's ability to complete range of motion. If an individual is unable to move a part through full range against gravity, the therapist may put the individual in a gravity-eliminated position to attempt the same movement. Finally, pain may be a limiting factor. This may particularly be seen in individuals with arthritis or changes in joint structure. Pain generally occurs in the end ranges of motion. Other options listed (proprioception and diadokinesis) may affect the quality of active movement or coordination but do not limit active or passive range of motion. See reference: Trombly: Evaluation of biomechanical and physiological aspects of motor performance.

70. (A) Pendulum exercises, icing, and active and passive range-of-motion exercises. The goal of treatment with an individual diagnosed with a frozen shoulder is to increase range of motion; therefore, treatment would include passive and active range-of-motion exercises. Pendulum exercises may be a part of this program. Icing may be helpful in reducing pain and inflammation. Strengthening activities would only be initiated once the full range is achieved. See reference: Cailliet: Reflex sympathetic dystrophy. In *Hand Pain and Impairment.*

71. (B) To wear noisy bracelets on the wrist or ankle as a reminder to visually scan toward the affected side. Although hazards may be removed from the environment, or padded, to prevent injury to an individual, use of these interventions is only feasible in a person's home. It is best to teach the individual visual scanning of the affected area and the environment, a technique that the person may use anywhere. An individual may avoid using sharp tools or extreme water temperature, but this avoidance does not teach him or her how to monitor the affected side visually, because it is a precaution that addresses only the problem with sensation. Noisy bracelets are one technique that may be used to accomplish compensation for both unilateral neglect and absence of sensation. Visual impairments that are not accompanied by sensory or perceptual deficits are more readily overcome with retraining. See reference: Trombly (ed): Quintana, LA: Remediating perceptual impairments.

72. (B) Permanent-press clothing. Use of a fabric that is wrinkle-resistant eliminates or decreases the amount of ironing needed for fabrics such as cotton or cotton blends. The side-loading washer is an example of household equipment adapted to eliminate excessive reaching from a wheelchair. An extended-handle dustpan eliminates the need for bending or stooping from a standing or sitting position; however, neither the dustpan nor the washer eliminates the work needed for the tasks. Good body mechanics are necessary to protect or maintain physical health, but they do not eliminate work either. See reference: Trombly: Retraining basic and instrumental activities of daily living.

73. (D) Incoordination. A person who has tremors or poor coordination could limit much instability by stabilizing the limb proximally before working distally. Stabilization adds a secure base of support from which to work. Reduced vision, poor endurance, and limited fine movement would not require stabilization when writing, but they would require stronger contrast of guiding lines or ink on paper, more frequent rests, or built-up writing tools. See reference: Trombly: Retraining basic and instrumental activities of daily living.

74. (A) Figure-ground discrimination. Figure-ground discrimination is the ability to distinguish an object from the background. A person with impaired figure-ground discrimination would have difficulty finding the sock despite its position on the bed. Other deficits that may be demonstrated by the person would be an inability to see the sock on one side of the bed (unilateral neglect), to find it in relation to the bed (position in space), and to know how to get back to the bed to look for the sock (cognitive mapping). See reference: Trombly (ed): Quintana, LA: Evaluation of perception and cognition.

75. (C) Topographic orientation. Topographic orientation is the ability to find or follow a familiar place or route. An example would be a person finding the therapy department from his or her room or a person going to the bathroom in the night without turning on the light. Position in space is the ability to find an object against a background. Visual closure is the ability to recognize an object when only part of it has been seen. See reference: Trombly (ed): Quintana, LA: Evaluation of perception and cognition.

76. (A) Joint approximation and slow stroking. Rood inhibition techniques are used to relax or decrease high muscle tone to improve positioning or posture. Some of the techniques are joint approximation, slow stroking, slow rolling, and neutral warmth. Other answers indicated included facilitatory techniques such as light touch, fast brushing, and slow icing. See reference: Trombly: Rood approach.

77. (C) Rood, Bobath, Brunnstrom, and PNF. All of these theorists are similar because they base their techniques on development or normal movement and posture in a brain-injured adult population. Ayres' treatment of sensory integration for children is based on developmental and neurophysiologic approaches. Mosey proposed that the theoretic foundation of a profession is laid through "frames of reference;" therefore, answers A, B, and D, which included Ayres and Mosey, are incorrect. See reference: Kielhofner: The motor control model.

78. (B) Exercises using the uninvolved arm to move the involved arm across the midline. Exercises involving bilateral use of the arms to move the involved arm across the midline are one treatment for unilateral neglect. Unilateral neglect treatment also includes stimulating the involved limb with ice, activities that cross the midline, and activities placed on the involved side. Activities that focus on the uninvolved side of the body only reinforce neglect of the involved side of the body. See reference:

Zoltan, Siev, and Freishtat: Body images and body scheme disorders.

79. (C) Flexor synergy and voluntary or associated reactions. While in stage 2 of muscle return, the individual's arm exhibits increased presence of synergy. Some of the characteristics of synergy may be elicited on a voluntary basis or as an associated reaction. Flexor synergy is characterized by shoulder abduction and external rotation, elbow flexion, wrist flexion, and finger flexion or extension. Association reactions are movements of the affected extremity that are elicited by forceful movements in other areas of the body. Brunnstrom defined the recovery of muscle function in six stages: (1) flaccidity, (2) development of synergy, (3) voluntary movement within synergies, (4) gross motor movement within synergy, (5) movement outside of synergy, and (6) near normal movement with isolated joint movement. Brunnstrom also defined three movements that are possible in stage 4. These are (1) placing the hand behind the back, (2) shoulder flexion at 90 degrees with the elbow fully extended, and (3) pronating and supinating the forearm. See reference: Trombly (ed): Mathiowetz, V, and Haugen, JB: Evaluation of motor behaviors.

80. (A) Successful for hypersensitivity. Hyposensitivity retraining cannot be accomplished when sensory system damage has occurred. Hypersensitivity retraining may be successful when the sensory system is intact and is most beneficial when the individual controls the stimuli. See reference: Trombly (ed): Bentzet, K: Remediating sensory impairment.

81. (A) A ratio of movement of 2:1 as the humerus moves on the scapula. This rhythm is accomplished as the arm is abducted. For every 20 degrees of movement in the humerus, 10 degrees of movement occurs in the scapula. See reference: Cailliet: The spastic hand. In *Hand Pain and Impairment.*

82. (B) Dressing apraxia. To some extent, dressing apraxia involves an impaired awareness of the affected side and the relation of body parts to the clothing, as well as assembly of the clothing onto the body. A difficulty with spatial relations involves awareness of self to another object, for example, underreaching or overreaching for an item. A person with anosognosia is unaware of any deficits. Figure-ground discrimination would be the ability to distinguish an object from its background. See reference: Trombly (ed): Quintana, LA: Evaluation of perception and cognition.

83. (D) Touch. The senses included in the somatosensory system are touch, movement, pain, and temperature. The auditory, olfactory, visual gustatory, and vestibular systems are special systems that directly give input into the brain. The somatosensory system has receptors located throughout the body (muscles, tendons, ligaments, joints, skin, and so forth). In the brain, receptors are located in the thalamus, cortex, and brain stem. Receptors also exist in certain tracts of the spinal cord. See reference: Trombly (ed): Woodson, AM: Stroke.

84. (D) Pressure marks or redness should disappear after 20 minutes. Many types of splints may be made with the fingers not flexed, or the thumb opposed and abducted—for example, an antispasticity ball splint or a dynamic splint for extension. Most splints are not worn at all times but are removed for activities such as self-care or exercise. A therapist issues a wearing schedule when a splint is fitted or given to a patient. All splints that are made or given to a patient are checked for correct fit by adjusting any areas that still have redness or pressure marks after the splint has been removed for 20 minutes. See reference: Trombly (ed): Linden, CA, and Trombly, CA: Orthoses: Kinds and purposes.

85. (D) A private treatment room with a dimmer light. A private treatment room with a dimmer light allows the therapist to incorporate additional environmental inhibition techniques of low lighting and fewer outside distractions, which improves the effectiveness of the Rood inhibition techniques. Answers A, B, and C are all incorrect because they all involve facilitating environmental stimuli, such as a busy clinic, a bright light, or a cool room. See reference: Pedretti (ed): McCormack, G: The Rood approach to the treatment of neuromuscular dysfunction.

86. (C) To both sides of the body. Answer C is correct because the individual needs to be able to transfer to both sides of the body at home, because the layouts of many home fixtures do not lend themselves to transferring the individual only from one side. If the transfers are not practiced to both sides, the individual may find it easy to transfer to the commode, but not from the commode. The family also needs to know the differences in the way the individual is handled, with more or less support. Thus, answers A (to the unaffected side), B (to the affected side), and D (to the side the commode will be approached) are all incorrect because they all involve transfer to only one side. See reference: Palmer and Toms: Wheelchairs, assistive devices and home modifications.

87. (A) Running horizontally with the end on the good side between the waist and the iliac crest. The wrap then goes around behind the individual's back, covers the end of the wrap, and then goes diagonally down toward the stump. A vertical wrapping (answer B) would not be performed, because it would not stay in place and shape the stump properly. Answer C, running diagonally from the crease of the hip, is incorrect because the stump would not be long enough for the wrapping to stay in place. Answer D, on the front of the leg running horizontally below the crease of the hip, is incorrect, because the wrapping would cut off circulation to the stump, or fall off because the stump would not be long enough to allow an adequate area to provide a secure wrap. See reference: Palmer and Toms: Wheelchairs, assistive devices and home modifications.

88. (C) Adaptations for pressure relief. A primary function of a power chair should be its offering adaptations for pressure relief to prevent the development of pressure sores. Answers A (a portable ventilator), B (arm troughs), and D (adjustable speed) are not features that every individual needs so these options are incorrect. An individual who spends more than a few minutes at a time in a wheelchair usually needs some assistance with pressure relief, which in a power chair is provided by a reclining back and special cushions. See reference: Palmer and Toms: Wheelchairs, assistive devices and home modifications.

89. (D) Decreased attention. An attention deficit would be discovered if the person recognizes the letter, marks it accurately throughout the page on the right and left sides, but misses letters in a random pattern. A visual field cut (answers A and B) would be evidenced by the missed letters appearing close together in one area. Functional illiteracy (answer C) would be determined before the test, during the interview before evaluation, or from the chart review, and a more appropriate test would be administered. The person with functional illiteracy may also be able to complete the task accurately, or mark additional letters, depending on the level of illiteracy. See reference: Trombly (ed): Quintana, LA: Remediating cognitive impairments.

90. (B) Good (4). The individual's "available" range is the range through which the joint may be moved passively. Therefore, if an individual is able to move the joint actively through the entire movement that is completed passively and then take maximum resistance, the grade is normal (5). Good (4) is the grade given when an individual is able to move a part through the available range against gravity and is able to sustain moderate resistance. Fair (3) is the grade given when an individual is able to move a part through the full range against gravity but lacks the strength for any resistance. Fair minus (3−) is the grade given when an individual moves a part against gravity through less than the full range of motion. Fair minus is the last graded range for movement against gravity. Grades poor and trace are for gravity-eliminated movements. See reference: Trombly: Evaluation of biomechanical and physiological aspects of motor performance.

91. (A) Hot is 40 to 45°C, cold is 5 to 10°C. Temperature levels are set so that there is a difference between the hot and cold levels, but not so extreme that they are painful or so slight that they are indistinguishable. (The temperature in degrees Fahrenheit are 105 to 114°F for hot and 40 to 50°F for cold.) See reference: Trombly (ed): Bentzel, K: Evaluation of sensation.

92. (A) Apply the stimuli distally to proximately. The general guidelines for sensation testing are that the person's vision should be occluded, that the stimuli should be randomly applied with false stimuli intermingled, that a practice trial should be performed before the test, and that the unaffected side or area should be tested before the affected side or area. Also, the amount of time a person has to respond should be established. See reference: Trombly (ed): Bentzel, K: Evaluation of sensation.

93. (C) Fair plus. A person with strength of fair or fair minus would be unable to tolerate resistance. A person with strength of fair plus during manual muscle testing can tolerate minimal resistance. A person whose strength is good minus can tolerate less than moderate resistance but more than minimal resistance. See reference: Trombly: Evaluation of biomechanical and physiological aspects of motor performance.

94. (A) Thumb against the tip of the index finger. The correct position for tip pinch is the thumb against the tip of the index finger. The thumb against the side of the index finger describes the position for lateral pinch. The thumb against the tips of the index and middle fingers describes the test position for three jaw chuck, or palmar pinch. The thumb against the tips of all the fingers is not a standard test position. See reference: Trombly: Evaluation of biomechanical and physiological aspects of motor performance.

95. (D) An aesthesiometer. An aesthesiometer is used to measure two-point discrimination. It has a gauge with a movable point and a stationary point. The distance between the two points is measured, as is the ability to discriminate between two points. A goniometer is used to measure joint range of motion. A dynamometer is used to measure grip strength, and a pinch meter is used to measure strength of opposition between a thumb and one or two fingers. See reference: Trombly (ed): Bentzel, K: Remediating sensory impairment.

96. (B) Continue the same positioning and splinting program as was indicated before discharge. It is necessary to continue positioning and splinting after discharge, because active scar development continues for many weeks, depending on the severity of the burn. The same positioning and splinting devices as were used at the hospital are used at home, with changes made as needed during follow-up visits. Individuals stay in the hospital until their conditions can be managed at home with outpatient visits to maintain status. Individuals are not kept until they are completely healed, which would be the only situation in which a home program would not be necessary. If an individual follows the home program only as he or she deems appropriate during the day or night, instead of as scheduled by the therapist, the position time may not be sufficient to prevent deformity from occurring. See reference: Trombly (ed): Alvarado, MI: Burns.

97. (A) A canister vacuum cleaner. A canister vacuum cleaner may be managed by someone with weakness and balance problems while sitting down. The hose is light enough to be easily pushed, and the canister is on wheels and may be moved by a seated person pushing it with the foot or having someone move it for him or her. An upright vacuum cleaner is too heavy for repetitive pushing and pulling, and can cause exhaustion or pull the person off balance. A self-propelled vacuum cleaner could also pull a person off balance by moving too fast for the person to respond with appropriate postural adjustments. A hand-held vacuum cleaner requires too much stooping to do anything but a very small area of the floor, because repetitive bending can cause fatigue quickly and challenges decreased balance. See reference: Trombly (ed): Stewart, C: Retraining housekeeping and child care skills.

98. (A) An electric razor. An electric razor is the safest for shaving because a rotary head or foil, instead of a blade, is in contact with the skin. Any shaving over the incision area or near it would not be recommended until the incision area is healed. The other razors have blades that could nick or cut the skin, which would need to be avoided until the patient is no longer treated with blood thinners and normal blood coagulation can occur. See reference: Trombly: Retraining basic and instrumental activities of daily living.

99. (A) Remove all throw or scatter rugs. Regardless of whether an individual with instability walks with the help of a walker, cane, or no equipment, the floor should be cleared of any obstacles that could cause him or her to slip or trip. Scatter or throw rugs may catch on a person's foot or on the tip of an assistive device. Rugs also may not be firmly taped down or secured with nonskid backing, or taped down, causing a safety hazard. Installing lever handles, a ramp, or a hand-held shower would make certain tasks easier for a patient, but they would not be necessary for safety. See reference: Trombly (ed): Versluys, HP: Facilitating psychological adjustment to disability.

100. (D) A tub bath using lukewarm water. A person with COPD would have difficulty breathing in hot, humid environments. A lukewarm tub bath would provide the lowest humidity by using the coolest water temperature combined with the method of dispensing water to keep evaporation at a minimum. See reference: Trombly (ed): Atchison, B: Cardiopulmonary diseases.

101. (C) Comprehensive Occupational Therapy Evaluation (COTE) Scale. All of the answers include the observation of behaviors. The COTE scale guides the therapist to rate behaviors in categories of general behaviors, interpersonal behaviors, and task behaviors. Answer A, MEDLS, assesses 21 daily living skills. Answer B, KELS, assesses self-care safety and health, money management, transportation and telephone, and work and leisure. Answer D, ACL, assesses levels of cognitive disability. See reference: Christiansen and Baum (eds): Bruce, MA, and Borg, B: Assessing psychological performance factors.

102. (A) The magazine picture collage. Although all methods are projective methods, the only instrument with protocol developed by and for occupational therapists is the magazine picture collage. The Rorschach and H-T-P tests are typically administered by psychologists. Proverb interpretation is a part of the mental status examination typically conducted by the psychiatrist. See reference: Christiansen and Baum (eds): Bruce, MA, and Borg, B: Assessing psychological performance factors.

103. (C) The ability to engage in superficial social conversation. The onset of most dementias is slow and progressive. Cognitive abilities such as reading and writing are most often initially affected. Sensorimotor abilities such as dressing tend to follow. Superficial social abilities are often preserved until the last stages of dementia and may often hide the earlier cognitive and sensorimotor changes. See reference: Bonder: Delerium and Dementia. In *Psychopathology and Function.*

104. (D) Parachek Geriatric Rating Scale. The Parachek Geriatric Rating Scale is a 10-item screening instrument that can be completed in approximately 5 minutes by those familiar with the individual's daily behaviors. The protocol for this assessment also contains suggested interventions appropriate for the score levels derived from this assessment. The BaFPE and COTE are direct observations of an individual's performance. The Role Checklist involves a self-assessment format. See reference: Christiansen and Baum (eds): Christiansen, C: Occupational performance assessment.

105. (C) Object relations. According to the psychoanalytic and object relations perspectives, the past is a determining influence on an individual's current functioning. Particularly important to these perspectives is that unconscious factors influence behaviors and are important to address in treatment. Occupational behavior, human occupation, and role acquisition are more concerned with the here-and-now adaptivity of behaviors, regardless of the past. See reference: Christiansen and Baum (eds): Bruce, MA, and Borg, B: Assessing psychological performance factors.

106. (A) Kohlman Evaluation of Living Skills (KELS). The KELS is the only item that was designed for acute care psychiatric settings. The MEDLS is most appropriate for long-term psychiatric treatment settings. The FIM indicates the severity of disability for individuals in rehabilitation programs. The Katz Index of ADL was developed for use with elderly and chronically ill individuals. See reference: Christiansen and Baum (eds): Christiansen, C: Occupational performance assessment.

107. (B) OT FACT. The abbreviation OT FACT stands for Occupational Therapy Functional Assessment Compilation Tool. It is a computer software program designed to organize and summarize occupational performance information obtained through a variety of evaluation strategies. The other items are instruments that provide specific evaluation results. The LDB can be administered through a computer, but it is not a summary of performance. See reference: Christiansen and Baum (eds): Christiansen, C: Occupational performance assessment.

108. (B) That there is a personality disorder or a prominent maladaptive personality feature. The *Diagnostic and Statistical Manual of Mental Disorders (DSM-IV)* uses a multiaxial system of classifying psychiatric disorders. Axis I indicates the primary psychiatric condition. Axis III indicates general coexisting medical conditions. See reference: Bonder: Psychiatric diagnosis and the classification system. In *Psychopathology and Function.*

109. (B) Attention-deficit hyperactivity disorder. Reports about interactions with peers and adults can tell us a great deal about the types of difficulties children with psychosocial problems experience. Autistic children's interactions tend to be lacking or involve engagement in repetitive speech patterns. Individuals with a personality disorder exhibit various interpersonal difficulties found in adults only. Childhood anxiety disorders are generally related to specific interactions that are avoided by the child. See reference: Bonder: Disorders of infancy, childhood, and adolescence. In *Psychopathology and Function.*

110. (D) The Mini Mental Status Examination. The ACL and LCL assess levels of cognitive disability. The Kitchen Task assesses initiation, sequencing, and organization. The Mini Mental Status Examination is a screening tool for orientation, calculations, and language skills. See reference: Christiansen and Baum (eds): Duchek, J: Assessing cognition.

111. (A) Counted cross-stitch needlework projects. Blurred vision is a common side effect of tricyclic antidepressants and small detailed activities can be quite difficult to work on. Food precautions are important with the use of monoamine oxidase inhibitors (MAOI). Precautions regarding the sun are important with the use of antipsychotics. Although blood pressure may change during gross motor activities, METS is a cardiac endurance-based grading method. See reference: Bonder: Fischer, PJ: Psychopharmacotherapy. In *Psychopathology and Function.*

112. (D) Cooperative group activity that both provides and elicits consistent and accurate feedback about interactions within the group. Because the underlying issues for most personality disorders are related to inaccurate perceptions of the self and others, the selected approach to treatment should directly address these problems. A group format offers a wider variety of feedback about the specific interactions that occur. The group activity should be based on a central goal of reducing misperceptions. Social skills groups (answer C) are often used to address the interaction difficulties experienced with cluster C personality disorders. The question does not specify that cluster C personality disorders are included in the group. Answer B is best used for problems with individuals, not groups. Answer A addresses decision making and not inaccurate perceptions. See reference: Bonder: Personality disorders. In *Psychopathology and Function.*

113. (A) Provide a variety of therapeutic sports, arts, crafts, music, and recreation activities to develop and reinforce healthy interest patterns. Differences among psychiatric service providers should be based on roles versus the media and types of treatment used. Answer B is the role of educational disciplines, answer C is the role of occupational therapy, and answer D is the role of vocational rehabilitation. Effective program planning is based on a clear understanding of the contributions of all the service providers within a team. See reference: Fidler: Program services.

114. (B) Each member of a small group is asked to draw a picture of himself or herself on a piece of paper. The occupational therapist then leads a discussion about body image concerns and links the discussion to the group's drawings. Adapting the procedures of one activity allows the therapist to use that single activity to address different treatment goals. Selecting an activity appropriate for eating disorders is based on a primary problem focus for this population: body-image distortions. Only answer B focuses on this problem area. Answer A focuses on cognitive deficits; answer C focuses on family dynamics problems; and answer D is an assessment task from the BaFPE. See reference: Denton: Treatment planning and implementation.

115. (A) The individual will initiate and complete laundry activities in his or her own laundry area while the caregiver provides verbal cues about matching colors and shapes and monitors the individual's performance for unanticipated problems. The role of the therapist, other caregivers, the individual, and the problem areas addressed vary among different frames of reference. The cognitive disabilities view is that the structure provided by others can enhance the performance of an individual's routine tasks. The cognitive disability frame of reference emphasizes changing the task versus changing the individual. Answer B is more consistent with the human occupation view. Answer C is more consistent with a sensorimotor view. Answer D is more consistent with functional performance views. See reference: Denton: Treatment planning and implementation.

116. (A) The therapist attributes an individual's problems to internal causes versus problems within the situation or environment. Answers B, C, and D are all recommended approaches to reduce therapist bias in the clinical reasoning process. Answer A describes a common tendency that can cloud the therapist's view because it involves ignoring potential causes of the individual's difficulties. See reference: Denton: Assessment.

117. (A) The amount of self-control demands, time-management demands, self-expression opportunities, and interest in the activity. Components that are primarily within the psychosocial areas and skills of occupational performance are most important when considering psychosocial populations. Answers B and C are performance components one generally analyzes when considering childhood populations. Answer D does not address performance components. See reference: Hopkins and Smith (eds): Simon, CJ: Use of activity and activity analysis.

118. (C) Mania and borderline personality disorder. Stabilizing the crisis that precipitated hospitalization is a common goal of short-term psychiatric treatment. The therapist's provision of consistent limit setting is an important stabilizing role for individuals whose judgment and impulsive behaviors are common admitting problems for mania and borderline personality. Limit setting concerning denial is more appropriate for alcoholism and anorexia, answer B. Depression and anxiety, answer A, usually involves limit setting concerning reassurance. Answer D, delirium and dementia, typically involve setting limits for decreased confusion. See reference: Hopkins and Smith (eds): Richert, GZ: Program planning, development, and implementation.

119. (D) Encouraging the individual to reconnect with his or her current and future personal life. Because the duration of a therapeutic relationship is linked to treatment plans and goals, the encouragement of the individual to focus on reconnecting to relationships that will be available outside of and after treatment is important. Behaviors listed in answers A, B, and C can be counterproductive to developing a therapeutic relationship. Answers A and B may be perceived as enhancing a friendship relationship. Answer C is appropriate for some specific situations rather than most therapeutic relationships. See reference: Bruce and Borg: The framework of therapy in occupational therapy. In *Frames of Reference in Psychosocial Occupational Therapy—Frames of Reference for Intervention.*

120. (A) Project group. Project groups should involve short-term tasks where the group participants are expected to share material or equipment and can cooperate in a shared task with limited amounts of competition. Groups in answers B, C, and D involve more interaction among the members and longer-term tasks and less involvement by the OTR. See reference: Mosey: Recapitulation of ontogenesis.

121. (D) Continuous reinforcement of correct responses. Continuous reinforcement is provided every time the correct behavior occurs. Continuous reinforcement is helpful with the learning of new behaviors. Time-based and intermittent reinforcement (answers A, B and C) are best for maintaining behaviors. See reference: Bruce and Borg: The behavioral frame of reference. In *Frames of Reference in Psychosocial Occupational Therapy—Frames of Reference for Intervention.*

122. (A) Social reinforcers. Social reinforcers such as verbal praise, a pat on the back, a smile, or a nod "yes" are least likely to interfere with the learning of the task. Providing consumable reinforcers (snacks, cigarettes, coffee, and so forth) or activity reinforcers (time alone or doing a favorite activity) would not be compatible with a continuous reinforcement schedule, which is needed for learning in a work environment. Punishment is designed to decrease behaviors. See reference: Bruce and Borg: The behavioral frame of reference. In *Frames of Reference in Psychosocial Occupational Therapy—Frames of Reference for Intervention.*

123. (B) Having the worker put only the last piece into the game package. Working backwards from the last (successful) step of a sequence is known as "backward chaining." Answer A represents the opposite of backward chaining. Answer C is more descriptive of shaping behaviors, and answer D is more descriptive of modeling behaviors. See reference: Bruce and Borg: The behavioral frame of reference. In *Frames of Reference in Psychosocial Occupational Therapy—Frames of Reference for Intervention.*

124. (A) Monitor and encourage the use of fine motor, tactile, figure-ground, and visuospatial functions; involve individual in expressive arts to focus on verbal-

ization of feelings; and provide leisure-time education. In general, there are three areas of focus with occupational therapy interventions for individuals identified with substance abuse problems. They are alternative leisure-time use, improved expression of feelings, and monitoring and encouraging return of central nervous system functions impaired by alcohol use. The approach described in answer B addresses the cognitive disability frame of reference approach. Answers C and D may address specific needs of the patient but not the overall needs of this population. See reference: Bonder: Substance related disorders. In *Psychopathology and Function*.

125. (B) A class about job-seeking strategies. The occupational therapist's remediation of identified deficits can be organized into three general approaches in psychosocial settings: enhancing the individual's skills and performance, assisting the individual in adjusting his or her perspective on skills and performance, and altering the environment. Teaching and training methods predominate the skill and performance remediation approach. Answer A is more consistent with object relations approaches; answer C with cognitive disabilities; and answer D with occupational behavior and human occupation approaches. See reference: Bonder: DSM-IV and occupational therapy. In *Psychopathology and Function*.

126. (D) Rice. There are many serious side effects with MAO inhibitors. Foods that are known to include aged proteins (smoked meats and aged cheese) should be avoided, and chocolate and coffee should be limited. See reference: Bonder: Fischer, PJ: Psychopharmacotherapy. In *Psychopathology and Function*.

127. (C) The precipitating conditions and events that elicit stress reactions. The conditions and events that elicit stress reactions are known as stressors. Stressors can be both short-term or long-term. The stress management terminology described by the other items are: Coping (answer A), stress (answer B), and adapta-tion (answer D). See reference: Christiansen and Baum (eds): Christiansen, C: Performance deficits as sources of stress—Coping theory and occupational therapy.

128. (B) Electromyography (EMG) biofeedback training combined with relaxation training. All of the answers describe stress management techniques. Electromyographic biofeedback provides the individual with information about his or her muscle tension levels, and relaxation techniques are strategies to reduce muscle tension. Answer A is for individuals who are unable to distinguish between assertive and aggressive behaviors and therefore do not respond assertively when necessary. Answer C is for individuals whose irrational beliefs and thought processes lead to maladaptive behaviors. Answer D is for individuals who have difficulty selecting effective solutions or identifying the source of their problems. See reference: Christiansen and Baum (eds): Christiansen, C: Performance deficits as sources of stress—Coping theory and occupational therapy.

129. (D) Measurability of activity performance. The potential to measure an activity's results is central to a be-

havioral frame of reference. Answer A is linked to developmental frames of reference. Answer B is linked to psychoanalytic frames of reference. Answer C is linked to sensory-integrative frames of reference. See reference: Hopkins and Smith (eds): Simon, CJ: Use of activity and activity analysis.

130. (C) 50 to 60 percent. In 1985, a study of practice revealed that 60% of therapists surveyed from a variety of treatment settings used groups to achieve treatment goals. Settings that were most likely to use groups were psychiatric hospitals and community mental health centers. Groups were used less often in schools, large general hospitals, and nursing homes. See reference: Howe and Schwartzberg: Current practice in occupational therapy.

131. (B) Activity-of-daily-living groups. Activity-of-daily-living groups are used by 17% of therapists who use a group format. This group format is most often used in psychosocial settings and rehabilitation centers. Concerns often addressed in these groups are self-care skill development and predischarge living skills. See reference: Howe and Schwartzberg: Current practice in occupational therapy.

132. (B) Remote memory. The ability to recall events from one's distant past is remote memory and is commonly assessed through verbal interviews and informal testing, such as this question about an individual's recall of childhood events. Retention is determined by giving the individual information and asking about the same information a few minutes later. Orientation is determined by asking about the current time and date. Recent memory is determined by asking about meals eaten that day. See reference: Christiansen and Baum (eds): Duchek, J: Cognitive dimensions of performance.

133. (C) Developing the group. Facilitating discussion based on similarities that are seen on the completion of an activity is an aspect of the development phase. The opening phase (answer A) generally includes introducing member names, group goals, and expected length of the group. Processing (answer B) is not a phase of group development. The term processing refers to reflections on the group with another therapist after the group session. Group closure (answer D) involves restating the purpose as well as giving and receiving feedback. See reference: Bruce and Borg: Throughput—The group as a system of change.

134. (B) Egocentric-cooperative groups. Structured learning activities that focus on beginning to use or encourage additional group roles (asking all to contribute briefly as experts), combined with the therapist's giving and asking for feedback, are consistent with an egocentric-cooperative developmental group. The therapist makes activity-based suggestions, if needed, in project groups. The therapist is an advisor in cooperative groups and a group member in a mature group. See reference: Mosey: Recapitulation of ontogenesis.

135. (C) Relationships with others. The primary problem area for most individuals with a personality disorder is their interactions with others. Specific personality disorder categories indicate that there is some variation among the types of relationships that are impacted. For example, authority relationships seem particularly dysfunctional with antisocial personality disorders whereas difficulty establishing relationships is linked to avoidant personality disorders. Answers A and B (ADL) are often problems with mood and thought disorder. Answer D is often a problem with schizophrenia. See reference: Bonder: Personality disorders.

136. (C) The focus of the group is to encourage here-and-now explorations of member behaviors and issues while promoting learning through "doing." Task groups as developed by Fidler focus on the here and now, involve learning through doing and activity and processing, and involve the development of daily living skills and work skills. Answer A describes an evaluative group; Answer B describes a topical discussion group, which is generally not a format exclusive to occupational therapy; and Answer D describes the developmental group levels proposed by Mosey. See reference: Mosey: Activity groups.

137. (D) Posttraumatic stress disorder. Posttraumatic stress disorder is an anxiety disorder that follows a traumatic event in a person's life. Answers A and B are mood disorders. Answer C is a psychotic disorder. See reference: Bonder: Anxiety disorders.

138. (A) When reminded to dress, and when clothing has been selected by another individual, the individual is able to put on his or her clothing. Allen asserts that different levels of cognitive disability are linked to different amounts of support provided by others for performance of daily living tasks. At level 3, performance, manual actions are used to manipulate material objects, but the effects of these manipulations are not recognized by the individual. The behaviors described in answer A reflect this level of functioning during a dressing task. Answer B behaviors are consistent with cognitive level 2. Answer C is consistent with level 4. Answer D is consistent with level 1. See reference: Allen: Independence and assistance in doing activities.

139. (A) Group size of less than 5 members. Group size strongly influences how members relate to one another. In general, an ideal group size is 7 to 10 members for the most interaction among members. Groups with less than 5 members tend to increase the focus on the leader in their interactions. Group membership of similar goals improves cohesiveness more than interactions. Differing ages is not known to have an impact on interactions. See reference: Howe and Schwartzberg: The group.

140. (D) The members are frustrated with an inability to successfully meet the demands of the group or activity. Frustration and trying to improve one's status within the group are often the cause of member fighting or engagement in conflict in a group. The causes linked to increased group apathy are described in answers A and B. Answer C often has an impact on group cohesion behaviors. See reference: Howe and Schwartzberg: The group.

141. (D) Rationalization. Making excuses for or justifying others' behaviors that are generally considered to be unacceptable is called "rationalization." Identification (answer A) occurs when one takes on the characteristics of another person. Projection (answer B) is the blaming of other people for performing the behaviors. Denial (answer C) is refusing to acknowledge that the behavior occurred. See reference: Bruce and Borg: Appendix E: Defense mechanisms. In *Frames of Reference in Psychosocial Occupational Therapy.*

142. (C) Tardive dyskinesia. Long-term use of antipsychotic medications can lead to tardive dyskinesia in approximately 15% of the individuals. Because the behavioral side effects described in this question can seriously impact the individual's daily living skill performance as well as his or her self-concept, the occupational therapist is responsible for knowing these side effects. Tremors, muscular weakness, and "rigid gait" are behaviors of Parkinsonian syndrome, sometimes seen as side effects of antipsychotic medications (answer A). Overdose symptoms (answer B) would vary according to the specific antipsychotic medication ingested. Lithium toxicity (answer D) is linked to antimanic medications. See reference: Bonder: Fischer, PJ: Psychopharmacotherapy. In *Psychopathology and Function.*

143. (D) Mood. Moods are pervasive and sustained emotions that influence an individual's perceptions of their situations. Affect (answer A) describes behaviors involved in expressing emotions. Anxiety (answer B) is a feeling of apprehension combined with tension. Ideas of reference (answer C) are feelings that situations have special meaning to the individual. See reference: American Psychiatric Association: Appendix C—Glossary of technical terms.

144. (B) The caregiver hands the individual a dust cloth and points to the location to dust. (The caregiver redirects the individual to continue dusting if the individual stops before finishing.) According to Allen's recent analysis of daily activities, the amount of caregiver assistance required with these answers would be graded B, A, C, or D (most to least assistance provided). The cognitive disabilities view is that individuals use manual action cues before they use cues from familiar simple tools. Cues about possible unseen effects and spatial relationships are considered to provide less assistance than manual actions and simple tools. See reference: Hopkins and Smith (eds): Levy, LL: Cognitive disability frame of reference.

145. (C) Coping strategies for continuing medication compliance. Studies designed to determine the factors related to frequent re-admissions for psychiatric individuals have found the major reason to be medication noncompliance. The other strategies listed are also important but are not the primary issue. See reference: Bonder: Fischer, PJ: Psychopharmacotherapy. In *Psychopathology and Function.*

146. (D) Sheltered workshop. Sheltered workshops are designed to help individuals master basic work skills.

Answers B and C are similar in that they incorporate actual job sites for developing work skills. Answer A focuses on work-related and leisure activities. See reference: Hopkins and Smith (eds): Humphry, R, and Jewell, K: Developmental disabilities.

147. (A) Paraphrasing. Paraphrasing is a response in one's own words of what someone said. Chitchat would be unrelated to what the individual said. Confrontation requires the individual to acknowledge difficult or painful issues. See reference: Denton: Effective communication.

148. (D) Work adjustment. Work adjustment programs are designed to address problems with valuing work and with behaviors in relating to others in the workplace. Competitive job placement, answer A, is rarely done by occupational therapists. Job coaching, answer B, is specific to one job setting and may not address interpersonal concerns. Supported employment, answer C, is for noncompetitive skills. See reference: Hopkins and Smith: Jacobs, K: Work assessment and programming.

149. (A) Partial hospitalization. Partial hospitalization is appropriate for individuals who are experiencing acute psychiatric symptoms and who have a place or family with whom to stay at night. Partial hospitalization offers most of the structure, staffing, and services available on an inpatient unit except for overnight provisions. Day treatment focuses on assisting individuals to adapt to their illness and develop daily living skills at the program site. Day treatment services are typically verbal activities and group therapy within a 3- to 6-month period. Day care is long-term care that provides structured daily activities and medications to maintain current levels of functioning. Community mental health centers provide a wide range of individual and outpatient services that address a variety of individual goals. See reference: Hopkins and Smith (eds): Richert, GZ, and Gibson, D: Practice settings.

150. (A) Milwaukee Evaluation of Daily Living Skills (MEDLS). The MEDLS was designed specifically for long-term psychiatric settings, whereas the KELS was designed for acute-care settings. The areas described in the question are contained in the MEDLS. The ACL is an indirect measure of self-care abilities. The Barthel Self-Care Index was designed for physically impaired individuals. See reference: Hemphill (ed): Leonordelli, C: The Milwaukee Evaluation of Daily Living Skills (MEDLS). In *Mental Health Assessment in Occupational Therapy—An Integrative Approach to the Evaluative Process.*

151. (A) Medicare. Medicare was established by Congress in 1965 as Title XVIII of the Social Security Act. The program consists of two parts. Medicare part A pays for inpatient hospitalization, skilled care, and hospice services. Medicare part B covers outpatient services along with physician and other professional medical services. Medicaid (answer B) provides health care for the poor and medically indigent. Third-party payors (answer C) represent the largest source of payment in the United States. These providers may either exist for profit or not for profit, and they adhere to state insurance codes that re-

quire set levels of coverage. With private pay (answer D), the patient is responsible for the financial payment of services rendered. See reference: Bair and Gray (eds): Scott, SJ, and Somers, FP: Payment for occupational therapy services.

152. (B) Criterion. Criteria are specific areas of the monitor that are to be assessed and recorded on a percentage of compliance with the corresponding statement. Thresholds (answer A) are levels at which the criteria are assessed if they fall below the measure. Norms (answer C) are a numerical measure of a permissible range. Monitors (answer D) are the areas that are to be analyzed. An example would be the following quality assurance plan:

Monitor = Feeding
Criteria = 1. Was patient assessed for feeding skills?
2. Was the patient issued appropriate feeding equipment?
3. Was the patient/family trained in the use of equipment if equipment was issued?
Threshold = 90%
Norms = 85% to 95%

See reference: Bair and Gray (eds): Joe, B: Quality assurance.

153. (D) Program evaluation. Program evaluations are various systems that measure the combined outcomes of patients and effectiveness of the program. These systems are designed to report information so that the facility may improve quality, increase organizational ability to plan and allocate resources, and justify to payors the outcomes and services. Quality improvement (answer A) is a systematic approach to monitoring patient care. Peer review (answer B) is a component of quality improvement. Cost accounting (answer C) is a method of tracking the costs of specific services or costs incurred by diagnosis-specific groups. See reference: Bair and Gray (eds): Scammahorn, G: Program planning.

154. (A) Patient-care monitoring. Quality improvement is a systematic and objective means of monitoring effective and efficient services. Mandated by the JCAHO, quality improvement encompasses all areas of patient care monitoring. This is inclusive of peer review and program evaluation. Cost accounting and health accounting systems also provide information that may be used as a part of an overall quality improvement plan. Therefore, the answer that is most inclusive of all areas of quality improvement is patient care monitoring. See reference: Jacobs and Logigian (eds): Cargill, L: Quality assurance.

155. (D) The title of the job, organizational relationships, essential job functions, and the job requirements. Job descriptions usually contain the title of the job, organizational relationships, essential job functions, work performed, job requirements, and environmental risks. Items that are not required but may compliment an individualized job description are personality characteristics, past experience requirements, and accomplishments. Answers A, B, and C include items that are NOT REQUIRED in a job description but are more appropriately located on a resume. See reference: Jacobs and Logigian (eds): Parisi, R: Managing human resources.

156. (B) Triage. "Triage" is a term used to describe a patient prioritization system for treatment. In a triage situation, those patients in the most need of treatment are seen. Techniques that may be implemented include (1) discharging patients who can no longer benefit from occupational therapy services and (2) treating those patients who may best benefit from occupational therapy services. In health care, it is unethical to provide services based on the patient's ability to pay; therefore, answer A is incorrect. Attrition (answer C) is the gradual reduction in personnel and thus is incorrect. The date of referral (answer D) may be useful in establishing priorities as a part of the triage process. However, the date of referral does not take into account acuity and the need for immediate treatment. See reference: Bair and Gray (eds): Scammahorn, G: Program planning.

157. (C) Analyzed the work flow. An organized work flow is one in which the employees and patients can move smoothly through the department. Environments with poor work flow may have areas that are "bottlenecks" or cause a congestion of individuals at one or more areas. Identifying the patterns in which work may most efficiently be completed is helpful in designing a new floor plan so that all areas may be optimized. Answers A, B, and D all occur in the space-planning process but were not correct based on the description. Elements critical to identifying a location (answer A) may include proximity to other physical medicine disciplines. However, the question indicated that the department was reallocating current space. Determination of equipment needs (answer B) may be accomplished by taking an inventory of current equipment compared with anticipated equipment. This procedure will identify items that may need to be purchased. Determining functional areas (answer D) is based on identification of the activity areas (clinic, offices, storage areas). See reference: Bair and Gray (eds): Leiter, P: Facility planning.

158. (A) Medicare Diagnosis-Related Groups (DRG) system. Introduced in April 1983, within the Prospective Payment System, diagnostic related groups (DRGs) were defined to establish the level of payment per diagnosis. The intent of the government was to impose constraints on health care spending for the beneficiaries of Medicare. Departmental charge structures (answer B) are designed to generate revenues for the provision of occupational therapy services. The fee for service structure (answer C) bills the patient for each procedure and is often more costly to the consumer. Per diem rates (answer B) are fees hospitals charge for a service per day. See reference: Jacobs and Logigian (eds): Logigian, M: Cost accounting.

159. (A) Specific measurable statements with time frames. Goals can be either short-term (meaning in the immediate future) or long-term (meaning over an extended period). The purpose of a goal is to provide a specific statement that is measurable and indicates what is to be accomplished. Patients and significant others play a vital role in working with the therapist to establish goals that are meaningful and realistic. Time frames (answer B) may be only a part of a measurable goal or objective. Specific measurements of the patient's skill and performance (answer C) is a part of the assessment information that assists the therapist in establishing appropriate goals and objectives for treatment. Activities to be completed that correspond with the goals (answer D) are part of the objective and treatment plan. See reference: Jacobs and Logigian (eds): Pagonis, J: Documentation.

160. (D) Statements of how the goals will be achieved. An objective is a statement of the plan for how a goal will be achieved. This statement is the vital link that connects a patient's status on admission to how he or she will make progress to meet the goals for discharge. Statements of what will be accomplished with time frames (answer A) are referred to as goals. Time frames of what will be accomplished (answer B) are the components that make goals measurable. Specific measurements of an individual's skill or performance (answer C) are part of the assessment portion of an evaluation or SOAP note that indicates his or her status. See reference: Jacobs and Logigian (eds): Pagonis, J: Documentation.

161. (A) Concise objective information. All medical documentation should be accurate, concise, and objective. Personal opinions and statements that are speculative, judgmental, or subjective are not appropriate to be included into the patient's chart. Therefore, answers B, C, and D are incorrect. See reference: Jacobs and Logigian (eds): Pagonis, J: Documentation.

162. (D) Summarizes the approach of management of an individual. The treatment plan or plan of care is a multidisciplinary approach to a patient's treatment. Each member of the treatment team contributes to the plan, which may be documented on a multidisciplinary form. Specific directions for the therapist in treatment (answer A), measurements of the patient's progress (answer B), and organization of the patient's priorities (answer C) are all pieces of information included in the occupational therapy departmental documentation. See reference: Jacobs and Logigian (eds): Pagonis, J: Documentation.

163. (C) All children with disabilities before they receive special education services. Also referred to as the IEP, the individual educational plan is required by the federal government to be written before the provision of special education services. This plan is written annually and is completed by all members of the team involved in a child's education. Continuing education plans (answer A) vary between therapists, employers, and states. Some state licensure boards do require CEUs (continuing education units) at the time of licensure renewal. A treatment plan or the plan of care would be the document written for individuals with head injuries (answer B) as a component of the rehabilitation program. Answer D is incorrect in that many families participate in education and training as part of the rehabilitation process. The training sessions as well as the family's ability to follow discharge plans are documented. Each rehabilitation unit establishes a form for documentation of services provided. See reference: Jacobs and Logigian (eds): Pagonis, J: Documentation.

164. (D) Quotes from the individual. SOAP is an acronym for *S*ubjective, *O*bjective, *A*ssessment, and *P*lan. The SOAP format is a common format for documentation in the medical fields. The subjective portion of the SOAP note contains information found in the chart, provided by the patient or family, or information communicated by other health professionals. Measurement results (answer A) are based on a patient's performance during the evaluation and are included in the objective section. Analysis of the measurements (answer B) is recorded in the assessment area of the SOAP note. Speculative information (answer C) is not included in the documentation under any area of the SOAP note. See reference: Hopkins and Smith (eds): Perinchief, J: Documentation.

165. (A) Functional performance levels. The objective portion of the SOAP format includes clinical findings of an evaluation. Analysis of measurements (answer B) is noted in the assessment component of documentation. Conclusions and assumptions of performance measures are included in the assessment portion of the SOAP format. Speculative information, answer C, is not included in the documentation under any area of the SOAP note. Quotes from the patient or family (answer D) are a part of the subjective portion. See reference: Hopkins and Smith (eds): Perinchief, J: Documentation.

166. (A) Collecting chart review information. Once a certified occupational therapist has demonstrated service competency, it is appropriate for him or her to complete data collection through record reviews, interviews, general observations, and behavior checklists. Answers B, C, and D require interpretive and analytical skills in which occupational therapists have received additional training. A certified occupational therapy assistant can collaborate with an occupational therapist but it is inappropriate to have a COTA complete these portions independently. See reference: Hopkins and Smith (eds): Entry Level Role Delineation Task Force for the Intercommission Council: Appendix F.

167. (D) Zero-based. In a zero-based budget process, the occupational therapy manager must justify and prioritize each expense for the coming budget period. Incremental budgeting (answer A) uses budget information from the previous year as a baseline. Projections are then made to take into account any changes in business or inflation anticipated for the coming year. Programmatic budgeting is a widely based budgeting plan that takes into account larger operational programs (e.g., Physical Rehabilitation versus an occupational therapy department). A cost accounting system (answer C) tracks information on the cost per procedure, or per patient's length of stay. It may also be possible to identify costs associated with a diagnostic group through cost accounting. See reference: Bair and Gray (eds): Laase, SM: Financial management.

168. (C) Planning, budgeting, monitoring, and controlling. The budgeting process is initiated with planning. The planning generally includes looking at the expenditures for the past year and gaining input from staff as to what future expense will need to be incurred to support departmental equipment and supplies. Once these activities have been completed, the next step of budgeting can occur. A budget projects the needed expenses for a specified time frame (usually referred to as a "fiscal year"). The third step is to monitor costs and revenues, which may be done by cost accounting to track the cost of a service. The final step is controlling the costs to keep them in line with the budget projections. See reference: Bair and Gray (eds): Laase, SM: Financial management.

169. (B) Generalization of learning. Generalization of learning occurs when a student exhibits a base of skills but must use that knowledge to complete an unfamiliar and more complex task. The basic educational principles are (1) meet the learner at his or her own level, (2) move from the familiar to similar but unfamiliar, (3) involve the learner in the instruction, (4) proceed from the simple to complex, (5) use spaced learning intervals, and (6) facilitate generalization or transfer of learning. See reference: Jacobs and Logigian (eds): Cohn, E: Designing fieldwork programs.

170. (B) 4 to 8 square feet per bed. This is the formula for identifying space needs that is used by Northern Indiana Health Systems Agency. Therefore, if a hospital has 100 beds, the occupational therapy department should have a size of 400 to 800 square feet. Answers A, B, and C are incorrect because they do not meet this standard. See reference: Bair and Gray (eds): Leiter, P: Facility planning.

171. (B) Cost shifting. Cost shifting is what occurs when a hospital increases its prices to all customers to make up for the shortfall of reimbursement. Prospective payment (answer A) is the plan that was signed into law in April 1983 and created a nationwide schedule of reimbursement based on diagnostic related groups (DRGs). Account billing (answer C) is a process within each facility in which the patient or the insurance company is billed for services rendered. Cost accounting (answer D) is an accounting system used to track and report expenses and revenues as they occur. See reference: Bair and Gray (eds): Lasse, SM: Financial management.

172. (C) CPT. The abbreviation CPT stands for Physicians *C*urrent *P*rocedural *T*erminology. A manual of CPT codes defines various medical services and procedures for billing purposes. The abbreviation UB-82 (answer A) stands for the Uniform Bill 82. This form is used under Medicare Part A for reimbursement. The HCFA 1450 (answer B) is an outdated form for reimbursement. This form was replaced by the UB-82. The abbreviation DRG (answer D) stands for Diagnostic Related Group, which belongs to the payment system used by Medicare. See reference: Bair and Gray (eds): Scott, SJ, and Somers, FP: Payment for occupational therapy services.

173. (A) Inpatient hospitalization. Medicare was established by Congress in 1965 as Title XVIII of the Social Security Act. The program consists of two parts. Part A pays for inpatient hospitalization, skilled care, and hospice services. Medicare part B covers answers B, C, and D. These are in home occupational therapy (psychiatric), outpatient occupational therapy, and comprehensive outpatient therapy. All of these services are physician services and other professional medical services. See reference: Bair and Gray (eds): Scott, SJ, and Somers, FP: Payment for occupational therapy services.

174. (C) Workers' compensation or Medicaid. Workers' compensation is a state-supported program fund into which employers pay. Medicaid is a joint state and federal program that provides coverage for the poor and medically indigent. Medicare (answer A) is a federal program for health care coverage for individuals 65 years or older, disabled individuals, or people in end-stage renal failure; therefore, answer A is incorrect. The Education for All Handicapped Children Act is assisted through the provision of state and federal grants; therefore, answers B and D are incorrect. See reference: Bair and Gray (eds): Scott, SJ, and Somers, FP: Payment for occupational therapy services.

175. (C) Worker's compensation. Workers' compensation is a state-supported program into which employers pay. Beneficiaries will receive coverage for those services that are identified to be covered within their respective state. Medicare (answer A) is a federal program for health coverage for individuals 65 years or older, disabled individuals, or people in the end stages of renal disease. Medicaid (answer B) is a joint state and federal program that provides coverage for the poor and medically indigent. The Education for All Handicapped Children Act (answer D) is assisted through the provision of state and federal grants. See reference: Bair and Gray (eds): Scott, SJ, and Somers, FP: Payment for occupational therapy services.

176. (A) Objectively assessing worker performance. Performance reviews are for the primary purpose of evaluating an employee's accomplishments. Answer B is incorrect because disciplinary problems are generally handled through the disciplinary process. Disciplinary processes usually include a verbal warning, written warnings, suspension, and termination. A merit increase (answer C) may accompany a performance appraisal but is not the purpose of the review. Answer D is also incorrect, because many times, goals and objectives are written for the upcoming year in addition to the performance review and are not a primary purpose of the review. See reference: Jacobs and Logigian (eds): Harel, B: Supervision.

177. (C) AC MRDD. The AC MRDD stands for Accreditation Council for services for the Mentally Retarded and other Developmentally Disabled persons. JCAHO (answer A) stands for the Joint Commission of Accreditation of Hospital Organizations. The JCAHO is an agency that reviews medical care of hospitals, psychiatric facilities,

hospices, long-term care agencies, and MR/DD programs seeking accreditation. CARF (answer B) stands for the Commission on Accreditation of Rehabilitation Facilities. CARF reviews programs in freestanding facilities as well as those that are part of a hospital system. The NLN/APHA stands for the National League for Nursing, American Public Health Association. The NLN/APHA surveys nursing homes. See reference: Bair and Gray (eds): Fine, SB, Bair, J, Hoover, SP, and Acquaviva, JD: Regulation and standard setting.

178. (D) NLN/APHA. The NLN/APHA stands for the National League for Nursing, American Public Health Association. JCAHO (Answer A) stands for the Joint Commission of Accreditation of Hospital Organizations. The JCAHO is an agency that reviews medical care of hospitals, psychiatric facilities, hospices, long-term care agencies, and MR/DD programs seeking accreditation and reimbursement. CARF (answer B) stands for the Commission of Accreditation of Rehabilitation Facilities. CARF reviews programs in freestanding facilities as well as those that are part of a hospital system. The AC MRDD (answer C) stands for Accreditation Council for services for the Mentally Retarded and other Developmentally Disabled persons. See reference: Bair and Gray (eds): Fine, SB, Bair, J, Hoover, SP, and Acquaviva, JD: Regulation and standard setting.

179. (C) Acting as a liaison between the academic setting, facility, and students. The academic fieldwork coordinator is a representative of the educational institution from which the student is attaining a degree. This individual oversees all of the students from the designated occupational therapy educational program. Responsibilities include identifying fieldwork sites, writing contracts with fieldwork sites, and maintaining a collaborative effort with the fieldwork sites. A fieldwork educator provides administrative and day-to-day supervision of the student program (answer A) and establishes objectives for the fieldwork site (answer D). "Fieldwork educator" is the official term used by the AOTA to refer to the direct supervisor (answer B). See reference: Jacobs and Logigian (eds): Cohn, E: Designing fieldwork programs.

180. (B) 60 percent. According to Logigian, the most common measure utilized used by management for staff productivity is 60%. This is the equivalent of approximately 5 hours of direct service per day or 20 15-minute sessions with patients. This percentage may be reduced for senior therapists who take on responsibilities above and beyond patient treatment. Therefore, answers A, C, and D are incorrect. See reference: Jacobs and Logigian (eds): Logigian, M: Cost accounting.

181. (B) Segmentation of the market into distinct groups with a focus on a specified area. The act of targeting a market is based on identifying one market to enter. Because a target market is specific, answer A is incorrect. Answers C and D are also incorrect. Answer C is a consumer analysis, and answer D is an environmental analysis. See reference: Jacobs and Logigian (eds): Jacobs, K: Marketing.

182. (C) CARF. The Commission on Accreditation of Rehabilitation Facilities is the regulatory agency for the provision of rehabilitation services. AOTA (answer A) was formed in March of 1917 as the National Society for the Promotion of Occupational Therapy. JCAHO (answer B) is the Joint Commission on Accreditation of Hospital Organizations. The JCAHO reviews the medical care provided by hospital organizations. The NBCOT (answer D) is the agency that develops and administers the examination for registration as an occupational therapist; therefore, answers A, B, and D are incorrect. See reference: Jacobs and Logigian (eds): Cargill, L: Quality assurance.

183. (A) Direct mailings. Advertising is the use of a paid message to attract a consumer to a product. Therefore, the only correct answer would be answer A. Answers B, C, and D are all "free" activities. See reference: Jacobs and Logigian (eds): Jacobs, K: Marketing.

184. (D) Occupational Therapy *Code of Ethics*. This writing was adopted by the AOTA in April 1977. A revised code was adopted by the Representative Assembly in April 1988. The Standards of Practice (answer A) were designed as a guideline for the provision of occupational therapy services. The Uniform Terminology System for Reporting Occupational Therapy Services, third edition (answer B) is a document that defines areas of practice and descriptors of services. Licensure boards (answer C) enforce state practice standards. See reference: Jacobs and Logigian (eds): Bloom, G: Ethics.

185. (A) The process of providing sufficient information so that an individual can make an informed decision about his or her own health care. Answer B is clinical reasoning, which is completed by the therapist in planning treatment. Answer C is acceptance of the job offer. Answer D is the result of the Americans with Disabilities Act, which was enacted in 1992. See reference: Jacobs and Logigian (eds): Bloom, G: Ethics.

186. (B) Mandatory certification. The NBCOT mandatory certification (government title control) recognizes those individuals who have achieved entry-level competence in occupational therapy. Malpractice insurance (answer A) is the payment of a fee to cover the therapist in the event of improper or negligent treatment of a patient that results in a settlement. Answer C is incorrect. Employers may require that occupational therapists be certified before employment but do not attribute employment to the completion of the items listed. Membership in the state association (answer D) is recommended for occupational therapists, but associations do not require proof of any of the items listed in the question. See reference: Bair and Gray (eds): Fine, SB, Bair, J, Hoover, SP, and Acquaviva, JD: Regulation and standard setting.

187. (B) "Tort" law. A tort law is a form of common law. Common laws are decisions enforced by the courts throughout the nation. As a subspecialty of common law, a tort is a "legal wrong committed upon a person or property independent of a contract." Restitution is usually made through assessment of monetary damages. Local ordinances (answer A) are statutes or regulations enacted by city governments. The NBCOT is responsible for the certification examination and the regulation and certification of occupational therapists. The NBCOT (answer C) is recognized by most state regulatory agencies. Licensure boards (answer D) enforce state practice standards, and individuals not in compliance with those standards may be fined or found guilty of a misdemeanor. See reference: Bair and Gray (eds): Fine, SB, Bair, J, Hoover, SP, and Acquaviva, JD: Regulation and standard setting.

188. (C) Created an increase in demand resulting in an inadequate supply of therapists. Recent trends in health care have caused an increased awareness of, and thus demand for, occupational therapy services. Federal and state regulations, as well as accrediting agencies, require the provision of occupational therapy services. In addition, the passage of the Americans with Disabilities Act in 1990 (enacted in 1992) has further enhanced the awareness of the rights of the disabled. Answers A, B, and D are incorrect because they do not convey the message of an increase in demand and a lack of supply. See reference: Jacobs and Logigian (eds): Parisi, RA: Recruitment and retention.

189. (A) Negotiate the contract. As the availability of therapists has declined, many occupational therapists have moved into consultation roles. The first step in the consultation process should include negotiation of the contract. This immediately establishes the general terms of agreement and a focus of the activities that are to be completed by the therapist. Answers B (establish trust), C (assess the environment), and D (identify problems), should follow once the contract has been negotiated. See reference: Jaffe and Epstein (eds): Jaffe, EG: Theoretical concepts of consultation.

190. (C) A benefits package. A benefits package is developed by human resources or personnel departments to provide for the needs of the employees of a facility or agency. These packages vary from one employer to another, but they generally cover child care, medical and dental insurance, long- or short-term disability (or both), and education assistance through continuing education and tuition assistance. A vacation package (answer A) is a part of the benefits package. Recruitment (answer B) is a process of bringing in job candidates to the facility and hiring the candidates. Orientation (answer D) is an activity of familiarizing the employee with the inner workings of the facility and department. Orientation is completed once the employee has accepted the position. See reference: Jacobs and Logigian (eds): Parisi, RA: Managing human resources: Recruitment and retention.

191. (D) Merit increases. A merit increase is based on demonstrated ability and performance. A merit increase typically is awarded following a performance review or assessment of an employee's demonstrated work skill (answer B). Disciplinary action (answer A) is a formal reproach taken in the occurrence of a violation of departmental, facility, or professional standards. Clinical education (answer C) is the responsibility of each occupational therapist and may be offered through employment as a benefit. See reference: Jacobs and Logigian (eds): Parisi, RA: Managing human resources: Recruitment and retention.

192. (B) A presentation to physicians. Personal selling is face-to-face communication with the customer. In occupational therapy, this most frequently occurs through open houses, presentations to professional or lay individuals, exhibiting at conferences, and attending professional meetings. A consumer analysis (answer A) assesses the potential of occupational therapy services in a geographic area. A self-audit (answer C) assesses the strengths, weaknesses, and future opportunities for growth of a department. Finally, the environmental assessment (answer D) encompasses the assessment of the geographic area, political trends, local regulations, and economic conditions. See reference: Jacobs and Logigian (eds): Jacobs, K: Marketing.

193. (C) Job tasks that are fundamental to the position. These tasks are required by law to be presented to potential employees. If a job candidate would be limited in completing a task, they are responsible for indicating the limitation and what possible accommodations may be made. Answers A, B, and D are incorrect because they all relate to accommodations or modifications being made to the work. See reference: Hopkins and Smith (eds): Jacobs, K: Occupational therapy assessment and treatment: Work assessments and programming.

194. (B) *Standards of Practice.* The *Occupational Therapy Standards of Practice* were approved in 1983 by the Representative Assembly. These standards are a guide in the provision and management of occupational therapy services. The *Uniform Terminology System for Reporting Occupational Therapy Services,* third edition, is a document that defines areas of practice and descriptors of services. This document assists in providing consistent documentation in occupational therapy throughout all areas of practice. Licensure regulations vary from state to state and are not always consistent in the guidelines for practice. The AOTA policies and procedures guide the activities of the organization but do not refer to the provision of services; therefore, answers A, C, and D are incorrect. See reference: American Occupational Therapy Association: System for Reporting Occupational Therapy Services.

195. (D) Correlation design. Many forms of research design exist. The experimental designs (answer A) are defined by random selection and manipulation of one independent variable. Quasi-experimental (answer B) research is like the experimental design except that it manipulates the independent variable to identify the effect on the dependent variable. Control or randomization is lacking in this design. Factorial designs (answer C) allow for investigation of the effects of two or more variables on the dependent variable. See reference: Bailey: Research designs.

196. (C) Completing a review of the literature. Review of the written material is necessary in preparing the design of the research project. The literature review helps the researcher to state the purpose clearly and establish boundaries. Stating the purpose and the hypothesis follows the identification of the research question; therefore, answer A is incorrect. The design of the research and the establishment of the boundaries are affected by information from the literature review; therefore, answers C and D are incorrect. See reference: Bailey: Reviewing the literature.

197. (C) PROs. PROs are state organizations that were established to ensure appropriate and cost-effective patient care. These organizations numerically assess unnecessary procedures, patient deaths, and substandard care. Answer A is incorrect because JCAHO (*J*oint *C*ommission on *A*ccreditation of *H*ospital *O*rganizations) is an agency that reviews medical care provided by hospitals, psychiatric facilities, hospices, long-term care agencies, and MR/DD programs. CARF stands for the *C*ommission of *A*ccreditation of *R*ehabilitation *F*acilities. CARF reviews freestanding rehabilitation facilities as well as those within hospital systems. ARA stands for the *A*merican *R*ehabilitation *A*ssociation. This organization was formerly known as NARF (*N*ational *A*ssociation of *R*ehabilitation *F*acilities). A majority of rehabilitation facilities belong to the ARA, which provides professional support services and information to its members. See reference: Bair and Gray (eds): Joe, B: Quality assurance.

198. (D) Joint Commission on Accreditation of Hospital Organizations. The JCAHO is an agency that reviews the medical care provided by hospitals seeking accreditation. The JCAHO was established in the 1950s when the American College of Surgeons linked with three different medical associations to set a standard for reasonable and necessary medical care. Beginning in 1965, the Federal Government required that hospitals participating in the Medicare program be accredited by the JCAHO. Answers A, B, and C were fabricated. See reference: Jacobs and Logigian (eds): Cargill, L: Quality assurance.

199. (C) A productivity report. Productivity information is the primary indicator for need of additional staff, according to Logigian. These data take into account the use of staff resources (productive hours versus nonproductive hours) compared with the services generated within a department. A cost-accounting report (answer A) is a compilation of all of the services provided to an individual. This report would include occupational therapy as well as any additional services provided. Because a cost-accounting report includes other departments, it is not a good source of data for justifying additional occupational therapy support. Answer B, a report of Relative Value Units, is often used as part of a cost-accounting system. It includes data of the services provided, the cost per unit for time and materials, and the variable cost per unit. A market analysis (answer D) is an assessment of a facility's ability to provide a service to a given population or region. See reference: Jacobs and Logigian (eds): Logigian, M: Cost accounting.

200. (B) The Education for All Handicapped Children Act. This bill was enacted in Congress in 1975. It requires that school systems receiving federal funds provide handicapped children with free appropriate education in the least restrictive manner. The Americans with Disabilities Act (answer A) was passed in 1990 and enacted in 1992 to provide accessibility to individuals with disabilities. Children's Protective Services (answer C) is an agency that investigates the home environment and removes children from families who neglect or abuse them. Medicare (answer D) was established by Congress in 1965 as Title XVIII of the Social Security Act. The program consists of two parts. Medicare part A pays for inpatient hospitalization, skilled care, and hospice services. Medicare part B covers outpatient services, physician services, and other professional medical services. See reference: Bair and Gray (eds): Scott, SJ, and Somers, FP: Payment for occupational therapy services.

SIMULATION EXAMINATION 2

> **Directions:** Circle the correct answer to the following questions. When you have completed this examination, check your answers against the answer key that follows. As you will see, an explanation is given for each answer along with a reference for further study. The book author is listed as well as the chapter author. See the bibliography for complete references. Study the areas in which your comprehension was low, then test yourself again by taking Simulation Examination 3.

PEDIATRIC QUESTIONS

Assessment of Occupational Performance

1. During the assessment of a 13-month-old child with congenital blindness, the child demonstrates a Moro reflex to loud noise and loss of position. This evaluation tells the occupational therapist (OTR) that:
   A. reflex maturation is occurring at a normal rate.
   B. reflex maturation is slightly delayed.
   C. reflex maturation is significantly delayed.
   D. reflex maturation is advanced for the child's age.

2. During assessment of a 10-month-old child with Down syndrome, the occupational therapist notes hyperextensibility of all joints. This term means that the child probably has:
   A. increased muscle tone.
   B. decreased muscle tone.
   C. anterior horn cell disease.
   D. muscle and joint disease.

3. A child diagnosed with autism is being evaluated by an occupational therapist. The child demonstrates a craving for tactile stimulation, rubbing objects on his arms and legs. He also avoids being touched by others. What sensory integration problem is he demonstrating?
   A. Poor modulation of tactile input
   B. Hypersensitivity to tactile input
   C. Hyposensitivity to tactile input
   D. Poor modulation of proprioceptive input

4. During an evaluation of a child's motor skills, the occupational therapist observes a 9-year-old child who is awkward at many gross motor tasks but is able to skip rope. When asked to skip backwards, the child is unable to complete this task after several attempts. For what problem should the therapist be particularly observant as the evaluation continues?
   A. Delayed reflex integration
   B. Inadequate bilateral integration
   C. Developmental dyspraxia
   D. Incoordination

5. A child referred for an occupational therapy evaluation has paralysis of both legs. Which of the following diagnoses would MOST likely result in paraplegia?
   A. Osteogenesis imperfecta
   B. Arthrogryposis
   C. Ankylosing spondylitis
   D. Myelomeningocele

6. During an assessment, the occupational therapist notes that a child responds to movement by falling backwards with abducted and extended arms. The reflex or reaction observed in this child is called:
   A. rooting.
   B. Moro reflex.
   C. flexor withdrawal.
   D. neck righting.

7. In a pediatric program, the occupational therapist would use a screening test for the following reason:
   A. it provides needed information for an occupational therapy consultation with teachers or parents.
   B. it tests a wide variety of developmental behaviors.
   C. it establishes an information base for the occupational therapy treatment plan.
   D. it determines the need for further occupational therapy evaluation.

8. The occupational therapist needs an appropriate screening tool to determine the need for Sensory Integration and Praxis Test (SIPT) referrals. Which of the following tests would BEST serve this purpose?
   A. Erhardt Developmental Test of Prehension
   B. Denver II Screening Test
   C. Ayres Clinical Observations of Sensory Integration
   D. Vineland Adaptive Behavior Scales

9. The occupational therapist has selected a standardized and norm-referenced test to screen 2½ to 5-year-old children for sensorimotor, cognitive, and verbal problems. This test is the:
   A. Erhardt Developmental Test of Prehension.
   B. Miller Assessment of Preschoolers Screening Test.
   C. Ayres Clinical Observation of Sensory Integration.
   D. Denver II Screening Test.

Development of the Treatment Plan

10. Occupational therapists can contribute their assessment and planning information to an "Individual Educational Plan," or IEP. In which of the following settings is an IEP used as the central plan for a child?
    A. Rehabilitation center
    B. Public school system
    C. Outpatient care center
    D. Home health agency

11. An occupational therapist is developing a treatment plan for a child with mild cerebral palsy who has difficulty with "in-hand manipulation." The skill that needs remediation is linear movement of an object from the palm to the fingers or fingers to the palm. Of the three types of in-hand manipulation, this type is called:
    A. translation.
    B. shift.
    C. rotation.
    D. stabilization.

12. A therapist who is planning treatment for a child with athetoid cerebral palsy is concerned about the child's inability to control flexion and extension of the arm when reaching for a toy. The child flexes too much or extends too much, which makes placement of the hand very difficult. The most appropriate goal for this type of problem in hand function would be:
    A. to improve ability to isolate movement.
    B. to improve ability to grade movement.
    C. to improve timing of movement.
    D. to improve bilateral integration of arm movements.

13. An occupational therapist is discharging a 4-year-old child with athetoid cerebral palsy from a rehabilitation setting to home. Instructions to the child's family for maintaining correct jaw control while being fed from the side include the following:
    A. jaw opening and closing are controlled with the adult's index and middle fingers; the adult's thumb is placed on the child's cheek.
    B. jaw opening and closing are controlled with the adult's index and middle fingers; the adult's thumb is placed on the child's larynx for stability.
    C. jaw opening and closing are controlled with the adult's whole hand on the child's jaw.
    D. jaw opening and closing are controlled with the adult's index and middle fingers; the adult's thumb is placed on the child's ear for stability.

14. Results of an occupational therapy evaluation show that a child has many tactile defensive behaviors. What activity would be the MOST appropriate for beginning a treatment plan?
    A. The therapist has the child play "sandwich" between heavy mats.
    B. The therapist applies a feather brush lightly to the child's arms and legs.
    C. The child is blindfolded and must guess where he or she is touched on the body.
    D. The therapist has the child play the "duck, duck, goose" circle game.

15. The most effective method of teaching children with moderate mental retardation to feed, groom, and dress themselves is:
    A. forward and backward "chaining."
    B. practice and repetition.
    C. demonstration.
    D. role modeling.

16. A 4-year-old child with an apparent learning disability is being seen by an occupational therapist in a preschool program. The teacher has asked for advice in teaching the child to identify forms and shapes. If the child is able to identify a circle shape, what shape would usually be expected to follow in developmental sequence?
    A. Square
    B. Cross
    C. Triangle
    D. Diamond

17. When using reflex-inhibiting patterns with a child who demonstrates extensor patterns of spasticity, an occupational therapist using the neurodevelopmental treatment (NDT) approach would:
    A. move the child into extension.
    B. facilitate righting and equilibrium reactions while the child is partially flexed.
    C. use a key point of control at the ankle.
    D. ask the child to hold a position of flexion.

18. When facilitating head control in a 2-year-old child with hypotonia, the most effective beginning activity (assuming the child is stabilized as needed) would be placement of the child:
    A. prone on a ball with forward movement.
    B. sitting on a ball with forward and side-to-side movement.
    C. quadruped on a tilting board with forward and side-to-side movement.
    D. supine on a mat and pulling him or her into a sitting position.

19. A 5-year-old child with athetoid cerebral palsy demonstrates a jaw and tongue thrust when a food-filled spoon is placed in his mouth. A treatment method that provides positioning to decrease this problem MOST likely includes:
    A. increased neck flexion.
    B. increased shoulder retraction.
    C. increased hip extension.
    D. increased neck extension.

20. If a child is on a puree diet because he is unable to chew food, the occupational therapist should:
    A. encourage the child to remove food from the spoon with his or her teeth.
    B. stimulate management of texture by using vegetable or beef soup.
    C. increase management of texture by using a baby food grinder.
    D. stimulate biting and chewing by placing a raisin between the child's teeth.

21. The treatment goal for a 4-year-old child with hypotonia is to improve grasp. Which of the following activities would be most appropriate to prepare the child's hand for grasp activities?
    A. Dropping blocks into a pail
    B. Placing pegs on a pegboard
    C. Weight bearing on hands
    D. Holding and eating a cookie

22. An occupational therapist who uses splints with children may find the most controversy over the use of hand splints for children who have:
    A. abnormal muscle tone.
    B. muscle weakness.
    C. traumatic injury.
    D. joint inflammation.

23. The adaptation on a chair that usually inhibits extensor tone or pattern and makes sitting in a chair possible is a:
    A. lateral trunk support.
    B. seat belt at the hips.
    C. wedge-shaped seat that is higher in front.
    D. lapboard.

24. A treatment goal for a child with athetoid cerebral palsy is self-feeding. Which piece of equipment would best solve the problem of food sliding off the plate when the child attempts to pick it up with a spoon?
    A. Swivel spoon
    B. Nonslip mat
    C. Mobile arm support
    D. Scoop dish

25. An occupational therapist is collaborating with a team in making a recommendation for a child to use a wheelchair for use at school. The child is 12 years old and has Duchenne's muscular dystrophy. Although he is able to use a manual chair for distances between classes, he is tired on arrival. What would be the best recommendation?
    A. Retain the manual chair to build up strength.
    B. Change to an ultralight sports model, because it requires less strength.
    C. Change to a power wheelchair to eliminate effort.
    D. Encourage walking with a walker to alternate mobility methods.

Implementation of the Treatment Plan

26. An occupational therapist is discussing normal child development with a parent. As a part of this discussion, the therapist explains that infants usually crawl in a four-point position (creeping):
    A. after they crawl on their bellies.
    B. before they sit with support.
    C. after they rise up independently to a standing position.
    D. before they lift their head in prone.

27. The BEST description of the occupational therapist's role with the parent would be:
    A. directive.
    B. substitute parent.
    C. partner.
    D. expert.

28. The occupational therapist is working with a child who has a condition characterized by joint inflammation and pain. This condition is:
    A. type I diabetes.
    B. patent ductus arteriosus.
    C. juvenile rheumatoid arthritis.
    D. tetralogy of Fallot.

29. The occupational therapist is working with a child who has a congenital abnormality in which the laminae of one or more vertebrae are incompletely closed. This condition is called:
    A. osteomyelitis.
    B. spina bifida.
    C. scoliosis.
    D. osteogenesis imperfecta.

30. The physician reports to the occupational therapist that the child referred to occupational therapy has a condition that is present in premature infants. The condition involves underdevelopment of the lungs. The physician would refer to this condition as:
    A. otitis media.
    B. Duchenne's disease.
    C. poliomyelitis.
    D. hyaline membrane disease.

31. An occupational therapist is attempting to attain certification beyond that of an entry-level therapist. Which one of the following tests requires advanced certification?
    A. Denver II Screening Test
    B. Hawaii Early Learning Profile (HELP)
    C. Southern California Sensory Integration and Praxis Tests (SIPT)
    D. Developmental Test of Visual Motor Integration (VMI)

32. If a child with cerebral palsy were placed in prone over a therapy ball, and if C-brushing were used over the deep back extensors to facilitate a pivot prone position, the therapist would be using a treatment approach developed by:
    A. Margaret Rood.
    B. Berta Bobath.
    C. Signe Brunnstrom.
    D. Knott and Voss (PNF)

33. According to public law, in order to qualify for special education (which includes occupational therapy), school-aged children with "learning disabilities" must have a disorder in:
    A. understanding or using language.
    B. motor function.
    C. intelligence.
    D. sensory acuity.

34. Occupational therapy in school systems:
    A. is a primary service for 5- to 21-year-old students.
    B. is provided to any child with a need for an occupational therapy evaluation.
    C. can be provided to any child receiving physical therapy service.
    D. must benefit the child's ability to participate in special education.

35. A child who has been diagnosed as having mental retardation enters the occupational therapy program at your agency. The primary functional problem of this diagnostic group in terms of daily life would be:
    A. abnormal motor functioning.
    B. below average intellectual functioning.
    C. psychologic and behavioral difficulties.
    D. presence of seizures.

36. When evaluating visual perceptual problems in a child who has cerebral palsy, the OTR should know that the following is true:
    A. acuity problems are seen in 10 percent of these children.
    B. cortical visual problems are usually caused by optic nerve damage.
    C. oculomotor problems are unrelated to the type of cerebral palsy.
    D. visual perceptual problems usually require a motor-free evaluation.

37. A therapist is discussing discharge plans for a 6-year-old child with her parents. The child has been receiving occupational therapy for developmental dyspraxia. The therapist is recommending additional activities to provide proprioceptive input. The most appropriate activity for this child would be to:
    A. walk barefoot on textured surfaces.
    B. rock over a large therapy ball.
    C. play in a large box full of styrofoam pellets.
    D. push or pull weighted objects while in a quadruped position.

38. Occupational therapists concerned about prevention should know that after the age of 1 year, the most common cause of mortality in young children is:
    A. malignancies.
    B. congenital malformations.
    C. accidents.
    D. infectious diseases.

39. When working within a school system to assist the mainstreaming of a child with spina bifida into a regular classroom, the occupational therapist consults with the classroom teacher. The uniqueness of the "consultation" relationship is best characterized by the following statement:
    A. The occupational therapist teaches the teacher.
    B. The occupational therapist provides therapy to the child.
    C. The occupational therapist directs the teacher.
    D. The occupational therapist does problem solving with the teacher.

40. Occupational therapists working with children who have been hospitalized for an acute illness need to understand that a child's reaction to hospitalization depends on his or her perception of his or her illness. The most common perception of the cause of sickness by young children is:
    A. a natural occurrence.
    B. a bacterial infection.
    C. separation from parents.
    D. punishment for bad behavior.

Evaluation of the Treatment Plan

41. The supine position provides a normal infant with the opportunity to work against gravity to develop the ability of:
    A. shoulder flexion and protraction.
    B. shoulder extension and retraction.
    C. development of head control.
    D. development of trunk control.

42. The prone position provides the infant with the opportunity to work against gravity to develop:
    A. retraction of the shoulders in weight bearing.
    B. stability of the head and neck.
    C. development of trunk flexion.
    D. mobility in the upper extremities.

43. Occupational therapists working with a child in whom a terminal illness has been diagnosed need to be aware of the child's and family's concerns. The following condition is more likely to include the diagnosis of a terminal illness during childhood years:
    A. Type I diabetes
    B. Acute lymphoblastic leukemia
    C. Hemophilia
    D. Otitis media

44. Eisenmenger complex is a life-threatening disorder that must be monitored in children who have the following medical condition:
    A. Rheumatic fever
    B. Ventricular septal defect
    C. Sickle cell anemia
    D. Asthma

45. An 11-month-old child who was born 3 months prematurely is being reevaluated through the occupational therapy outpatient clinic. The child's abilities in all areas should be compared with those of a normal child of:
    A. 11 months.
    B. 14 months.
    C. 8 months
    D. 10 months.

Discharge Planning

46. The occupational therapist is preparing to discharge a 6-year-old child who was initially referred for treatment for developmental dyspraxia. The child's new teacher asks, "What does 'dyspraxia' mean?" The best description would be:
    A. a problem with learning new motor skills.
    B. a sensory integration problem.
    C. a lack of development of higher-order reflex reactions.
    D. a problem of poor balance.

47. A 5-year-old child diagnosed with autism is being discharged to a school program for children with severe emotional impairments. The occupational therapist is recommending a preparatory vestibular activity to be used in the classroom. This activity will decrease arousal so that this child will be able to concentrate on simple activities. A therapeutic activity that would meet this criterion would be:
    A. bouncing while sitting on a large therapy ball.
    B. manual rocking while in prone on a therapy ball.
    C. spinning in supine while on a hammock swing.
    D. rolling down a large wedge.

48. At the time of discharge, the parents of a handicapped child with feeding problems ask the occupational therapist the purpose of "jaw control." The therapist responds, "Jaw control actually serves two purposes during feeding . . .
    A. strengthening and providing external stabilization of the jaw."
    B. controlling opening and closing and providing external stabilization of the jaw."
    C. strengthening and controlling opening and closing of the jaw."
    D. decreasing tactile defensiveness and stimulating swallowing."

49. A child with poor oral-motor organization is being discharged with a home feeding program. The parents need instruction in food consistency that will help the child to organize her oral-motor mechanism. Which of the following food textures would be most difficult for this child?
    A. Smooth semisolids (pureed bananas)
    B. Lumpy semisolids (cottage cheese)
    C. Liquid/solid combinations (minestrone soup)
    D. Thickened liquids (malted milk)

50. When planning to discharge an infant from an occupational therapy program in a neonatal intensive care unit, reevaluation of home therapy should:
    A. be done on a regular basis.
    B. be done at the end of 1 year.
    C. be scheduled as the parent finds time.
    D. be done if the child is not making progress.

PHYSICAL DISABILITY QUESTIONS

Assessment of Occupational Performance

51. According to the manual muscle test system of letters and numbers, the word that would be the equivalent of grade 1 would be:
    A. absent.
    B. trace.
    C. good.
    D. normal.

52. The instrument used to measure the strength of three jaw chuck is:
    A. an aesthesiometer.
    B. a pinch meter.
    C. a dynamometer.
    D. a volumeter.

53. One method of measuring total finger flexion without recording in degrees is to:
    A. measure the passive flexion at each joint and total the numbers.
    B. measure the distance from the fingertip to the distal palmar crease with the hand in a fist.
    C. measure the active flexion at each joint and total the measurements.
    D. measure the distance between the tip of the thumb and the tip of the fourth finger.

54. An individual who is suspected of having carpal tunnel syndrome is tested by the therapist for Tinel's sign. The position of the wrist for test purposes should be:
    A. ulnar deviation.
    B. radial deviation.
    C. extension.
    D. flexion.

55. During measurement of active range of motion at the metacarpophalangeal (MCP) joints, stabilization is provided:
    A. above the MCP joints.
    B. below the MCP joints.
    C. at the wrist.
    D. on top of the MCP joints.

56. The common body landmark that is used to evaluate the functional movements of shoulder abduction and internal rotation is:
    A. the back of the neck.
    B. the top of the head.
    C. the lower back.
    D. the opposite shoulder.

57. An individual with arthritis has a total range of shoulder flexion from 0 to 90 degrees. During manual muscle testing of the pain-free range, the individual is able to take moderate resistance. The individual's manual muscle grade is:
    A. poor.
    B. fair.
    C. good.
    D. normal.

58. During measurement of an individual who wears a hip brace for a wheelchair, the seat should be:
    A. two inches wider than the widest point across the individual's hip while he or she wears the brace.
    B. two inches wider than the widest point across the individual's hips.
    C. two inches more than the distance from the back of the bent knee to the buttocks.
    D. the same as the distance from the back of the bent knee to the buttocks.

59. The best time of day to schedule an individual with arthritis for an evaluation would be:
    A. early morning (8 to 10 AM).
    B. afternoon.
    C. late morning (10 to 11 AM).
    D. early morning and again in the afternoon.

Development of the Treatment Plan

60. The purpose of using adaptive equipment with an individual who has arthritis would be to:
    A. preserve joint integrity.
    B. correct deformity.
    C. simplify work.
    D. decrease independence.

61. The primary goal of the occupational therapist when treating an individual who was recently diagnosed with rheumatoid arthritis would be to:
    A. increase strength with resistive exercises.
    B. provide positioning and adaptive equipment.
    C. provide emotional support.
    D. prepare for surgical intervention.

62. An individual with functionally impaired shoulder abduction and external rotation would have difficulty performing which of the following self-care activities?
    A. Buttoning a shirt
    B. Combing the hair
    C. Tucking in a shirt in the back
    D. Tying a shoe

63. The part of a treatment objective that describes the level of performance the individual is expected to achieve is the:
    A. terminal behavior.
    B. condition.
    C. criterion.
    D. plan.

64. An individual with an injury to the nondominant right cerebral hemisphere often has difficulty understanding:
    A. written information presented on the right side of the body.
    B. facial expressions.
    C. concrete verbal instructions.
    D. visual stimulation on the right side of the body.

65. An area that is frequently overlooked in the treatment of brain-injured individuals is:
    A. speech.
    B. ambulation.
    C. self-care activities.
    D. sexuality.

66. What is the condition in the following treatment objective? "The individual will increase sitting tolerance to 10 minutes while propping on upper extremities bilaterally."

A. "The individual"
B. "Increase sitting tolerance"
C. "10 minutes"
D. "Propping on upper extremities bilaterally"

67. **The part of a treatment objective that describes the circumstances under which an individual performs an activity is:**
    A. the terminal behavior.
    B. the condition.
    C. the criterion.
    D. the plan.

68. **The rehabilitation team member who is typically responsible for educating an individual with a below-knee amputation about wrapping for compression and shaping of the stump is the:**
    A. nurse.
    B. prosthetist.
    C. physical therapist
    D. occupational therapist.

69. **The rehabilitation team member who is typically responsible for sexual/marital counseling of a brain injured individual and his or her significant other is:**
    A. a physiatrist.
    B. a rehabilitation nurse.
    C. a rehabilitation psychologist.
    D. an occupational therapist.

70. **Proper use of body mechanics when lifting objects from the floor would be a primary goal for individuals who have:**
    A. chronic obstructive pulmonary disease.
    B. fibromyalgia.
    C. carpal tunnel syndrome.
    D. a low back injury.

71. **An individual with weak grip strength and poor endurance wishes to bake something for a family member's birthday. The therapist wishes to work on grasp and release for 5 minutes without exhausting the individual. Which activity is appropriate for these goals?**
    A. Mixing blueberry muffins from scratch using a hand-powered mixer and scooping them into muffin tins with a cup
    B. Mixing an angel food cake from a box mix using an electric mixer and pouring the mix into a pan
    C. Mixing cold chocolate chip cookie dough using a spatula with a built-up handle and dropping dollops onto a tray using an ice cream scoop
    D. Slicing a prepared roll of sugar cookies at room temperature and placing them on a tray using a spatula

72. **After a radial nerve injury, an individual initially had trace muscle strength in elbow extension. One week later, strength is noted to have increased to poor minus. The individual is ready for strengthening exercises at which level?**

A. Passive range of motion
B. Active assisted range of motion with gravity eliminated
C. Active range of motion against gravity
D. Active resistive range of motion with gravity eliminated

73. **To allow tenodesis to develop in a quadriplegic hand, the wrist is kept in which position during passive range of motion of the fingers?**
    A. Neutral position for finger flexion and extension
    B. Flexion for finger flexion and extension
    C. Extension wrist for finger flexion and flexed wrist for finger extension
    D. Flexion for finger flexion and extended for finger extension

74. **Keeping a diary or log when a person has memory problems is called:**
    A. problem solving.
    B. retraining.
    C. substitution.
    D. compensation.

75. **To perform a sliding board or shoulder depression transfer, an individual's wheelchair must have:**
    A. detachable footrests.
    B. detachable arms.
    C. anti-tip bars.
    D. brake handle extensions.

76. **An occupational therapy program designed to teach an individual to compensate for poor handwriting would most likely involve the individual's:**
    A. learning to type.
    B. practicing fine motor coordination exercises.
    C. practicing letter or shape formations.
    D. strengthening the finger flexors and extensors.

77. **The neck position that would most likely be used in positioning an individual for feeding is:**
    A. thirty degrees of head extension.
    B. ten degrees of head extension past the midline.
    C. ten degrees of head flexion from the midline.
    D. thirty degrees of head flexion.

78. **The position of the wrist that should be avoided for individuals with mild carpal tunnel syndrome is:**
    A. extension.
    B. flexion.
    C. ulnar deviation.
    D. radial deviation.

Implementation of the Treatment Plan

79. **The most common cause of amputation in the lower extremity is:**
    A. trauma.
    B. metastasizing tumor.

C. peripheral vascular disease.
D. congenital defects.

80. **The movement of shoulder flexion occurs in which plane?**
A. Sagittal
B. Coronal
C. Frontal
D. Transverse

81. **The anatomic landmark of the body that is used to center the fulcrum of the goniometer when measuring elbow flexion is the:**
A. lateral epicondyle of the humerus.
B. posterior aspect of the acromion process.
C. xiphoid process in the midline of the thorax.
D. olecranon process.

82. **The adapted utensil that aids self-feeding in an individual with poor supination is a:**
A. rocker knife.
B. spork.
C. spoon with a built-up handle.
D. swivel spoon.

83. **Which of the following activities could result in median nerve compression?**
A. Pounding nails while holding the hammer with the wrist in neutral
B. Washing a table top with the wrist extended
C. Writing with the wrist extended
D. Using a vibrator with the wrist ulnarly flexed

84. **An individual complains of perspiration that caused his resting hand splint to be uncomfortable. The therapist would most likely:**
A. recommend putting talcum powder in the splint.
B. line the splint with moleskin.
C. fabricate a new resting hand splint with perforated material.
D. provide a stockinette for the individual to wear inside the splint.

85. **Which of the following activities is considered to be facilitory by Margaret Rood when a therapist performs it on an individual?**
A. Fast rocking while the individual is inverted over a barrel
B. Slow rocking in a rocking chair
C. Slow rolling in bed
D. Pressure to the tendon insertions on a spastic arm

86. **What positioning is recommended during sexual intercourse when the person has left side hemiplegia with spasticity?**
A. Lying on the left side while propped with pillows
B. Lying on the right side while propped with pillows
C. Lying in supine
D. Lying in prone

87. **When performing a stand pivot transfer with an individual, the therapist would most likely:**
A. move slowly, twisting the body from the trunk.
B. keep feet shoulder width apart, lifting with the arms.
C. keep knees bent and feet planted when moving.
D. maintain a normal curve of the back, slowly shifting feet as the turn is completed.

88. **A therapist transferring an individual from the wheelchair to a mat table using a stand pivot transfer would verbally cue the individual with mild hemiparesis to:**
A. push up from the mat.
B. scoot forward to the edge of the wheelchair.
C. unfasten a rear-locking seat belt.
D. position the wheelchair so that it directly faces the mat table.

Evaluation of the Treatment Plan

89. **The therapist is reevaluating an individual's passive range of motion for elbow flexion by completing three consecutive measurements. A 10-degree discrepancy exists between the first two measurements and the third. The therapist would most likely:**
A. check the alignment of the goniometer.
B. use a larger goniometer.
C. use a smaller goniometer.
D. attempt to force the individual's arm further into flexion.

90. **When a therapist updates an individual's treatment plan, activities are continued when:**
A. the individual is unable to complete the task after several repetitions.
B. the individual is easily able to complete the task.
C. the individual continues to be motivated toward improving performance.
D. the individual lacks motivation to improve performance on the task.

91. **A primary reason to revise a treatment plan for an individual is:**
A. modification of the plan to discharge the individual from therapy.
B. a change in the individual's status.
C. completion of the evaluation.
D. ensuring that the individual continues to make progress toward a goal.

92. **An individual on a puree diet has demonstrated a gurgle or wet voice after swallowing a second time. The diet had not been difficult for the individual until this instance. This individual would benefit from:**
A. a videofluoroscopy.
B. a diet change to include thin liquids.
C. a tracheostomy.
D. a regular diet.

93. An individual with dysphagia wants to progress from thickened liquids to thin liquids. Before the therapist could upgrade the individual's status, the individual's swallow must be:
   A. more than 3 to 5 seconds.
   B. 3 to 5 seconds.
   C. 1 second.
   D. a normal swallow.

94. What form of arthritis is characterized by chronic inflammation of the joints in the cervical area of the spine and the extremities, with periods of remissions and exacerbations?
   A. Osteoarthritis
   B. Rheumatoid arthritis
   C. Ankylosing spondylitis
   D. Systemic lupus erythematosus

95. A degenerative arthritis of the noninflammatory type that may affect any joint is referred to as:
   A. osteoarthritis.
   B. rheumatoid arthritis.
   C. ankylosing spondylitis.
   D. juvenile rheumatoid arthritis.

Discharge Planning

96. The occupational therapist is performing a home evaluation for an individual with arthritis. This individual exhibits severe hand weakness as a result of her arthritis. Which of the following activities would the individual need to be able to demonstrate for safety?
   A. the ability to work locks and latches on doors or windows.
   B. the skill in manipulating built-up utensils while eating.
   C. the ability to demonstrate energy conservation techniques.
   D. the skill in manipulating fasteners on clothing for easy donning and doffing.

97. Before an individual with a splint is discharged home, the individual or family, or both, should be able to:
   A. identify landmarks on the hand or arm to align the splint.
   B. discontinue use of the splint if redness occurs.
   C. describe in general terms the wearing schedule.
   D. remove and replace the splint with verbal cues from the therapist.

98. When performing exercises at home, a person with inflamed arthritis should be instructed to perform exercises:
   A. with brisk passive range of motion.
   B. with weight as tolerated.
   C. isotonically.
   D. with gentle active range of motion.

99. What wheelchair feature is necessary for an individual who will be traveling by car with the family to community outings and bringing their wheelchair?
   A. A lightweight folding frame
   B. A one-arm drive
   C. An amputee frame
   D. A reclining backrest

100. An individual's family wants to build a ramp to the primary entrance of the home. The proper grade for the ramp should be:
   A. 1 inch of ramp for every foot of rise in height.
   B. 1 foot of ramp for every inch of rise in height.
   C. 10 inches of ramp for every 2 inches in height.
   D. 1 foot of ramp for every foot of rise in height.

PSYCHOSOCIAL QUESTIONS

Assessment of Occupational Performance

101. The occupational therapist has completed the facility's assessment protocol, which includes a chart review, an interview, and a performance measurement, with an individual referred for psychiatric services. In writing the summary of the assessment results, the therapist will rely on the interview information to address:
   A. the individual's diagnosis.
   B. the individual's current medications.
   C. the individual's ability to concentrate and solve problems.
   D. the individual's view of the problem and overall goal.

102. The best performance measure for the occupational therapist observing an adult's performance and determining that individual's sensorimotor functions in a psychosocial setting is the:
   A. Bay Area Functional Performance Evaluation (BaFPE).
   B. Schroeder Block Campbell (SBC).
   C. Southern California Sensory Integrative Test (SCSIT).
   D. Comprehensive OT Evaluation Scale (COTE).

103. The occupational therapist is working within a behavioral frame of reference in a psychosocial treatment setting. The therapist wants to obtain data about the individual's interests. The best assessment strategy to select is:
   A. to use an interest checklist that identifies the individual's past, present, and future interests as well as the level of satisfaction with interests.
   B. to present the individual with activities through which the individual's knowledge and skill are determined.
   C. to ask the individual to identify the interests that evoke the strongest feelings.

D. to use an interest checklist that compares the individual's current involvement with the past 6 months.

104. **The occupational therapist uses an object relations frame of reference in treatment. When offering an individual the choice between the moderately structured activities of kneading bread dough and making a collage of his or her current interests, the occupational therapist is assessing the individual's:**
    A. id.
    B. superego.
    C. ego.
    D. libido.

105. **The best assessment instrument to obtain data about an individual's stressors is:**
    A. biofeedback equipment to determine changes in muscle tension.
    B. the Holmes-Rahe Life Change Index.
    C. Axis V of *DSM-IV.*
    D. The Type A Behavior scale.

106. **The occupational therapist works with an entry-level COTA on an inpatient psychiatric unit. They each work 4 days a week, overlapping schedules only on Mondays. The task that would be inappropriate for the OTR to ask the COTA to do is:**
    A. to lead the daily craft group.
    B. to begin the assessment process when individuals are admitted on the weekends. The OTR will finish the assessment on Monday.
    C. to assist individuals in carrying out their activities of daily living (ADLs) on Saturday and Sunday mornings.
    D. to lead a leisure planning group on Saturday afternoon.

107. **The statement that best describes the Vineland Adaptive Behavior Scale is:**
    A. The format of this assessment is an interview or questionnaire.
    B. This assessment instrument is a screening tool that usually takes 15 minutes or less to administer.
    C. This instrument should not be used with individuals who are visually or hearing impaired.
    D. This assessment does not require any special training to administer.

108. **Which assessment instrument addresses most of the important areas of concern to occupational therapists working with adolescents with psychiatric disorders?**
    A. Vineland Adaptive Behavior Scale
    B. Visual Motor Integration Test (VMI)
    C. Takata's Play History
    D. Neuropsychiatric Institute Interest Checklist (NPI)

109. **The best overall approach for evaluating adolescents with psychiatric problems is:**
    A. to determine the level of function in play, social behavior, and visual motor skills.
    B. to determine the level of function in socialization, task performance in daily living skills, time management, and visual motor skills.
    C. to determine the level of interest in work, leisure, and self-care.
    D. to determine the level of function in play and social behaviors in overall development and in visual motor skills.

Case Example for Question 110

> *Individual 1:* **"This is really stupid! Why are we doing this collage anyway?"**
> *OT Group Leader:* "As I already told you before we started, . . . this activity will help you to identify what is important or interesting to you."
> *Individual 2:* **"Should I tear from the magazine or use scissors?"**
> *OT Group Leader:* "I want you to tear the pages out of the magazines and then use the scissors to cut out the pictures or words you want to use."
> *Individual 1:* (Tears out two whole pages from the magazine nearest to him and quickly pastes the pages onto the paper provided.) **"OK. I'm finished. I'm going back to my room now."**

110. **Based on the case example, which patient-therapist variable from the Lerner Collage Scoring System should the therapist use to score individual 1:**
    A. Seeks repetition of directions:
      a. yes   b. no
    B. Seeks reassurances of doing it correctly:
      a. yes   b. no
    C. Time taken to complete the collage:
      a. 0 to 15 minutes
      b. 16 to 30 minutes
      c. 31 minutes to 1 hour
    D. Number of pictures or cuttings:
      a. 1   b. 2 to 5   c. 6 to 10
      d. 11 to 15   e. 16 and over.

Development of the Treatment Plan

111. **The therapist is planning a series of groups for social skill development with adults. The therapist uses the following sequence of activity sessions: introductions, identifying topics of mutual interest, and focus on listening skills. This sequencing strategy is known as:**
    A. normal developmental sequencing.
    B. normal activity sequencing.
    C. chronologic sequencing.
    D. role acquisition sequencing.

112. The therapist is planning a fourth social skills activity for the sequence described in question 111. The best theme for a fourth session is:
    A. recognizing emotions.
    B. expressing age-appropriate emotions.
    C. giving and receiving feedback to supervisors in work-related situations.
    D. exiting conversations.

113. Why does the occupational therapist decide to respond to an individual by paraphrasing?
    A. To refocus or redirect an individual's comments
    B. To show acceptance and understanding to the individual
    C. To repeat what an individual has said
    D. To encourage an individual to give additional information

114. Which patient problems are occupational therapists working in mental health most likely to address?
    A. Adjustment disorders
    B. Affective disorders
    C. Alcohol use disorders
    D. Anxiety disorders

115. An individual's assessment reveals that assertiveness is new and quite difficult for her. Which teaching method is most appropriate to use with this individual who is working toward developing assertiveness skills?
    A. Provide a diary or log book in which the individual records the interactions during which she was passive
    B. Role-play assertiveness skills in simulated situations that are proposed by the occupational therapist
    C. Guide the individual in applying the problem-solving process to the nonassertive behaviors
    D. Demonstrate the techniques of "broken-record" and "I" statements to the individual and asking the individual to imitate these techniques

116. For which of the following side effects of neuroleptic medications would the therapist want to take precautions when planning a community outing in the summer that involves walking outdoors between the bus stop, the bank, a utility company, and a grocery store?
    A. Hypotension
    B. Photosensitivity
    C. Excessive perspiration
    D. Weight gain

117. In psychosocial areas of occupational therapy, the therapist's relationship with an individual is best described as:
    A. the central focus of occupational therapy treatment.
    B. a therapeutic device in helping.
    C. a friendship.
    D. sympathy for the individual's problems.

118. The primary disadvantage in implementing a group format for occupational therapy services provided in an acute care psychiatric setting is that:
    A. the other group members provide feedback.
    B. a greater number of individuals can be treated by fewer occupational therapists.
    C. cohesiveness is difficult to achieve.
    D. each person's individual goals can be met.

119. The therapist is working with a group of individuals who are diagnosed with major depression. The therapist is focusing on issues related to being ready for discharge. What would be the most helpful approach for the therapist to take?
    A. The therapist should be upbeat, positive, and cheerful when encouraging the individuals to discuss their discharge plans.
    B. The therapist should allow more time for the individuals to respond to questions about discharge plans.
    C. The therapist should remain silent and still while the individuals are describing their feelings about discharge.
    D. The therapist should allow the individuals to structure the group discussion.

120. The therapist is deciding which activity will (1) allow the individual to experience success (after using a messy process) and (2) delay gratification. The activity process that best provides this experience is:
    A. working in a group of three other individuals.
    B. selecting the design pattern for a tile trivet.
    C. applying grout to a tile trivet and waiting for it to dry.
    D. encouraging the individual to clean off the table at the end of the group session.

121. The therapist is working with an individual who was admitted to an inpatient psychiatric program for major depression. This individual is also diagnosed as having AIDS in stage 4. The best major focus of treatment to pursue would be to:
    A. restore and maintain functional performance of self-chosen occupations that enhance competent performance of valued occupational roles.
    B. increase physical endurance and maintain desired self-care tasks.
    C. facilitate resolution of current and anticipated losses through the grieving process.
    D. restore and maintain functional performance of the individual's primary work role.

122. When using a health promotion approach, stress-management interventions are an example of:
    A. primary prevention.
    B. secondary prevention.
    C. tertiary prevention.
    D. intermediate prevention.

123. The therapist is working with individuals who have eating disorders. Overall, the most important treatment direction that the therapist should pursue in the discharge planning phase is to:
    A. provide information about times and days of Overeaters Anonymous meetings held at the treatment facility.
    B. make recommendations or referrals for family therapy.
    C. make recommendations for adapting the kitchen area of the individual's residence to decrease binge eating.
    D. make recommendations or referrals to agencies or programs that help individuals get and maintain appropriate jobs.

124. The occupational therapist is selecting a game to use with a group of individuals who have psychosocial problems. Which type of game is contraindicated for a paranoid individual?
    A. A game that requires some people to hide their eyes while others keep their eyes open
    B. A game that requires game players to sit in a circle
    C. A game that requires members to work in pairs
    D. A game that requires members to take turns

125. The following-stress management technique is contraindicated for individuals who are diagnosed with schizophrenia and are actively hallucinating:
    A. Aerobic exercise
    B. Communication skills training
    C. Mental imagery
    D. Deep breathing

Implementation of the Treatment Plan

126. Which food preparation activity is the simplest?
    A. Preparing a can of soup
    B. Preparing a casserole
    C. Preparing brownies from a box mix
    D. Preparing a meal with two side dishes and an entree

127. An individual who is HIV positive cuts his finger while doing copper tooling. To follow universal precautions, the therapist should take this action:
    A. Throw the piece of copper tooling into the trash can, and get the individual a new piece of copper to use.
    B. Obtain the clinic's first aid kit and put an adhesive bandage on the individual's cut finger.
    C. Locate a puncture-resistant container that the copper piece could be placed into before disposing of it.
    D. Wipe up any blood that is on the counter top with a paper towel.

128. The therapist is working with an individual being treated for anxiety. The medication the therapist would expect to see in the individual's home during an outreach home visit is:
    A. Tegretol.
    B. Tranxene.
    C. Trilafon.
    D. Tofranil.

129. The therapist is working with a 16-year-old female with depression. The primary problem identified is her socialization with peers. Her strength is in the area of task skills. Which of the following treatment goals is best for this individual?
    A. The individual will increase socialization with peers during participation in task groups.
    B. The individual will select and teach two peers a craft activity that she enjoys.
    C. The individual will be provided with the opportunity to interact with peers while she demonstrates a familiar craft activity.
    D. The individual will select and demonstrate a craft activity to the therapist and provide two positive comments about her demonstration.

130. The primary reason that a laissez-faire style of leadership is contraindicated in working with groups is that:
    A. cooperation among members is increased.
    B. problem solving among members is increased.
    C. anxiety and withdrawal are increased.
    D. indecisiveness is increased.

Treatment Example for Question 131

Section I.
   Time: 45 minutes, three times per week
   Size: three to six individuals
Section II.
   This group assists individuals who have psychotic and organic impairments in reorganizing behavior to a basic level of competence in a supportive environment.
Section III.
   1. Increase initiation of activity.
   2. Follow one- to two-step verbal instructions on task projects.
   3. Increase the frequency of appropriate verbal responses.
Section IV.
   1. Can imitate or follow one direction at a time
   2. Has difficulty initiating interactions with others
   3. Often unaware of needs of others
Section V.
   1. Knowledge of and ability to analyze cognitive components of tasks.
   2. Knowledge of and ability to adapt and structure activities for functional levels of members.

131. The information provided in the treatment example is an example of a(n):

A. treatment plan.
B. group protocol.
C. session planner.
D. activity analysis.

132. **Based on the information from the treatment example, which diagnosis would be an appropriate referral for this treatment?**
 A. Schizophrenia
 B. Adjustment disorder
 C. Psychogenic fugue
 D. Bulimia nervosa

133. **Based on the treatment example for question 131, which section contains the criteria for individual selection?**
 A. Section II
 B. Section III
 C. Section IV
 D. Section V

134. **An individual with schizophrenia who is newly admitted to the hospital is asked by the therapist to tell about what brought him or her to the hospital for admission. The individual responds by saying, "I took a cab." This response is an example of:**
 A. delusional thinking.
 B. a distractible response.
 C. a concrete response.
 D. an insightful response.

135. **The therapist is organizing a group to get ready for a picnic outing to a park. The therapist wishes to take precautions for neuroleptic side effects of medications and would:**
 A. encourage members to use PABA-free sunblock and to wear a hat.
 B. encourage members to change positions slowly from sitting to standing.
 C. encourage members to use an antiperspirant and wear light-colored clothing.
 D. take along low-calorie snacks, such as carrot and celery sticks.

136. **Which craft sequence is an example of an adapted sequencing method?**
 A. The individual kneels in front of the supply cabinet to obtain the craft kit; the individual proceeds to sitting in a chair with the assembly materials placed to the right and left of the midline; and the individual is asked to stand up and press down on the craft that is positioned on the table.
 B. The small craft pieces are precut by the occupational therapy (OT) aide; a template for cutting the large straight-edged pieces is available to the individual; step-by-step directions with photographs are available to the individual.
 C. The individual measures and saws all the needed pieces, sands the pieces, assembles the pieces

with glue, resands the pieces, assembles the craft, and applies a coat of stain.
 D. the first step requires gross motor movements with sawing, and then gross elbow movements with a sanding block, and fine motor grasps and movements during the final painting.

137. **After administering the NPI interest checklist, the therapist documents that the individual identifies a few casual solitary leisure interests and no interests involving others. Based on this information, what is the best activity to use in the next session of a leisure-awareness group?**
 A. The Leisure Activities Blank
 B. A leisure values clarification activity
 C. A magazine picture collage
 D. a calendar of community leisure activities for the first week after discharge

138. **The most important feature to consider in selecting computer software for individuals with behavioral disorders is:**
 A. the availability of simulations of interactional skills.
 B. "teacher options" that allow the therapist to adjust the individual's number, type, and frequency of attempts.
 C. the requirements for cooperative efforts of two or more persons providing input in a game format.
 D. the capacity to assess aptitudes and abilities.

139. **The occupational therapist in a psychosocial treatment setting is deciding whether to use a group or a one-to-one approach with an individual. The MOST appropriate individual for a one-to-one approach is the individual who:**
 A. has difficulty with socialization.
 B. has daily living skill deficits.
 C. is new to the program and needs to be assessed.
 D. is easily distracted.

Evaluation of the Treatment Plan

140. **The occupational therapist is working with an individual in a psychosocial partial hospitalization program. The individual is having difficulty making decisions. The occupational therapist's response that is MOST LIKELY to facilitate better decision making is:**
 A. "I think baking would be a helpful activity to try. Baking something you like offers you several choices and decisions. You wanted to bake cookies today, didn't you?"
 B. "I think baking would be a helpful activity to try. Baking something you like offers you several choices and decisions. Why do you want to bake?"
 C. "I think baking would be a helpful activity to try. Baking something you like offers you several choices and

decisions can help you feel more positive about making other decisions. You can choose a cake mix or a cookie mix. Which would you like?"
D. "I think baking would be a helpful activity to try. Baking something you like offers you several choices and decisions. These choices and decisions can help you feel more positive about making other decisions. Do you want to bake cookies?"

141. **The occupational therapist who functions primarily as a role model, teacher, and provider of motivation and feedback reinforcement during treatment sessions is functioning from the:**
A. human occupation perspective.
B. object relations perspective.
C. behavioral perspective.
D. cognitive behavioral perspective.

142. **In carrying out inpatient treatment groups for individuals with schizophrenia, the occupational therapist should routinely:**
A. encourage the individuals to disclose themselves in the groups.
B. encourage the individuals to express negative feelings that come up in the groups.
C. offer practical advice and skill enhancement in the groups.
D. confront the individuals' difficulty in expressing their anger.

143. **When implementing the reality orientation approach with individuals with dementia, the therapist should focus on:**
A. the individual's plans for the future.
B. the name of the individual's family members who visited earlier in the day.
C. the name of the current U.S. president.
D. the name of the occupational therapist.

Discharge Planning

144. **The following treatment program format emphasizes discharge planning in addressing mental health problems:**
A. Club house
B. Community mental health center
C. Acute care hospitalization
D. Quarterway house

145. **The therapist is working with an individual on a goal of enhancing the individual's self-esteem. The individual is diagnosed with depression. This person refuses to participate in the treatment activities today. Which form of refusal is MOST LIKELY linked to acute depression?**
A. "I can't."
B. "I don't know how."
C. "I'm just too tired."
D. "I'm waiting for my visitors to come."

146. **To which of the following community vocational services are adults with mental retardation most likely to be referred?**
A. Adult activity centers
B. Supported employment
C. Job coaching
D. Sheltered workshops

147. **The occupational therapist working within a behavioral frame of reference should document an individual's progress by:**
A. using a narrative description of progress.
B. using charts and graphs of changes from the baseline.
C. using the Occupational Case Analysis and Interview Rating Scale (OCAIRS).
D. using the Adaptive Skills Developmental Chart.

148. **The therapist is talking with a group of individuals in the inpatient psychiatric occupational therapy program. The individuals are describing to the therapist why they attend occupational therapy groups. The reason the individuals are MOST likely to give is:**
A. "I attended occupational therapy to decrease my boredom and the sitting around and doing nothing."
B. "Occupational therapy groups helped me to work out my problems."
C. "Occupational therapy groups helped me to learn new skills."
D. "Occupational therapy groups gave me a chance to be around others."

149. **The occupational therapist is working in an acute care, inpatient psychiatric program with children who are between 6 and 12 years old. The therapist would recommend to parents of an 8-year-old child who is being discharged at the end of the week:**
A. to encourage the use of board games in which the parents focus on "playing only by the rules."
B. to encourage the use of board games in which the parents do not interfere with the variety of rules modifications made by the children playing the game.
C. to encourage participation in organized competitive sports.
D. to pursue involvement of the child in Girl or Boy Scouts.

150. **When an individual's discharge from a psychiatric inpatient service is delayed, he or she may risk:**
A. disruptions in the continuity of care.
B. countertransference.
C. ineffective coping skills.
D. regression.

ADMINISTRATION AND MANAGEMENT QUESTIONS

Organize and Manage Services

151. In most states, acute care orders for occupational therapy services must come from:
    A. a patient's self-referral.
    B. a physician's referral.
    C. a referral from a significant other.
    D. a referral from physical therapy.

152. It is a Joint Commission on Accreditation of Hospital Organizations (JCAHO) requirement that occupational therapy policies and procedures should be:
    A. reviewed and updated annually.
    B. reviewed and updated on years in which JCAHO surveys are performed.
    C. reviewed and updated when new occupational therapy managers take over a department.
    D. reviewed every other year.

153. Quality-improvement plans include a model for identifying quality indicators or areas that should be monitored. An area that should be monitored regardless of reaching 100% compliance would be one:
    A. with high volume.
    B. with high risk.
    C. with high incidence.
    D. that is problem-prone.

154. The institution that requires employers to institute practices that protect employees from bloodborne pathogens is the:
    A. Federal Drug Administration (FDA)
    B. Environmental Protection Agency (EPA)
    C. JCAHO
    D. Occupational Safety and Health Administration (OSHA)

155. OSHA requires that all work areas have an accessible copy of material safety data sheets (MSDS) so that employees may:
    A. be aware of hazardous chemicals in the work environment, side effects, and cleansing procedures for the chemicals.
    B. be aware of work procedures and practices for inventory of departmental materials.
    C. gain further knowledge of appropriate body mechanics to use in the workplace.
    D. document workplace injuries for collection of workers' compensation.

156. The most frequently used universal precaution is:
    A. the wearing of goggles.
    B. the wearing of a mask.
    C. frequent hand washing.
    D. wearing of a gown over work clothes.

157. Materials that require universal precautions as listed by OSHA are:
    A. nasal secretions and blood.
    B. sputum, nasal secretions and blood.
    C. blood, semen and saliva from dental procedures.
    D. urine, vomitus, and nasal secretions.

158. The occupational therapist is working with a patient on an acute care floor when the patient's intravenous (IV) equipment disengages, splashing the therapist in the eye with the medication and IV "backwash" fluid. The therapist's first response should be to:
    A. rub the eye and continue treatment.
    B. rinse the eye with an eye wash or water immediately.
    C. write an incident report.
    D. cover the eye with a bandage and contact the immediate supervisor.

159. General supervision is defined by the American Occupational Therapy Association (AOTA) as:
    A. contact with supervisor once a day.
    B. contact with supervisor once a week.
    C. contact with supervisor once a month.
    D. contact with supervisor as needed.

160. Close supervision is defined by the AOTA as:
    A. contact with supervisor once a day.
    B. contact with supervisor once a week.
    C. contact with supervisor once a month.
    D. contact with supervisor as needed.

161. An occupational therapist with 6 years of experience in psychiatry is beginning to work in a rehabilitation center. Based on the *Occupational Therapy Roles*, this therapist would be functioning in the physical disability setting at:
    A. an entry level.
    B. an intermediate level.
    C. an advanced level.
    D. an educator's level.

162. A therapist has been working in the area of mental health for 3 years and meets with her supervisor every other week. This therapist has gained mastery of basic role functions and assists in the education of other personnel to her service area. Based on the *Occupational Therapy Roles*, this therapist is functioning as:
    A. an entry-level therapist with close supervision.
    B. an intermediate therapist with minimal supervision.
    C. an advanced therapist with routine or general supervision.
    D. an intermediate therapist with routine or general supervision.

163. The term that best describes the relationship between an occupational therapist and a certified occupational therapy assistant (COTA) is:

A. dependent.
B. independent.
C. collaborative.
D. intuitive.

164. **An occupational therapist and a certified occupational therapy assistant share and coordinate therapy for a caseload. One of the roles that the COTA may assume would be to:**
    A. complete the chart reviews.
    B. complete the nonstandardized portions of the evaluation.
    C. interpret the results gained from the nonstandardized portions of the evaluation.
    D. independently design a treatment plan for the individual.

165. **A COTA may independently administer standardized tests:**
    A. as a level I student affiliate.
    B. once service competency has been established.
    C. once licensure has been received.
    D. when certification from the National Board for Certification in Occupational Therapy (NBCOT) is received.

166. **Quality improvement is:**
    A. a process of complying with regulatory agency guidelines.
    B. an objective system for measuring appropriateness of patient care.
    C. medical credentialing to validate skill in compliance with regulatory agencies.
    D. research to test validity and reliability of treatment approaches.

167. **A COTA with 10 years of experience is working in a rehabilitation unit. He has refined his skills and can contribute knowledge to others as well as act as a resource person. This person will most likely be functioning at an:**
    A. advanced level with minimal supervision.
    B. intermediate level with routine or general supervision.
    C. entry level with close supervision.
    D. entry level with routine or general supervision.

168. **Occupational therapy departments should keep information regarding indicators of the quality of services provided, improvements documented in the provision of service, and cost effectiveness and efficiency. This information is most likely to be included in the:**
    A. quality-improvement plan.
    B. policy and procedures.
    C. safety manual.
    D. utilization review.

169. **A written plan that identifies problems, provides objective assessment of the problems, determines whether an intervention worked,** reassesses interventions, and develops information that describes a program's effectiveness is most likely contained within a:
    A. quality-improvement plan.
    B. peer review.
    C. utilization review.
    D. program evaluation.

170. **In the quality-improvement plan, "measures" are:**
    A. the degree to which objectives are achieved.
    B. the results a program aims to achieve.
    C. characteristics according to severity.
    D. the standards with which outcomes are compared.

171. **The law that expanded the rights of individuals with physical or mental disabilities for employment, housing, public accommodations, public service, public transportation, and telecommunications is:**
    A. the Architectural Barriers Act of 1969.
    B. the Federal Rehabilitation Act of 1973.
    C. the Fair Housing Amendment Act of 1988.
    D. the Americans with Disabilities Act of 1990.

172. **The primary purpose of licensure is to:**
    A. delineate roles between occupational therapists and certified occupational therapy assistants.
    B. protect consumers of occupational therapy.
    C. ensure continued levels of competency of therapists.
    D. justify occupational therapy services for Medicare and Medicaid reimbursement.

173. **Student objectives for fieldwork:**
    A. vary in each facility.
    B. are standardized for all facilities.
    C. are written by the NBCOT.
    D. must meet state licensure requirements.

174. **Defining a possible outcome for a research project before it is initiated is referred to as:**
    A. a hypothesis.
    B. a question.
    C. a rationale.
    D. a theory base.

Promote Professional Practice

175. **The primary emphasis of occupational therapy services since the early 1900s has been:**
    A. skill acquisition.
    B. compensation for deficits.
    C. skill attainment.
    D. reinforcement and enhancement of performance.

176. **NBCOT regulations and state licensure regulate the provision of occupational therapy. Regarding the relationship between these two sets of guidelines:**

A. State licensure laws supersede NBCOT guidelines in the practice of occupational therapy.
B. NBCOT guidelines supersede individual state licensure laws regarding the practice of occupational therapy.
C. NBCOT and state licensure laws are viewed equally and enforced equally.
D. NBCOT guidelines are recommended but are not enforceable. However, state licensure guidelines are enforceable.

177. **Trends for providing occupational therapy services to older adults are:**
A. remaining stable.
B. expanding.
C. diminishing.
D. fluctuating.

178. **Trends are changing in the provision of health care in society and will cause:**
A. a reduction in home health services.
B. an increase in the amount of hospitalizations.
C. a reduction in the need of nursing homes.
D. an increase in the amount of services available on an outpatient basis.

179. **Based on the service need, the role of the occupational therapist may vary. A therapist who is called to give expert witness testimony on behalf of a claimant in an Americans with Disabilities Act (ADA) lawsuit would be acting as:**
A. a therapist.
B. a consultant.
C. a consumer.
D. a counselor.

180. **The term used to describe the negotiation of HMO's to pay a preestablished rate per diagnosis is:**
A. fee for service.
B. capitation.
C. cost shifting.
D. cost control.

181. **The occupational therapy setting that MOST requires a therapist to find creative alternatives for providing treatment equipment and overcoming professional isolation is:**
A. acute care hospitals.
B. nursing homes.
C. home care.
D. rehabilitation hospitals.

182. **Occupational therapists most frequently see individuals with the diagnosis of:**
A. cerebrovascular accident.
B. cerebral palsy.
C. developmental delay.
D. neuromuscular disorders.

183. **Therapists employed in community settings are most likely employed in:**
A. private practice.
B. school systems.
C. home health agencies.
D. residential care facilities.

184. **A research design that can be done both across behaviors, and across subjects or settings is:**
A. the multiple baseline design.
B. the withdrawal design.
C. the randomization treatment design.
D. the multi-element treatment design.

185. **After a question or problem has been identified and a literature review completed, the researcher should:**
A. refine the question and develop the background.
B. decide on methodology.
C. establish boundaries for the study.
D. collect and analyze qualitative data.

186. **The area of research in which the researcher may most benefit assistance from a statistician would be:**
A. in refining the question and developing the background.
B. in deciding on the methodology.
C. in establishing boundaries for the study.
D. in collecting and analyzing qualitative data.

187. **When writing the results of a research project, the researcher should include:**
A. writing conclusions in the results section.
B. writing qualitative and quantitative facts in the results section.
C. writing subjective information in the results section.
D. interpretive and analytical information in the results section.

188. **Individuals who are over the age of 65 or have renal failure usually have their primary health care costs covered by:**
A. Medicare.
B. Medicaid.
C. third party payors.
D. private pay.

189. **The concept of the federal government making a standard payment for health care services for individuals in diagnostic categories is known as:**
A. DRGs
B. PROs
C. UB-82s
D. Cost shifting

190. **Volunteers used in an occupational therapy setting will MOST likely:**
A. independently transport patients to and from therapy.

B. independently work with a patient once the therapist has set up the activity.

C. assist with stock and inventory control.

D. complete chart reviews.

191. The manager of an occupational therapy department is approached with an ethical dilemma by an occupational therapist. In using The Savage Model of Ethical Contemplation, the manager's first response will be to:
    A. identify problems to be solved.
    B. sort decisions to be made.
    C. ascertain facts and impressions.
    D. verify information with key players.

192. An occupational therapist is confronted with an ethical decision when she takes a rehab patient out of the hospital to complete a home evaluation. While en-route to the home, the hospital vehicle carrying the patient sustained a flat tire on the highway. (The therapist was travelling in her own vehicle behind the hospital vehicle.) The driver indicates that fixing the tire will take approximately half an hour. By hospital policy, the therapist is not allowed to transport the patient in her own car. However, the only other two alternatives were to have the patient remain with the taxi until it was repaired or to send for another vehicle which will take at least another 20 minutes. The therapist decides to drive the patient in her personal vehicle to the home since it is only another 5 minutes, leaving directions with the driver to meet them at the home after the tire of the vehicle is repaired. While in the above situation, the form of ethical tension involved was:
    A. ethical uncertainty.
    B. ethical distress.
    C. an ethical dilemma.
    D. unethical behavior.

193. The NBCOT investigates allegations of misconduct against occupational therapists. The least punitive form of action which is possible for misconduct is:
    A. a reprimand.
    B. a censure.
    C. probation.
    D. revocation.

194. The most severe sanction that may be taken by the NBCOT against an occupational therapist who has demonstrated misconduct is:
    A. a reprimand.
    B. a censure.
    C. probation.
    D. revocation.

195. The section of the Occupational Therapy Code of Ethics that addresses credentialing and continuing education is:

A. beneficence/autonomy.
B. competence.
C. compliance with laws and regulations.
D. public information.

196. The Occupational Therapy Code of Ethics was developed as:
    A. a guide to promote the highest standards of behavior.
    B. guidelines to assist the occupational therapist in the provision of services.
    C. a guide to assist the practitioner in identifying career options and developing career plans.
    D. a document to assist therapists in applying medical terminology.

197. The Occupational Therapy Roles document was developed as:
    A. a guide to promote the highest standards of behavior.
    B. guidelines to assist the occupational therapist in the provision of services.
    C. a guide to assist the practitioner in identifying career options and developing career plans.
    D. a document to assist therapists in applying uniform terminology.

198. The purpose of the Uniform Terminology, second edition, document is:
    A. to provided a written standards of behavior.
    B. to assist the occupational therapist in defining appropriate service interventions.
    C. to be used by the practitioner in identifying career options and developing career plans.
    D. to provide standard language for the description of occupational therapy services.

199. The profession of occupational therapy is continually evolving and developing. As health care changes through the next century, the focus will move more toward health status and away from health care. The occupational therapists role in this trend to enhance wellness through education, behavioral change, and cultural support is called:
    A. occupational behavior.
    B. synchrony.
    C. self efficacy.
    D. health promotion.

200. Studies that support the benefit of occupational therapy based on a comparison of the outcomes with the costs incurred are referred to as:
    A. efficacy studies.
    B. quality improvement studies.
    C. market survey studies.
    D. expenditure studies.

ANSWERS FOR SIMULATION EXAMINATION 2

1. (C) Reflex maturation is significantly delayed. The Moro reflex should be integrated before 5 to 6 months of age. Because this child is 13 months, this represents a significant delay. Answer A is incorrect because the child has not integrated a reflex at 13 months that should have been absent by 6 months. Answer B is incorrect because an 8-month delay in reflex maturation is a significant delay. Answer D is also incorrect since all primitive reflexes (including the motor reflexes) should have been integrated by 6 months. Therefore reflex integration could not be "advanced" when primitive patterns are still present at 13 months. See reference: Hopkins and Smith (eds): Simon, CJ, and Daub, MM: Human development across the life span.

2. (B) Decreased muscle tone. Decreased muscle tone is usually characterized by joints that are lax and hyperextensible. Low muscle tone and joint hyperextensibility are also frequent characteristics of Down syndrome. Answer A is incorrect because loss of range of motion would be the joint characteristic of increased muscle tone. Answers C and D are incorrect because they are diagnoses that cannot be made on the basis of joint laxness, even though instability at the joint may occur with either of these conditions. The observation of joint hyperextensibility is merely an indication of below normal muscle tone, and not necessarily the indication of a specific condition or disease process. See reference: Hopkins and Smith (eds): Simon, CJ, and Daub, MM: Human development across the life span.

3. (A) Poor modulation of tactile input. This is the only answer that describes both his hypersensitive and hyposensitive responses to tactile input. The child with autism may be unpredictable in terms of response to sensory stimuli, but avoiding and craving stimulation at various times. Answers B and C are incorrect because they describe only one part of the problem. Answer D is wrong because he appears to be craving deep pressure or proprioceptive input in order to modulate the tactile system. See reference: Hopkins and Smith (eds): Kinnealey, M, and Miller, LJ: Sensory integration/learning disabilities.

4. (C) Developmental dyspraxia. The motor problem described as it occurs during the evaluation is characteristic of developmental dyspraxia. Children with dyspraxia often learn tasks such as jumping rope with great difficulty, effort, and considerable practice. However, when the task is altered, such as in this case by asking the child to skip backwards, the child is unable to adapt the task for a long while. Answer A is incorrect because the child with delayed reflex integration would have difficulty with all aspects of the task. Answer B is incorrect because a problem of bilateral integration would affect both aspects of this task. Answer D is also incorrect because incoordination would not necessarily be the determining factor between performance of each aspect of the task. See reference: Hopkins and Smith (eds): Kinnealey, M, and Miller, LJ: Sensory integration/learning disabilities.

5. (D) Myelomeningocele. Myelomengiocele is the most severe form of spina bifida, which is characterized by protrusion of meninges, spinal fluid, and a portion of the spinal cord through an opening in the spine. This usually results in paraplegia. Osteogenesis imperfecta, often called "brittle bone" disease usually does not interfere with spinal cord function. Arthrogryposis is a severe orthopedic problem that is characterized by deformed joints or absent muscle groups. Ankylosing spondylitis or Strumpell-Marie disease is characterized by progressive ankylosing of the spine, which makes it into a mass of bone. Answers A, B, and C do not generally cause a destruction of the spinal cord, which results in paraplegia. See reference: Case-Smith, Allen, and Pratt (eds): Gordon, CY, Schanzenbacher, KE, Case-Smith, J, and Carrasco, RC: Diagnostic problems in pediatrics.

6. (B) Moro's reflex. Moro's reflex is characterized by extension of the head, back, and arms in response to a dropping of the head in the young infant. The rooting reflex involves turning of the head to tactile stimulation near the mouth. Flexor withdrawal reflex is characterized by flexion of an extremity to a painful stimuli, and neck righting reaction involves body alignment in rotation following turning of the head. The Moro is the only reflex that causes an extension movement. See reference: Hopkins and Smith (eds): Simon, CJ, and Daub, MM: Human development across the life span.

7. (D) It determines the need for further occupational therapy evaluation. The purpose of using a screening test is to determine whether further assessments are needed, and if so, which tests would be appropriate for that child. A screening test is not designed for planning programs, consultation, nor does it test any skill in a comprehensive way. See reference: Dunn: Collier, T: The screening process.

8. (C) Ayres Clinical Observations of Sensory Integration. The Ayres Clinical Observations generally look at similar components of function, in the area of sensory integration and at the same age level (5 to 8 years) as the SIPT. The other tests either screen children of a younger age, or screen all areas of development without specifically focusing on sensory integration. See reference: Dunn: Collier, T: The screening process.

9. (B) Miller Assessment of Preschoolers Screening Test. The Miller Assessment of Preschoolers Screening Test is standardized and norm-referenced for children 2.5 to 5 years of age. The other tests are not norm-referenced or they do not specifically address the sensory-motor area of development. See reference: Dunn: Collier, T: The screening process.

10. (B) Public school system. Answer B is correct as the Individual Education Plan (IEP) is the required plan for children receiving special education in public school systems. It is a document that incorporates the child's needs and the occupational therapist contributes his or her evaluation of the child as well as educational objectives. Answers A, C, and D are incorrect because they each have different methods of coordinating a plan for a child, none of which are called an IEP. See reference: Hopkins and Smith (eds): Kaufmann, NA: Occupational therapy in school systems.

11. (A) Translation. The linear movement of the object from the palm to fingers is called "translation." Answer B, "shift," is incorrect because this type of in-hand manipulation is the movement of an object between or among the fingers. Answer C, "rotation," is incorrect because this type of in-hand manipulation rolls the object horizontally or end-over-end between the finger pads. Answer D, "stabilization," is incorrect because it is not one of the three types of in-hand manipulations. See reference: Case-Smith, Allen, and Pratt (eds): Exner, CE: Development of hand skills.

12. (B) To improve ability to grade movement. The "grading of movement" goal best addresses difficulty with control of the midrange of a movement pattern (common with athetosis). Answer A is incorrect as this goal would be appropriate for a child who cannot break up a flexion or extension pattern during a movement. Answer C is not correct because this goal is appropriate for a child who has difficulty with an arm or hand movement being too fast or too slow (graded movements are also too fast). Answer D is incorrect because this goal is appropriate for a child who has difficulty bringing both arms to midline and using them effectively together. See reference: Case-Smith, Allen, and Pratt (eds): Exner, CE: Development of hand skills.

13. (A) Jaw opening and closing are controlled with adult's index and middle fingers; the adult's thumb is placed on the child's cheek. The correct position of the adult's hand for jaw control is as described in Answer A when the child is fed from the side. Answers B and D are incorrect because the thumb should be placed on the cheek to provide joint stability. Answer C is incorrect because controlling the child's jaw movement with the adult's whole hand provides less control of the child's jaw than the recommended method. Placing the adult's thumb on the ear (answer D) is also incorrect because of discomfort for the child, as well as thumb placement should be near the fulcrum of jaw movement (temporomandibular joint). If the child is fed from the front the adult's thumb is placed on the chin, with middle finger under the chin to control opening and closing of the jaw. The index finger then rests on the side of the child's face to provide stability. See reference: Case-Smith, Allen, and Pratt (eds): Parham, LD, and Mailloux, Z: Sensory integration.

14. (A) The therapist has the child play "sandwich" between heavy mats. The "sandwich" activity provides heavy pressure over the child's body, which can inhibit the child's protective reactions to light touch. Answer B is incorrect because light use of a feather brush stimulates the light touch system, which is already impaired and would be extremely uncomfortable for a child with tactile

defensiveness. Answer C is not correct because the use of a blindfold when a child is already reacting to unexpected touch would most likely create a fearful response in a child with tactile defensiveness. Finally, Answer D, although not using a blindfold, also has unexpected touch from the back as a characteristic of the game, and this would also be aggravating to the child's existing problem. Answer A, the use of proprioceptive input to break through the protective response to light touch, will initially treat the child's defensiveness problem instead of stimulating further reaction. See reference: Hopkins and Smith (eds): Kinnealey, M, and Miller, LJ: Sensory integration and learning disabilities.

15. (A) Forward and backward "chaining." Chaining with the child who demonstrates a cognitive disability shows the entire process of a task with all sequences. Initially, the child performs only the beginning or end of the task. Thus, the child concentrates on only a small part of the task but gradually increases participation in all sequences in their correct order. Answers B, C, and D are other methods that can be used, but forward and backward chaining are instructional methods that have been particularly successful with individuals who are mentally retarded. See reference: Hopkins and Smith (eds): Humphrey, R, and Jewell, K: Mental retardation.

16. (A) Square. The square follows the circle in developmental order. Answer B, the cross, follows the square, followed by the triangle, and lastly, the diamond. See reference: Case-Smith, Allen, and Pratt (eds): Amundson, SJ, and Weil, M: Prewriting and handwriting skills.

17. (B) Facilitate righting and equilibrium reactions while the child is partially flexed. Although all treatment is individually adapted to the needs of a certain child, the general approach of this method would be to use a reflex-inhibiting pattern, which will inhibit the extensor tone. At the same time, righting and equilibrium reactions should be elicited through the therapist's handling of the child to assist him/her toward automatic motor responses, which will eventually take over. Answer A is incorrect because a reflex inhibiting pattern is the opposite of the child's abnormal pattern, and therefore partial flexion would be reflex inhibiting for this child. Answer C is incorrect because most often the key point of control for a total pattern would be at the neck, trunk, or hips. Finally, answer D is incorrect because the neurodevelopmental treatment (NDT) approach emphasizes automatic (subcortical) responses on the part of the child. See reference: Hopkins and Smith (eds): Erhardt, RP: Cerebral palsy.

18. (B) Sitting on a ball with forward and side-to-side movement. Answer B is correct because the position of the child requires the least resistance to gravity. By tilting the child in this position, the therapist controls how much the child will work against gravitational pull. Answers A and D are incorrect because they would require that the child lift his or her head directly against gravity. Answer C is also incorrect because the head is positioned against gravity in the quadruped position, and the child probably could not hold a quadruped position if head control is extremely poor. See reference: Hopkins and Smith (eds): Er-hardt, RP: Cerebral palsy.

19. (A) Increase neck flexion.   Answer A is correct because this method will decrease the abnormal extension pattern that is influencing the oral-motor patterns. Jaw and tongue thrust are part of an overall extension pattern. Answers B, C, and D would only increase the abnormal pattern in the mouth because they are part of an extension pattern. See reference: Case-Smith, Allen, and Pratt (eds): Case-Smith, J, and Humphry, R: Feeding and oral motor skills.

20. (C) Increase management of texture by using a baby food grinder.   This method offers a gradual increase in texture that will encourage chewing. Answer A is not correct because scraping food off of a spoon with the child's teeth does not encourage any voluntary oral-motor control. Answer B is incorrect because it combines liquid with pieces of food (soft and chewy) and this combination of textures will be too unpredictable for a child who is having difficulty organizing oral-motor skills to manage food. Answer D is incorrect because a raisin is too large of a step in terms of texture from pureed food. See reference: Case-Smith, Allen, and Pratt (eds): Case-Smith, J, and Humphry, R: Feeding and oral motor skills.

21. (C) Weight bearing on hands.   This is the only activity that will facilitate hand function in the preparation phase. Weight-bearing on the hands gives deep pressure to the surface of the hand and facilitates wrist and arm extension, as well as shoulder cocontraction, to prepare the arm for reach and stabilization of the hand for grasping. The other answers all provide different types of grasp activities that could be used as therapy. See reference: Case-Smith, Allen, and Pratt (eds): Wright-Ott, C, and Egilson, S: Mobility.

22. (A) Abnormal muscle tone.   The literature addresses splinting for adults with abnormal tone, but only a few articles have been written about children. More articles have been written about splinting of children's hands where (B) muscle weakness, (C) traumatic injury and (D) joint inflammation exist. See reference: Case-Smith, Allen, and Pratt (eds): Wright-Ott, C, and Egilson, S: Mobility.

23. (C) Wedge-shaped seat that is higher in front.   A wedge-shaped seat insertion will increase hip flexion more than 90 degrees, which is inhibitory to an extensor pattern. Answer A is incorrect because lateral trunk supports will support the trunk from sideward movement only. Answer B is incorrect because a seat belt at the hips will hold a child in a chair, but cannot inhibit an extension pattern. Answer D is incorrect because although it may contribute to holding a child in a chair, it does not affect the angle of the hip joint, which is necessary to decreasing extensor tone in sitting. See reference: Case-Smith, Allen, and Pratt (eds): Shepherd, J, Procter, SA, and Coley, IL: Self-care and adaptations for independent living.

24. (D) Scoop dish.   This is the most correct answer because the sides of the scoop dish will provide a shape that aides the scooping movement. A high back to the plate provides a surface to push the food against to aide in getting the food onto the spoon. Answer A is not correct because the swivel spoon helps primarily when supination is limited. Answer B is not correct because the nonslip mat helps stabilize the plate itself. Answer D is incorrect because the mobile arm support positions the arm and helps weak shoulder and elbow muscles to position the hand. See reference: Case-Smith, Allen, and Pratt (eds): Shepherd, J, Procter, SA, and Coley, IL: Self-care and adaptations for independent living.

25. (C) Change to a power wheelchair to eliminate effort.   Considering the progressive nature of the child's disease, as well as strength and endurance, the best recommendation would be to change to a power wheelchair. The child would be better able to participate in the cognitive tasks of school if less effort was used toward mobility. Answer A, retaining the manual chair, would be counter-productive to functioning well at school, and strength will not be improved with this child's condition. Answer B might make mobility a little easier, but will not solve a long-term problem of decreasing strength and endurance. Answer D would still make demands on strength and energy that would appear unwise considering the nature of Duchenne's dystrophy. The team's recommendation should also be integrated with the family's needs. See reference: Case-Smith, Allen, and Pratt (eds): Johnson, J: School-based occupational therapy.

26. (A) After they crawl on their bellies.   Infants crawl or creep in a four-point position after they crawl on their bellies. Answer B is not correct because infants often sit with support at the same time as they crawl. Answer C is not correct because infants crawl before they rise up independently to stand. Answer D is not correct because infants crawl long after they have lifted their head in a prone position. See reference: Case-Smith, Allen, and Pratt (eds): Case-Smith, J, and Shortridge, SD: The developmental process: Prenatal to adolescence.

27. (C) Partner.   The occupational therapist working with children needs to be accepting of parents in order to develop successful working relationships. Answer A is incorrect because a strong authoritarian approach may intimidate parents and decrease effective communication. Answer B is incorrect because therapists should strengthen the parent-child relationship and not compete with parents. Answer D is incorrect because one of the major roles in working with parents is to share information about the child so that the child's problems and function are clearly understood. See reference: Case-Smith, Allen, and Pratt (eds): Humphry, R, and Case-Smith, J: Working with families.

28. (C) Juvenile rheumatoid arthritis.   Juvenile rheumatoid arthritis is the only condition listed that is a joint disorder causing joint inflammation and pain. Type I diabetes (answer A) is incorrect because it is an endocrine disorder. Answer B and D are incorrect because they are both conditions of the cardiovascular system. See reference: Case-Smith, Allen, and Pratt (eds): Gordon, CY,

Schanzenbacher, KE, Case-Smith, J, and Carrasco, RC: Diagnostic problems in pediatrics.

29. (B) Spina bifida. Spina bifida is characterized by incomplete closure of the spinal vertebrae. Osteomyelitis is an infection in the bone (answer A is incorrect). Scoliosis is a curvature of the spinal column (answer C is incorrect). Osteogenesis imperfecta, often called "brittle bone" disease, does not affect the closure of vertebrae during fetal development (answer D is incorrect). See reference: Case-Smith, Allen, and Pratt (eds): Gordon, CY, Schanzenbacher, KE, Case-Smith, J, and Carrasco, RC: Diagnostic problems in pediatrics.

30. (D) Hyaline membrane disease. Hyaline membrane disease is a condition of prematurity causing underdevelopment of the lungs. Answer A, otitis media, is incorrect because this is a common infection of childhood where blockage of the eustachian tube causes formation of fluid in the middle ear. Duchenne's disease is a neuromuscular condition (answer B) and symptoms usually begin between the second and sixth year of life. Poliomyelitis (answer C) is a viral disease that can occur at any time after birth. See reference: Case-Smith, Allen, and Pratt (eds): Gordon, CY, Schanzenbacher, KE, Case-Smith, J, and Carrasco, RC: Diagnostic problems in pediatrics.

31. (C) Southern California Sensory Integration and Praxis Tests (SIPT). In order to administer the SIPT, a therapist must complete a series of courses to become certified. The Denver II, Hawaii Early Learning Profile (HELP), and the Developmental Test of Visual-Motor Integration (VMI) may be administered by entry level therapists. See reference: Case-Smith, Allen, and Pratt (eds): Parham, LD, and Mailloux, Z: Sensory integration.

32. (A) Margaret Rood. The use of C-brushing for facilitation of the pivot prone position was developed by Margaret Rood. Answer B is not correct because Berta Bobath did not describe brushing "pivot prone;" however, she would describe reflex-inhibiting patterns along with facilitation of higher order reactions. Answer C is not correct since Signe Brunnstrom techniques are applied primarily to the adult hemiplegic with an emphasis on upper limb synergies. Answer D is incorrect because PNF usually includes the assistance of manual contacts and auditory commands; PNF is also usually described in the context of treatment of an adult. See reference: Trombly: Neurophysiological and developmental treatment approaches.

33. (A) Understanding or using language. Answer A is correct according to the definition of a "learning disability" in Public Law 94-142. A learning disability is "a disorder in one of the more basic psychological processes involved in understanding or in using language, spoken or written, which may manifest itself in an imperfect ability to listen, think, speak, read, write or do mathematical calculations." Answer B is not correct because, although children with learning disabilities may in fact have problems with motor function, this does not qualify them for

service. Answer C is not correct because children with learning disabilities, by definition, have average or above average intelligence. Answer D is not correct because sensory acuity (blindness or deafness) cannot be the reason for the child's academic problems. See reference: Case-Smith, Allen, and Pratt (eds): Gordon, CY, Schanzenbacher, KE, Case-Smith, J, and Carrasco, RC: Diagnostic problems in pediatrics.

34. (D) Must benefit the child's ability to participate in special education. Answer D is correct because the present public law (IDEA—Individuals with Disabilities Education Act) requires that any related service be provided to children who are receiving special educational service or "specialized instruction," and the related service can improve their educational performance. Answer A is incorrect because occupational therapy is not a primary service, but a "related service" that is related to special education services. Answer C is incorrect because physical therapy is also a related service and follows the same guidelines as occupational therapy in that the child must have been receiving special education and educational performance will probably be improved by the provision of physical therapy service. See reference: Case-Smith, Allen, and Pratt (eds): Johnson, J: School-based occupational therapy.

35. (B) Below average general intellectual functioning. Answer B is correct because it describes the essential feature of the diagnosis of mental retardation. Other factors such as answer A, abnormal motor functioning, answer C, psychosocial and behavioral difficulties, and answer D, the presence of neurologic impairments such as seizures, may be present and associated with the diagnosis. Approximately 80% of retarded children have additional problems. See reference: Hopkins and Smith (eds): Humphrey, R, and Jewell, K: Mental retardation.

36. (D) Visual perceptual problems usually require a motor-free evaluation. Children with cerebral palsy and normal intelligence usually score lower than a normal child on motor-free visual perceptual tests. This suggests that many of these children may have visual perception problems and, since these children have motor disabilities, using a motor-free test will provide the therapist with the most accurate assessment of visual perception alone. Answer A is not correct because 75 percent of children with cerebral palsy have visual refractive errors. Answer B is not correct because cortical visual problems reflect damage to the visual cortex of the central nervous system. Answer C is not correct because the oculomotor problems usually reflect the type of motor dysfunction seen throughout the child's body. See reference: Hopkins and Smith (eds): Erhardt, RP: Cerebral palsy.

37. (D) Push or pull weighted objects while in a quadruped position. Answer D is correct because it is the only activity that provides resistance of additional weight, which will give added proprioceptive input needed to improve body awareness. Answers A and C are not correct because they emphasize additional tactile input. Answer B is not correct because it emphasizes slow vestibular input. See reference: Hopkins and Smith (eds): Kinnealey, M, and Miller, LJ: Sensory integration/learning disabilities.

38. (C) Accidents. Answer C is correct because after the age of 1 year, accidents (especially car accidents) are the most common cause of death in children. Answer A, malignancies, are the second cause of death in children from 4 to 18 years of age. Congenital malformations, answer B, are the second cause of death before four years of age. Infectious diseases, although common in childhood, seldom cause death or leave sequelae. Occupational therapists need to be aware of and participate in the prevention aspect of conditions that cause disability or death in children. See reference: Case-Smith, Allen, and Pratt (eds): McIlroy, MA, and Koranyi, KI: General pediatric health care.

39. (D) The occupational therapist does problem solving with the teacher. Answer D is correct because the consultation relationship in the school is based on a shared relationship with the school staff for whom the occupational therapist is hired to consult. Answer A is incorrect as the teaching role is usually associated with monitoring type of service. Answer B is incorrect as a provision of therapy is direct service. Answer C is incorrect because it describes an authoritarian approach, which would take away the teacher's commitment to solving the problems of mainstreaming a child with a disability. Answer D reflects one of the essential tenets of consultation—that the consultee, by sharing in problem solution, will become committed to a child's program. See reference: Hopkins and Smith (eds): Kauffman, NA: Occupational therapy in the school system.

40. (D) Punishment for bad behavior. Answer D is correct as young children most frequently see the cause of illness as being punishment for bad behavior. Answer A is incorrect because children find hospitalization to be a very difficult experience and not a natural occurrence. Answer B is incorrect because children are unable to understand the actual and real causes of disease, such as a bacterial infection. Answer C is incorrect because, although infants and toddlers suffer from separation from parents, they still may see the cause of the illness as punishment for something they have done. The infant and very young child may also see themselves as "bad" because they seem to disturb their parents. See reference: Case-Smith, Allen, and Pratt (eds): Barnstorff, MJ: The dying child.

41. (A) Shoulder flexion and protraction. Answer A is correct because the infant changes from extensor influences on posture to development of flexion in supine. This includes the ability to flex and protract the shoulders against gravity in order to reach forward and upward to grasp toys. Answer B is not correct because shoulder extension and retraction are part of the extensor tone and pattern seen in early infancy, which is replaced by development of shoulder flexion and protraction. Answers C and D are not correct because most activities of looking and grasping can be accomplished without using head or

trunk control against gravity in supine. See reference: Kramer and Hinojosa: Colangelo, CA: Biomechanical frame of reference.

42. (B) Stability of the head and neck. The correct answer is B because the prone position allows the child to vertically right the head against gravity and develop the alternating flexion and extension control that provides head and neck stability. Answer A is not correct because the infant begins to protract, rather than retract the shoulders, and hip extension develops during prone positioning in normal development. Answer C is not correct because the prone position provides the infant with the opportunity to develop trunk extension rather than trunk flexion. Answer D is not correct because the prone position per se, during weightbearing on the upper extremities, provides the opportunity to develop stability or co-contraction in the arms. See reference: Kramer and Hinojosa: Colangelo, CA: Biomechanical frame of reference.

43. (B) Acute lymphoblastic leukemia. Answer B is correct because of all the medical conditions listed, a terminal diagnosis could be present or feared by the child and family with acute lymphoblastic leukemia. Prognosis has significantly improved over recent years with many patients going into remissions of more than 5 years. Although life span may be shortened by the presence of type I diabetes, answer A, and hemophilia, answer B, they do not generally involve a sudden onset of an acute illness which can be life threatening during childhood years. These two conditions therefore do not usually require consideration of issues of death and dying with treatment planning. Otitis media, answer D, although it is a common medical problem (ear infection) during childhood, is not a life-threatening condition. See reference: Case-Smith, Allen, and Pratt (eds): Gordon, CY, Schanzenbacher, KE, Case-Smith, J, and Carrasco, RC: Diagnostic problems in pediatrics.

44. (B) Ventricular septal defect. Answer B is correct as Eisenmenger's complex is the pooling of blood in the right ventricle as a result of the heart's inability to pump against a pulmonary vascular obstruction. The latter occurs because of prolonged exposure to the increased blood flow and high pressure associated with the presence of a ventricular septal defect. Children with a severe defect need to be monitored when in therapy for the possibility of the occurrence of this life-threatening situation. None of the other conditions listed (rheumatic fever, sickle-cell anemia, or asthma) include a heart defect that can create an Eisenmenger's complex. See reference: Case-Smith, Allen, and Pratt (eds): Gordon, CY, Schanzenbacher, KE, Case-Smith, J, and Carrasco, RC: Diagnostic problems in pediatrics.

45. (C) 8 months. This is correct because 3 months (number of months premature) are subtracted from the child's chronological age to adjust for prematurity. This child is then given the benefit of time lost because of a shorter gestation period. See reference: Dunn, W: Cook, DG: The assessment process.

46. (A) A problem with learning new motor skills. A is the correct answer because it describes the central problem of dyspraxia—difficulty in performing skills not previously mastered where motor planning is required. Answer B is not correct because, although developmental dyspraxia is considered a sensory integration problem, it does not explain what problems the child faces, which are praxic in nature. Answers C and D are incorrect because, although reflex integration and balance problems may be present with developmental dyspraxia, they are not problems of praxis or motor planning. Answers C and D are automatic motor activities, and dyspraxia is a problem of mastering activities that must be learned. See reference: Case-Smith, Allen, and Pratt (eds): Parham, LD, and Mailloux, Z: Sensory integration.

47. (B) Manual rocking while in prone on a therapy ball. Answer B is correct because it employs slow, regular vestibular input in a comfortable and safe position, which is inhibitory. Answers A, C, and D are vestibular activities, but they involve fast or irregular movements, which will increase the level of arousal. See reference: Hopkins and Smith (eds): Kinnealey, M, and Miller, LJ: Sensory integration/learning disabilities.

48. (B) Controlling opening and closing and providing external stabilization of the jaw. Answer B is correct because it incorporates the two reasons for use of jaw control techniques when feeding a handicapped child: (1) to control opening and closing the jaw, and (2) to provide external stabilization of the jaw. Answers A and C are incorrect because strengthening of the jaw does not occur, but increased control does. Answer D, is not correct because this technique may be difficult for children who have tactile defensiveness around the mouth and jaw. Additionally, although jaw closure will facilitate the swallow, jaw control techniques are used to provide and develop the child's control of the jaw. See reference: Case-Smith, Allen, and Pratt (eds): Case-Smith, J, and Humphry, R: Feeding and oral motor skills.

49. (C) Liquid/solid combinations (minestrone soup). Answer C is correct because it combines two food consistencies. Liquids are very difficult for children with poor oral-motor organization to manage in eating. When solids are added into the liquid the child will have difficulty managing two different forms of food. Answers A, B, and D, depending on the child's oral-motor skills, will be easier to move and manage within the mouth. See reference: Case-Smith, Allen, and Pratt (eds): Case-Smith, J, and Humphry, R: Feeding and oral motor skills.

50. (A) Be done on a regular basis. Answer A is correct because treatment goals change considerably within the first year of life, and this will ensure appropriate home management and parental education and support. Answer B is incorrect because the child's development changes rapidly before the end of 1 year, and treatment goals and activities would not be appropriate if 1 year is the time of re-evaluation. Answer C is incorrect, because the parents' schedules should not be the only determining factor in the decision for re-evaluation of treatment, but change in the

infant's status. This needs to be followed regularly by the therapist who can observe change and need for new treatment activities. Answer D is incorrect because it is not only a lack of progress that determines changes in treatment goals, but progress itself that changes the need for introduction of new goals and activities. See reference: Case-Smith, Allen, and Pratt (eds): Case-Smith, J, and Humphry, R: Feeding and oral motor skills.

51. (B) Trace. Trace muscle equals a one on the numerical scale of muscle testing. The other answers would be incorrect, since answer A, absent strength would equal zero, answer C, good strength would equal a four, and answer D, normal strength would equal a five. See reference: Pedretti and Zoltan (eds): Pedretti, L: Evaluation of muscle strength.

52. (B) A pinch meter. A pinch meter is used to measure the strength of a three jaw chuck grasp (also known as palmar pinch), in addition to key (lateral) pinch and tip pinch. These tests are performed with three trials that are averaged together and then compared with a standardized norm. The other answers are incorrect because, answer A, the aesthesiometer measures two point discrimination, answer C, the dynamometer measures grip strength and answer D, the volumeter measures edema in the hand. See reference: Pedretti (ed): Kasch, M: Acute head injuries.

53. (B) Measure the distance from the fingertip to the distal palmar crease with the hand in a fist. The distance from the fingertip to the distal palmar crease with the hand fisted may be measured in either inches or centimeters. This measures how close the finger tip comes to the palm. A person who has full flexion would have a measurement of zero. Answers A and C are incorrect as actively or passively measuring the flexion at each joint and totaling them are measurements taken with a goniometer and recorded in degrees. Answer D, measuring the distance between the tip of the thumb and the fourth phalanx, is incorrect because it is a measurement of opposition. See reference: Hunter, Schneider, Mackin, and Bell (eds): Cambridge, C: Range of motion measurements of the hand.

54. (D) Flexion. Answer D describes the test position for the Tinel's sign, which is when the wrists are held in a flexed position for 1 minute and the therapist taps from the fingertips to the palm. The individual indicates any sensory changes such as tingling or an electric shock feeling. The positions indicated in answers A, wrists ulnarly deviated, B, wrists radially deviated, and C, wrists extended, would not provide compression to the median nerve to elicit such a sensory change. See reference: Hunter, Schneider, Mackin, and Bell (eds): Baxter-Petralia, P: Therapist's management of carpal tunnel syndrome.

55. (B) Below the MCP joints. The MCP joints are stabilized proximally, or below the MCP joints, to isolate the joint movement being measured and to eliminate any combined movements. Answers A, above the MCP joints, and C, at the wrist, would allow combined movements of the joints and would invalidate the individual joint measurements. Answer D, on top of the MCP joints, would block joint movement and make any individual joint measurements incorrect. See reference: Norkin and White: Procedures.

56. (C) The lower back. Touching the lower back requires shoulder abduction and internal rotation by a person. Answers A, back of the neck, and B, top of the head, are incorrect because they would require external shoulder rotation. Answer D, opposite shoulder, is also incorrect because horizontal adduction is required. See reference: Trombly: Evaluation of biomechanical and physiological aspects of motor performance.

57. (C) Good. The person has good muscle strength because moderate resistance is taken in the pain-free range. An individual with arthritis should always be tested in the pain-free area of their active range of motion, because testing at the end of the active range causes pain to inhibit the effort the individual is able to give against resistance. This gives a false assessment of the individual's functional strength and also could be damaging to the arthritic tissues. Answers A, poor, or B, fair, refer to an inability to sustain any resistance in the pain free range. Answer D, normal strength, demonstrates the ability to take full resistance against gravity in the pain free range. See reference: Trombly: Evaluation of biomechanical and physiological aspects of motor performance.

58. (A) Two inches wider than the widest point across the individual's hip while he or she wears the brace. By measuring the individual with the brace on and adding 2 inches, as in answer A, allows the individual to easily get in and out of the chair, while preventing pressure areas to the individual's sides. Answer B measures only the hips and would not allow enough room for the individual to sit or move easily in the chair while wearing the brace. Answers C and D are both incorrect measurements for seat length, as both would have the seat too deep for the individual's leg length. The correct length of the seat should be two inches shorter than the distance from the back of the bent knee to the back of the buttocks. See reference: Pedretti (ed): Pedretti, L, and Stone, G: Wheelchairs and wheelchair transfers.

59. (D) Early morning and again in the afternoon. The individual with arthritis would need to be evaluated at both times to assess the functional abilities of the individual during and after morning stiffness. To evaluate the individual only in the morning (answers A and C) or in the afternoon (answer B), would only accurately reveal the individual's functional level at one time of day. This would be incorrect as an individual with arthritis would have many changes in functional status after the morning stiffness has disappeared. See reference: Trombly (ed): Feinberg, JR, and Trombly, CA: Arthritis.

60. (A) Preserve joint integrity. It is very important to preserve joint integrity in the individual with arthritis by using adaptive equipment to avoid or reduce the wear and tear stresses on fragile joints. Adaptive equipment would

not correct deformities, as deformities are only corrected by surgery or with orthotic devices which reposition the joints in correct alignment. Adaptive equipment allows activities to be completed, but would not simplify work by eliminating steps to an activity. Another reason adaptive equipment is used is to increase independence. See reference: Hopkins and Smith (eds): Spenser, EA: Functional restoration—Neurologic, arthritic, orthopedic, cardiac, and pulmonary conditions.

61. (B) Provide positioning and adaptive equipment. Positioning and adaptive equipment are necessary to maintain the integrity of the musculoskeletal system to prevent deformity. An individual with rheumatoid arthritis would not want to perform any resistive exercises because the excessive force would result in stress deformities by over-stretching and tissue breakdown. An individual would need some emotional support (answer C) from the therapist, but the primary method of support would be through the family or a support group. Surgical intervention (answer D) would not be needed in the early stages of rheumatoid arthritis but as a corrective measure for long standing deformities. See reference: Hopkins and Smith (eds): Spenser, EA: Functional restoration—Neurologic, arthritic, orthopedic, cardiac, and pulmonary conditions.

62. (B) Combing the hair. The shoulder abducts and externally rotates when combing the hair. Shoulder abduction is not required for buttoning a shirt (answer A) or tying a shoe (answer D). Shoulder abduction is needed for tucking a shirt in the back (answer C), but it also requires internal rotation to perform that activity. See reference: Cailliet: Tissue sites and mechanisms of pain. In *Shoulder Pain.*

63. (C) Criterion. The criteria is the method by which the level of an individual's performance will be measured in the treatment objective. The terminal behavior (Answer A) is the change an individual must demonstrate through performance or behavior. The condition (Answer B) is the circumstances under which the individual will perform. The plan (Answer D) is the approach used to reach a treatment objective. See reference: Pedretti: Treatment planning.

64. (B) Facial expressions. An individual with an injury to the right nondominant cerebral hemisphere will have difficulty understanding facial expressions and body gestures. The individual will often have neglect to the left side of the visual field. Answers A, presenting written information on the right side and D, visual stimulation on the right side, are incorrect as the individual is able to see to the right, but not to the left side. Answer C, concrete verbal instructions, is incorrect because the individual is able to understand concrete instructions, but not abstract information which includes information obtained from body language or voice inflections. See reference: Griffith and Lemberg: Neurological impairments relating to sexuality.

65. (D) Sexuality. Sexuality is a frequently overlooked area of human behavior, because many professionals receive little training in this area and do not feel comfortable approaching it with an individual. Also, the focus of hospitalization is to stabilize the individual medically and to provide treatment to return the individual to the family to manage or to a longer term facility for further treatment. Answers A, speech, B, ambulation, and C, self-care activities, are all treated as a primary function of speech, and of physical and occupational therapies, and are always addressed. Sexuality is frequently not a primary focus for any member of the rehabilitation team, and is only addressed when the individual's behavior requires it. See reference: Griffith and Lemberg: Sexuality and the person with traumatic brain injury.

66. (D) Propping on upper extremities bilaterally. The condition under which sitting tolerance will be performed is propping on upper extremities bilaterally. The individual describes who will change sitting tolerance, not the condition. Answer B is incorrect because it describes the behavior or performance skill to be changed, which is sitting tolerance. Answer C is incorrect because it describes the criterion of the terminal objective, which is measured by 10 minutes. See reference: Pedretti: Treatment planning.

67. (B) The condition. The condition is the circumstances under which an individual will perform. This includes adaptive equipment, assistance, or the type of environment. The terminal behavior is the change in performance or behavior demonstrated by the individual. The criterion is the method used to measure an individual's performance. The plan is the approach to be used to achieve a treatment objective. See reference: Pedretti: Treatment planning.

68. (C) Physical therapist. The physical therapist is concerned with properly preparing the stump prior to the individual being fitted with a prosthetic device and would educate the individual frequently regarding stump wrapping and shaping. Throughout the treatment day, the nurse is primarily concerned with the proper healing and care of the incision following surgery. The prosthetist is concerned with providing a prosthetic device which fits correctly for the individual's ambulation. The primary role of the occupational therapist is to train the individual for as much independence in self care as possible. This includes stump wrapping, which is completed as a part of the dressing skills one to two times per day. See reference: Palmer and Toms: Amputations and Prosthetics.

69. (C) A rehabilitation psychologist. The rehabilitation psychologist provides sexual and marital counseling to the individual and family, as well as coordinates behavior programs and cognitive retraining to decrease undesired behaviors. The physiatrist, answer A, is incorrect because the team treatment as a whole is often coordinated by this person. The rehabilitation nurse, answer B, assists in carrying out the team plan and is responsible for the education of the individual and family regarding continence, medication, and so on. The occupational therapist, answer D, is also incorrect because they would be responsible for

training regarding sensation and perception, and as a team member, work on self care and cognitive skills. See reference: Griffith and Lemberg: Management.

70. (D) A low back injury. A lower back injury would require training to prevent further injury to the area and to allow healing. Answers A, chronic obstructive pulmonary disease, and B, fibromyalgia, are diseases that would cause the individuals to be primarily in need of energy conservation techniques to prevent further depletion of their limited energy. Answer C is incorrect because an individual with carpal tunnel syndrome would need to implement positioning of the wrist and only lift items that are light weight because of weakened grip strength and pain in the wrist. See reference: Pedretti (ed): Roozee, S: Low back pain.

71. (D) Slicing a prepared roll of sugar cookies at room temperature and placing them on a tray using a spatula. The sugar cookie dough would be soft enough to provide minimal resistance without causing immediate fatigue and to provide isotonic contractions during the repetitive grasp and release of the knife and the spatula. While muffin and cake batter provide the least amount of resistance, the hand is using sustained isometric grasp on the electric or hand powered mixer, which combined with the minimal resistance of the batter and mixer weight is fatiguing. The chocolate chip cookie dough is resistive whether it is warm or cold and to maintain an isometric grasp while mixing with a spatula or scooping with an ice cream scooper would cause the individual to fatigue before the activity is finished. If the individual becomes fatigued while performing any of the activities, only the sugar cookies or the chocolate chip cookies would allow the individual time to rest without affecting the final product. See reference: Trombly (ed): Stewart, C: Retraining housekeeping and child care skills.

72. (B) Active assisted range of motion with gravity eliminated. Muscles with poor minus strength would only be able to move a body part through partial range of motion in a gravity eliminated position. The individual would then need assistance to complete the range of motion while using what strength is available in the body part. Passive range of motion would not provide resistance of the muscle against anything to improve strength since the muscle does not contract. A muscle with poor minus strength would be unable to move against gravity or to take any resistance, even with gravity eliminated. See reference: Trombly: Evaluation of biomechanical and physiological aspects of motor performance.

73. (C) Extension wrist for finger flexion and flexed wrist for finger extension. The method used to maintain tenodesis in a quadriplegic hand is to keep the wrist extended during finger flexion and the wrist flexed during finger extension. This allows the finger flexor tendons to shorten so that tenodesis action can occur. The other methods would stretch the tendons too much, which would not allow a tenodesis grasp. See reference: Trombly: Hollar, L: Spinal cord injury.

74. (D) Compensation. Compensation techniques are used to work around a deficit area, by using alternative methods to accomplish the same task. An example of compensation is using elastic shoe laces or velcro closures on shoes for someone unable to reach the feet or unable to tie shoes. Retraining and substitution continue to use skills to accomplish the same task, where compensation techniques may avoid that activity entirely. Problem solving would be the ability to organize information to reach a solution, for example how a person decides to handle his or her memory problems. See reference: Zoltan, Siev, and Freishtat: Body image and body scheme disorders.

75. (B) Detachable arms. Armrests will need to be removed to allow the individual to move sideways out of the chair. Footrests (answer A) may be swung away, but do not need to be detached to perform a transfer. Antitip bars (answer C) prevent a wheelchair from tipping over backwards, such as when performing a wheelie or when going up or down a step, but not when transferring. Brake-handle extensions (answer D) allow the brakes to be locked more easily, but would be in the way of a sliding board transfer. See reference: Palmer and Toms: Wheelchairs, assistive devices, and home modifications.

76. (A) Learning to type. Typing would allow the individual to communicate legibly in writing, while circumventing the individual's poor handwriting skills. Answers B, fine motor coordination exercises, and C, practicing letter or shape formations, are both ways to improve control of the writing utensils by improving coordination through exercises which will provide a greater smoothness to the writing. Answer D, exercises or activities for strengthening flexors and extensors in the finger, also allow improved use of the writing utensil by providing enough strength to properly position the writing tool. However, answers B, C, and D do not bypass the individual having to perform handwriting with a pen or pencil. See reference: Fisher, Murray, and Bundy (eds): Cermak, S: Somatodyspraxia.

77. (C) Ten degrees of head flexion past midline. When an individual's neck is kept at 10 degrees of flexion past midline, this closes the passage to the lungs, but allows food to easily pass down the esophagus. Answers A and B both involve extension of the neck, which should be avoided as this opens the passageways to the lungs and may cause choking or aspiration. Answer D, extreme flexion of the head, narrows the passageway to the stomach and causes a feeling of food sticking in the throat. See reference: Kovich and Bermann (eds): Van Dam-Burke, A, and Kovich, K: Self-care and homemaking.

78. (B) Flexion. Flexion at the wrist, especially while grasping or pinching, should be avoided. Repetitive flexion and extension movements also cause compression of the median nerve. Answers A, extension, C, ulnar deviation, and D, radial deviation do not cause inflammation to the area surrounding the median nerve by repetitive compression or a static hold to that area of the wrist. See reference: Hunter, Schneider, Mackin, and Callahan (eds): Baxter-Petralia, P: Therapist's management of carpal tunnel syndrome.

79. (C) Peripheral vascular disease. The highest percentage of amputations result from peripheral vascular disease, primarily as a result of diabetes or atherosclerosis, which both restrict peripheral circulation. Answers A, trauma, B, metastasizing tumor, and D, congenital defects all result in amputations at times. However, they are in a vast minority when compared with peripheral vascular disease. See reference: Palmer and Toms: Amputations and prosthetics.

80. (A) Sagittal. The sagittal plane goes through the body from front to back, which divides the body into right and left sides. Answer B, coronal, refers to the coronal axis which is what joints moving in the sagittal plane rotate around during motion. Answer C, the frontal plane, goes through one side of the body to the other, dividing the body into front and back. Answer D, the transverse plane, divides the body into the upper and lower halves. See reference: Norkin and White: Introduction to goniometry.

81. (A) Lateral epicondyle of the humerus. The lateral epicondyle of the humerus is the bony prominence located on the radial side of the elbow. Answers B, posterior aspect of the acromium process, and D, the olecranon process, are incorrect because they describe, respectively, the bony landmarks used in the measurement of shoulder abduction, shoulder extension, and internal and external rotation. The xiphoid process, answer C, is a bony landmark used for identifying correct hand placement while performing cardiopulmonary rescusitation. See reference: Norkin and White: Upper extremity testing.

82. (D) Swivel spoon. A swivel spoon would allow the handle to remain in one position while allowing the head of the spoon to rotate, thus compensating for poor supination. A rocker knife, a spork, and a spoon with a built-up handle all have the heads of the utensils fixed to the handles, which would allow no swiveling to compensate for decreased supination while bringing the utensil to the mouth. See reference: Trombly (ed): Feinberg, JR, and Trombly, CA: Arthritis.

83. (D) Using a vibrator with the wrist ulnarly flexed. Using a tool that vibrates, flexing the wrist, or holding an object with the wrist ulnarly deviated all contribute to median nerve compression. Answer A, pounding nails, does not provide a continuous vibrating force to the arm, and avoids a flexed position. Answers B, washing a table with extended wrist, and C, writing with wrist extended, are both activities that avoid flexion at the wrist, ulnar deviation, and use of vibrating tools. See reference: Hunter, Schneider, Mackin, and Callahan (eds): Baxter-Petralia, P: Therapist's management of carpal tunnel syndrome.

84. (D) Provide a stockinette for the individual to wear inside the splint. A stockinette liner when worn inside the splint keeps the perspiration from irritating the skin by absorbing the perspiration and keeping the skin away from the damp plastic. A stockinette liner is inexpensive enough to have several, so the individual may always have a clean one available. Answer A, putting talcum powder in a splint, works well with a small splint, but in a large splint would require a larger amount, and feel muddy when an individual perspires. Answer B, moleskin as a liner, does not clean well after wearing for a short time, and although it may be comfortable, it usually is discarded because of the soiled appearance and smell. Answer C, an individual using a splint made with perforated material, will continue to have perspiration and will need to use another method to keep the damp plastic from irritating the skin. See reference: Trombly (ed): Linden, CA, and Trombly, CA: Orthoses: Kinds and Purposes.

85. (A) Fast rocking while the individual is inverted over a barrel. Fast rocking while inverted over a barrel combines two facilatory techniques, which are inversion and fast rocking. When the therapist performs slow rocking, slow rolling, or pressure to tendon insertions, he or she is using an inhibitory technique, which involves slow movement or maintained stretch and pressure. See reference: Pedretti (ed): McCormack, G: The Rood approach to the treatment of neuro- muscular dysfunction.

86. (A) Lying on the left side while propped with pillows. This positioning allows the unaffected right extremities to remain free and provides weight bearing to the affected side to assist with tone reduction. The pillows behind the individual allow support and the individual may lean against the pillows to also provide pressure relief as needed to the affected side, since sensation may be reduced on that side along with movement. Side-lying on the right (answer B) would not provide any tone reduction, which is needed during a stressful activity such as sexual intercourse and also impairs the movement of the unaffected extremities, which would be needed for activities involving foreplay or applying contraceptive devices. Lying supine (answer C) or lying prone (answer D) are not positions that provide tone reduction to an individual with spasticity and may be uncomfortable without many pillows to assist with positioning comfortably. Also an individual lying prone has less mobility than when lying on the right side. See reference: Griffith and Lemberg: Neurological impairments relating to sexuality.

87. (D) Maintain a normal curve of the back, slowly shifting feet as the turn is completed. A correct transfer is performed slowly with the knees bent and the feet a shoulder width apart, while the normal curve of the back is maintained and the lifting is performed with the legs. The body should not be twisted at the trunk (answer A), as this could injure the back. Lifting with the arms (answer B), instead of the legs also could injure the therapist's back. Another way of injuring the back during a transfer is to keep the feet planted when moving (answer C) because this causes twisting of the back and may damage the knees. See reference: Palmer and Toms: Body mechanics and guarding techniques.

88. (B) Scoot forward to the edge of the wheelchair. When the therapist has the individual scoot forward to the edge of the wheelchair, this helps the individual position the body over the feet and causes the weight to shift forward during a transfer. The individual is much easier to transfer when the weight is shifted forward. If the weight is shifted back during a transfer, the individual may require more than one person to assist with the transfer or it may be a total lift by one or more individuals. If the individual attempts to push up from the mat using his or her arms and legs to lift (answer A), the body weight has shifted too far forward, making it difficult for the individual to push up effectively and maintain his or her balance. If the individual pushes off from the wheelchair seat while using only one arm and one leg to lift himself or herself during a transfer, the individual would have more difficulty rising from a seated position than if both arms and legs were used to lift himself or herself. The individual would need to pivot away from the mat in order to position himself or herself using the least amount of movements to the mat table from the wheelchair. If the therapist is in front of the individual during the pivot toward the mat table, the therapist would either be placed between the individual and the mat or forced to reposition his or her hand holds on the individual, so the therapist would cue the individual to pivot facing away from the mat table before sitting down. See reference: Palmer and Toms: Body mechanics and guarding techniques.

89. (A) Check the alignment of the goniometer. If the goniometer is not aligned correctly, any joint measurements will demonstrate a discrepancy. A variability of 5 degrees is normal between two different evaluators, and maybe that much less on a retest by the same therapist. Changing the size of the goniometer to larger (answer B) or smaller (answer C) during measurements could make the discrepancy greater, because it could make aligning the arms of the goniometer with the landmarks more difficult. It is much faster to check the alignment of the goniometer first when using one of the proper length for the job. Forcing the individual's arm further into flexion (answer D) would be painful to the individual because measurements are taken at the end of the individual's full range of motion and the joint would be unable to go further. See reference: Norkin and White: Procedures.

90. (C) The individual continues to be motivated toward improving performance. An activity is only continued with an individual when that individual has motivation to improve on the task. An activity that is too difficult (answer A) or too easy (answer B) does not inspire the proper motivation of the individual to perform at their best. When an individual is unmotivated (answer D), there will be no improvement on the task. See reference: Fisher, Murray, and Bundy (eds): Koomar, J, and Bundy, A: The art and science of creating direct intervention from theory.

91. (B) A change in the individual's status. Revising the treatment plan is a continuous process to allow the treatment to be updated to match the individual's needs. Answers A, discharge from therapy, C, completion of the evaluation, or D, continuing to make progress towards goals, are all situations where a revision to the treatment plan would not be necessary. When an individual is discharged, the treatment plan has ended, and if the individual is seen again, a new one would need to be written. The treatment plan is current when the evaluation is completed and would only need to be updated when the goals have been met or individual status has changed. An individual who continues to make progress toward a goal would find the treatment plan still appropriate. See reference: Pedretti: Treatment planning.

92. (A) A videofluoroscopy. A videofluoroscopy should be performed when it is suspected that the individual is aspirating. An individual who suddenly has a wet voice when there was no prior difficulty may have had a sudden change in medical status causing aspiration. He or she should be re-evaluated to determine if there is aspiration into the larynx or trachea. Answers B, a change to thin liquids, and D, a regular diet, would be inappropriate for an individual who does not have a normal swallow or who may be aspirating, because they are too difficult to control. Answer C, a tracheostomy tube, is usually in place prior to the initiation of a feeding program, because the individual was having difficulty with breathing, not swallowing or wet voice qualities. See reference: Pedretti (ed): Nelson, K: Dysphagia: Evaluation and treatment.

93. (B) 3 to 5 seconds. A swallow delay of 3 to 5 seconds may be adequate for an individual to handle a bolus of thick liquids before it loses shape. A swallow delay of over 3 to 5 seconds (answer A) would be too slow and a bolus of thick liquids would disperse, causing a risk of aspiration. Answers C, 1 second, and D, a normal swallow, are the same thing, as a normal swallow would be able to handle any liquid consistency presented in 1 second. However, the individual would need to perform well at the next level consistency (thinner liquid) before being tried with thin liquids. See reference: Pedretti (ed): Nelson, K: Dysphagia: Evaluation and treatment.

94. (B) Rheumatoid arthritis. Rheumatoid arthritis is a chronic inflammation of the peripheral joints and cervical spine that has periods of remission and exacerbation. Answer A, osteoarthritis, is incorrect because it is a noninflammatory disease that can affect any joint. Answer C, ankylosing spondylitis, is also incorrect because it affects primarily the axial joints in the spine, shoulders, and hips. Answer D, systemic lupus erythematosus, is incorrect because it is an inflammatory disease that affects the organ systems. See reference: Trombly (ed): Feinberg, JR, and Trombly, CA: Arthritis.

95. (A) Osteoarthritis. Osteoarthritis is a degenerative, noninflammatory type of arthritis, which may affect any joint. Answers B, rheumatoid arthritis, C, ankylosing spondylitis, and D, juvenile rheumatoid arthritis, are all incorrect because they are types of inflammatory arthritis. Rheumatoid arthritis, both adult and juvenile, affects the peripheral joints, which are located in the extremities and the cervical area of the spine. Ankylosing spondylitis affects primarily the axial joints of the spine, hips, and shoulders. See reference: Trombly (ed): Feinberg, JR, and Trombly, CA: Arthritis.

96. (A) The ability to work locks and latches on doors or windows. Checking the individual's ability to work the locks and latches at home on the doors and windows needs to be assessed because the style and stiffness of them vary from any available in the clinic. The locks and latches may not be maintained in the same way and may be stiffer or smoother to work. The ability to work the locks and latches is also a safety concern, as the individual may not be able to open them to let family into their home or close them to keep intruders from entering. Answers B, built up handles, C, energy conservation techniques, and D, adaptations to clothing fasteners, are all adaptations or activities that could be easily performed in the clinic, because clothing and utensils are able to be transported to the clinic and energy conservation may be incorporated into treatment activities. See reference: Trombly (ed): Feinberg, JR, and Trombly, CA: Arthritis.

97. (A) Identify landmarks on the hand or arm to align the splint. The individual or family must be familiar with the landmarks on the hand and arm in order to align the splint when replacing it correctly. If redness occurs, the splint would not be remolded if the redness lasts less than 20 minutes after the splint has been removed. The splint is usually unable to be remolded after the initial application of straps. A heat gun may be used to spot adjust the splint in any area where it causes pressure marks. The wearing schedule needs to be specifically known by the individual in order for the splint to be worn appropriately so as to receive maximum benefit. Also, the individual or family needs to be able to remove or replace the splint independently prior to discharge, since the therapist will not be present at all times to provide verbal cueing. See reference: Trombly (ed): Linden, CA, and Trombly, CA: Orthosis: Kinds and purposes.

98. (D) With gentle active range of motion. Gentle active range of motion allows the individual to control the movement and avoid over stretching to inflamed joint tissues. Answers A, brisk passive range of motion, B, weight as tolerated, and C, isotonic exercises, are all incorrect, as they would over stretch the joint by increased resistance or movement. This causes further damage to the joint by increasing the stress, which results in more inflammation. In therapy, the individual must be taught of the importance of joint protection during exercise. See reference: Trombly (ed): Linden, CA, and Trombly, CA: Orthosis: Kinds and purposes.

99. (A) A lightweight folding frame. A lightweight folding frame is needed when a wheelchair will be frequently lifted in and out of a car trunk or back seat, and folded to fit into the space. This is much easier on the individual or family member who will be lifting the wheelchair. Answers B, a one-arm drive, C, an amputee frame, on a wheelchair that is taken out into the community; however, they add a great deal of weight and bulk, which makes the wheelchair much more difficult to lift in and out of the car. This in turn may cause an individual or family member to be more reluctant to go on a community outing. See reference: Trombly (ed): Feinberg, JR, and Trombly, CA: Arthritis.

100. (B) 1 foot of ramp for every inch of rise in height. A foot of ramp for every inch of rise in height provides a gentle slope, which may be independently and safely navigated by an individual. Answers A, 1-inch ramp for every foot of rise, C, 10 inches of ramp for every 2 inches of height, and D, 1 foot of ramp for every foot of rise, would all make extremely short and steep ramps, which would be either unsuitable or unsafe for an individual independently entering or exiting a home. See reference: Pedretti (ed): Stone, G, and Pedretti, L: Wheelchairs and wheelchair transfers.

101. (D) The individual's view of the problem and an overall goal. The interview is generally the component of the assessment process where the occupational therapist asks about the individual's goals for treatment and gains an understanding of the problems from the person's perspective. Answers A and B are most often found in a review of the chart. Ability, answer C, is determined through performance measures. See reference: Denton: Assessment.

102. (B) Schroeder Block Campbell. The only evaluation method in the list that assesses adult sensory motor functions is the Schroeder Block Campbell. The BaFPE and COTE assess a variety of task skills. The SCSIT is used only with children. See reference: Denton: Assessment.

103. (D) To use an interest checklist that compares the individual's current involvement with the past 6 months. A behavioral perspective focuses on obtaining data that identifies current problems. Comparing current and past involvement can identify problems related to interest involvement. Information about past interests can identify potential reinforcers. Answer A describes a model of human occupation perspective that examines personal satisfaction with interests in addition to patterns of involvement. Answer B describes a cognitive-behavioral focus on skills. Answer C describes an object relations perspective focus on affective meanings. See reference: Bruce and Borg: The behavioral frame of reference. In Frames of Reference in Psychosocial Occupational Therapy.

104. (C) Ego. Improvement of ego function is one of the functions of activity in occupational therapy with this frame of reference. The ego helps make choices, set priorities, postpone gratification, and could be addressed by choosing between activities. The id and libido are less conscious and would be addressed with expressive media and directions to "make whatever you want to." The superego could be addressed by exploring the "rules" or self evaluations used by the individual during an activity.

See reference: Bruce and Borg: Object relations frame of reference. In Frames of Reference in Psychosocial Occupational Therapy.

105. (B) The Holmes-Rahe Life Change Index. Answers A, C, and D are all designed to identify an individual's responses or reactions to stressors. Stressors are the triggers to the reactions, not the reactions. The Holmes-Rahe lists major social and environmental stressors. See reference: Hopkins and Smith (eds): Neistadt, ME: Stress management.

106. (B) To begin the assessment process when individuals are admitted on the weekends. The OTR will finish the assessments on Monday. The primary role of the COTA is to implement treatment such as that described in answers A, C, and D. 1990 AOTA guidelines about supervising a COTA state that a COTA may not independently evaluate patients. Working on weekends, the COTA would be independently initiating evaluations. See reference: Hopkins and Smith (eds): Entry Level Role Delineation Task Force for the Intercommission Council: Appendix F.

107. (A) The format of this assessment is an interview or questionnaire. This assessment uses interview or questionnaire formats. Administration time varies with the format selected but generally ranges between 20 and 90 minutes. There are norms provided for individuals who are hearing and hearing impaired. The interview format requires training to administer. See reference: Hopkins and Smith (eds): Entry Level Role Delineation Task Force for the Intercommission Council: Appendix F.

108. (A) Vineland Adaptive Behavior Scale. The Vineland provides information about daily living skills, communication, socialization, motor skills, and maladaptive behaviors. The VMI and NPI provide information about one area of function. The Play History is appropriate for the preschool age group. See reference: Hopkins and Smith (eds): Florey, LL: Psychiatric disorders in childhood and adolescence.

109. (A) To determine the level of function in play, social behavior, and visual motor skills. The purposes of evaluation vary according to the age of the client in childhood and adolescence in addressing psychiatric disorders. Answer B is the overall purpose for school-age children. Answer D is the purpose for toddlers and preschool children. Answer C is more consistent with adult populations. See reference: Hopkins and Smith (eds): Florey, LL: Psychiatric disorders in childhood and adolescence.

110. (C) Time taken to complete the collage:

    a. 0 to 15 minutes   b. 16 to 30 minutes
    c. 31 minutes to 1 hour

Individual 1's quickly tearing and pasting pages provides the therapist with information about answer C. It is individual 2's comments that provide the therapist with information about answer A. There is no information about answer B from either individual in this situation.

Answer D is a collage variable, not a patient-therapist variable. See reference: Hemphill: Lerner, CJ: The magazine picture collage. In The Evaluative Process in Occupational Therapy.

111. (B) Normal activity sequencing. The presentation of activities can be organized according to several sequences. Answer B is an example of normal sequencing of activities related to social skills. Sequencing according to normal development would involve crawling and sitting before standing. Chronologic and role acquisition (answers C and D) are not sequencing approaches for activities. See reference: Denton: Treatment planning and implementation.

112. (D) Exiting conversations. Beginning social skills are based on initiating conversations, identifying mutual interests, and exiting conversations. Answers A, B, and C are social skills that are linked to more intimate or ongoing relationships such as friendships and dating. See reference: Denton: Treatment planning and implementation.

113. (B) To show acceptance and understanding to the individual. The therapist's response was an example of paraphrasing. Paraphrasing is used to clarify and relay acceptance of what an individual has communicated. Paraphrasing is in the therapist's own words versus repeating what the individual stated. Answer A is the purpose of clarifying whereas answer D is the purpose for probing. Answer C describes the paraphrasing technique and is not a purpose. See reference: Denton: Treatment planning and implementation.

114. (B) Affective disorders. Affective disorders are problem areas addressed by 22 percent of mental health occupational therapists. Adjustment disorders, answer A, and alcohol use disorders, answer C, make up approximately 5 percent of the problems treated. Anxiety disorders, answer D, are a problem area with less than 1 percent of the patients. See reference: Hopkins and Smith (eds): Richert, GZ, and Gibson, D: Practice settings.

115. (D) Demonstrate the techniques of "broken-record" and "I" statements to the individual and asking the individual these techniques. Demonstration and imitation of desired performances is particularly useful when individuals are learning new and difficult behaviors. The therapist should be aware of a need to supplement this strategy with techniques that provide generalization after skills are developed. Answer A is appropriate when the goals are self evaluative versus skills training. Answer B is effective for testing out new skills. Answer C is effective for helping the patient to generalize their skills to other situations. See reference: Denton: Treatment planning and implementation.

116. (B) Photosensitivity. Photosensitivity is a side effect of neuroleptic medications that increases the reactions one has to the sun. Answers A and D are also known to be side effects of neuroleptic medications but would generally not be problematic for a community outing. Answer C is not a side effect of these medications. See reference: Denton: Treatment planning and implementation.

117. (B) A therapeutic device in helping. How the occupational therapist uses "the self" is a tool in the therapy process but is not the central focus of the therapy. The therapeutic use of self has a few qualities of a friendship but also requires the therapist to understand and manage some of their reactions. Empathy, not sympathy, is recommended in the therapeutic relationships. See reference: Hopkins and Smith (eds): Scwartzberg, SL: Therapeutic use of self.

118. (C) Cohesiveness is difficult to achieve. The development of cohesiveness is negatively influenced by the ongoing addition and subtraction of members in a group in acute care settings. Answer A and B are advantages of a group format. Answer D is an advantage of individual treatment. See reference: Denton: Treatment planning and implementation.

119. (B) The therapist should allow more time for the individuals to respond to questions about discharge plans. Depression slows patients' responses, so allowing them more time to respond is important. Both silence and a cheerful approach can be perceived as unaccepting or insincere. The therapist needs to provide the structure as initiating and maintaining discussions is often difficult for depressed individuals. See reference: Hemphill: Shaw, C: The interview process in occupational therapy. In Mental Health Assessment in Occupational Therapy—An Integrative Approach to the Evaluative Process.

120. (C) Applying grout to a tile trivet and waiting for it to dry. Activities provide a variety of opportunities for therapeutic gains. The process of grouting a tile trivet involves covering the individual's tile design with the grout mixture and is a messy step. The individual then sees that the tile pattern is emphasized with the addition of the grout. Waiting for the grout to dry requires an individual to delay gratification. See reference: Hopkins and Smith (eds): Simon, CJ: Use of activity and activity analysis.

121. (A) Restore and maintain functional performance of self-chosen occupations that enhance competent performance of valued occupational roles. The depression is likely to be in reaction to the individual's AIDS disease and major loss of functioning at Stage 4. Stage 4 of AIDS generally means severe physical and neurologic changes. Because the change of function can be broad, answer A is the most comprehensive approach. Answers B, C, and D are too restrictive to be a "major focus." Also, restoration of work is typically unrealistic at Stage 4 of AIDS. See reference: Hopkins and Smith (eds): Pizzi, M: HIV infection and AIDS.

122. (A) Primary prevention. Primary prevention strategies are designed to prevent occurrences before symptoms occur. Secondary and tertiary prevention focus on interventions for emerging and existing symptoms. Intermediate prevention is not a type of prevention. See reference: Hopkins and Smith (eds): Levy, LL: The health care delivery system today.

123. (D) Make recommendations or referrals to agencies or programs that help individuals to get and maintain appropriate jobs. Most individuals with an eating disorder have not entered the work environment or have had difficulty making appropriate work choices. This is a long range goal that is usually best continued after the person's eating disorder has been stabilized. Referrals to Overeater's Anonymous meetings should be located near the person's residence. Family therapy referrals are typically performed by other disciplines on the team. Adapting the individual's environment is an external control strategy that is in conflict with most programs' focus on developing internal controls. Hopkins and Smith (eds): Beck, NL: Eating disorders—Anorexia nervosa and bulima nervosa.

124. (A) A game that requires some people to hide their eyes while others keep their eyes open. When analyzing games before selection, the therapist should determine if the game is appropriate for all of the members. Having some individuals hide their eyes would be very difficult for those who are paranoid. See reference: Posthuma: Group activities.

125. (C) Mental imagery. Individuals with schizophrenia generally have difficulty with abstract concepts or approaches. Also, they have difficulty accurately perceiving reality. Because imagery involves both abstracting and relies on the individual developing alternate perceptions, this strategy is contraindicated. All the other listed stress management techniques would be generally appropriate. See reference: Hopkins and Smith (eds): Niestadt, ME: Stress management.

126. (A) Preparing a can of soup. Grading activities according to complexity is an important part of the therapist's selection of appropriate activities for an individual's abilities. Complexity increases as the number of steps, number of different ingredients or tools used, and time to complete the task increases. Answers B, C, and D all require more steps, materials, and time than preparing a can of soup. See reference: Bruce and Borg: Appendix I. In Psychosocial Occupational Therapy—Frames of Reference for Intervention.

127. (C) Locate a puncture-resistant container that the copper piece could be placed into before disposing of it. Answer C is the only action that is consistent with universal precautions guidelines. Answers A and D do not dispose of blood-exposed items in a manner that would protect others from contact. Answer B does not include any blood exposure protection for the person applying the bandage. See reference: Hopkins and Smith (eds): Pizzi, M: HIV infection and AIDS.

128. (B) Tranxene. Tranxene is considered to be an antianxiety medication. Tegretol is an anticonvulsant medication, and Trilafon is an antipsychotic medication. Tofranil is classified as an antidepressant. See reference:

Hopkins and Smith (eds): Gibson, D, and Richert, GZ: The therapeutic process.

129. (B) The individual will select and teach two peers a craft activity that she enjoys. Answer B is the only option that is measurable and builds upon the strengths of the individual to address problem areas. Answer A is an appropriate goal direction but it is difficult to measure the individual's attainment or progress. Answer C describes the therapist's methods. Answer D does not address the problem area of peer socialization. See reference: Hopkins and Smith (eds): Florey, LL: Psychiatric disorders in childhood and adolescence.

130. (C) Anxiety and withdrawal are increased. The laissez-faire style of leadership involves minimal direction from the leader. The main problem with a laissez-faire approach is increased anxiety among the members and withdrawal from the group. Contraindications are unwanted effects; therefore, A and B are not the correct answers. Indecisiveness may occur among some of the members, but generally leadership behaviors are encouraged by this type of leadership. See reference: Bruce and Borg: Appendix I. In Psychosocial Occupational Therapy—Frames of Reference for Intervention.

131. (B) Group protocol. Group protocols describe the content and structure of treatment groups that are developed for treatment programs for specialized patient populations. Group protocols should contain the overall structure, goals, criteria for patient selection, leadership qualifications, and evaluation formats and frequency. See reference: Hopkins and Smith (eds): Appendix I—Guidelines for occupational therapy documentation.

132. (A) Schizophrenia. Schizophrenia is the only diagnosis listed that is considered to be a psychotic disorder. There are no organic disorders listed in this question. Bulimia nervosa is an eating disorder. Psychogenic fugues are dissociative disorders. Adjustment disorder is a category of many disorders. See reference: Bonder: Appendix A—DSM IV classification.

133. (C) Section IV. Criteria for patient selection should list the abilities and functional limitations that indicate or describe patients who are appropriate for the group format and content. Section II includes the group process. Section III includes the specific goals of the group. Section V describes the abilities needed by the group leader. See reference: Hopkins and Smith (eds): Appendix I—Guidelines for occupational therapy documentation.

134. (C) A concrete response. Literal and concrete responses to general inquirie indicate the difficulty that people with schizophrenia have in understanding questions with several possible meanings. Delusional responses would most likely be completely off topic. A distractable response would change the topic or stop in the middle of responding. An insightful response would include reasons that led up to being hospitalized. See reference: Hemphill, BJ: Shaw, C: The interviewing process in occupational therapy. In Mental Health Assessments in Occupational Therapy—An Integrative Approach to the Evaluative Process.

135. (A) Encourage members to use PABA-free sunblock and to wear a hat. The precautions for photosensitivity are related to protecting the patient from the sun. The precautions described in answer B are helpful to the individual experiencing hypotension but this was not the side effect indicated in the question. Answers C and D are not linked to the side effects of neuroleptic medications. See reference: Hopkins and Smith (eds): Gibson, D, and Richert, GZ: The therapeutic process.

136. (B) The small craft pieces are precut by the occupational therapy (OT) aide; a template for cutting the large straight-edged pieces is available to the individual; step-by-step directions with photographs are available to the individual. Adapted sequencing involves using steps that have been adapted to enhance success or completion. Precutting pieces decreases the number of steps required while using templates, and picture directions simplify the task. Answers A and D are examples of developmental sequencing. Answer C is an example of normal sequencing. See reference: Denton: Treatment planning and treatment implementation.

137. (B) A leisure values clarification activity. The individual's values are still not known and a values clarification activity would help to understand the values that underlie the individual's past and present interests. This individual's leisure interests are already known, so the answer A would be a duplication of information you already have. Magazine picture collages could be adapted to further examine interests and values, but this answer (answer C) does not describe such an adaptation. Answer D is premature at this point as the individual has not identified any goals around which to plan future leisure activities. See reference: Hopkins and Smith (eds): Simon, CJ: Use of activity and activity analysis.

138. (B) "Teacher options" that allow the therapist to adjust the individual's number, type, and frequency of attempts. The use of computer applications within psychosocial settings is linked to the overall goals of treatment. In the treatment of behavioral disorders, behavior management and reinforcement are overall goals. Answer B is the software features that best enable the therapist to grade and adapt reinforcement. Answers A and C are criteria that are important for individuals with interactional skill deficits. Answer D can provide feedback that can best be used in working with personality disorders. See reference: Hopkins and Smith (eds): Simon, CJ: Use of activity and activity analysis.

139. (D) Is easily distracted. Individuals who are easily distracted, as well as those needing constant supervision, are two common indicators for a one-to-one approach. Socialization and daily living skill deficits are well suited to group approaches. Many psychosocial assessments do not require a one-to-one administration. See reference: Hopkins and Smith (eds): Richert, GZ: Program planning, development, and implementation.

140. (C) "I think baking would be a helpful activity to try. Baking something you like offers you several choices and decisions. These choices and decisions can help you feel more positive about making other decisions. You can choose a cake mix or a cookie mix. Which would you like?" Answer C limits options as well as provides the rational for the choices. Answer A is a leading question that really offers only one "choice." Answer B does not provide any options. Answer D is a closed question, offering no real "choice for the individual." See reference: Denton: Effective communication.

141. (C) Behavioral perspective. Although the teacher role is also linked to the cognitive behavioral perspective, the other roles described in the question are consistent with a behavioral perspective. The therapist's role within the occupation behavior perspective is that of mutual problem solver and coplanner. Object relations perspective therapists serve as guides who develop a collaborative relationship with the individual. See reference: Bruce and Borg: The behavioral frame of reference. In Psychosocial Occupational Therapy—Frames of Reference for Intervention.

142. (C) Offer practical advise and skill enhancement in the groups. Intense treatment milieus that focus on insight development, self disclosure, confrontation, and the open expression of anger have been found to be contraindicated in the inpatient treatment of individuals with schizophrenia. Structured, supportive milieus with an emphasis on enhancing positive skills have been found to be helpful. See reference: Bonder: Schizophrenia and other psychotic disorders.

143. (B) The name of the individual's family members who visited earlier in the day. The emphasis is on names, places, events, and time. In prioritizing which area to focus on, the individual's memory and focus on their ongoing relationships would take priority over staff names or the names of individuals the individual is not in contact with. See reference: Bruce and Borg: Holistic frames of reference. In Psychosocial Occupational Therapy—Frames of Reference for Intervention.

144. (C) Acute care hospitalization. The emphases of acute care hospitalization are symptom reduction, medications, and discharge planning. The club house treatment format emphasizes belonging and security. Community mental health centers focus on medication management, crisis intervention, and outpatient therapy. Quarterway houses emphasize increasing autonomy and decreasing supervision. See reference: Hopkins and Smith (eds): Richert, GZ, and Gibson, D: Practice settings.

145. (C) "I'm just too tired." One of the main symptoms of severe depression is decreased energy, therefore the response of "I'm too tired" indicates fatigue. Answers A and B are responses reflecting the individuals perceptions of their ability or competence. Answer D is a response reflecting interests or values that conflict with the proposed activity. See reference: Bonder: Mental disorders.

146. (D) Sheltered workshops. Sheltered workshops are the most available vocational service for adults with mental retardation. Although supported employment and job coaching may be preferred, they are not commonly available. Adult activity centers do not emphasize vocational goals. See reference: Hopkins and Smith (eds): Humphrey, R, and Jacobs, K: Mental retardation.

147. (B) Using charts and graphs of changes from the baseline. A graphical display of progress is consistent with a behavioral frame of reference perspective. Answers C and D are documentation methods for recording assessment findings from the model of human occupation and the recapitulation of ontogenesis frames of reference, respectively. Answer A is not related to any particular frame of reference. See reference: Bruce and Borg: The behavioral frame of reference. In Psychosocial Occupational Therapy—Frames of Reference for Intervention.

148. (A) "I attended occupational therapy to decrease my boredom and the sitting around and doing nothing." A recent study found that individuals' reasons for attending occupational therapy groups focused on escaping the hospital routine. The individuals' responses were also found to be quite different from the therapist's perception of what was helpful about therapeutic groups. It is important for occupational therapists to understand the different perceptions and to clearly and routinely provide individuals with the therapeutic goals and purposes of all therapeutic activities. See reference: Polimeni-Walker, I, Wilson, KG, and Jewers, R: Reasons for participating in occupational therapy groups—Perceptions of adult psychiatric inpatients and occupational therapists. Can J Occup Ther 59:241–247, 1992.

149. (D) To pursue involvement of the child in Girl or Boy Scouts. Parents of children with severe psychiatric conditions tend to either over or under estimate their child's play and social interaction skills. It is important for OTs to provide education to parents about realistic age-related expectations. Organized activities that are peer focused, for example Scouts, are often important to 8- and 9-year-old children. Competition is more appropriate for 10 to 12 year olds and would be an "overestimation" of skills. Board games with rule changes and focusing on playing by the rules are examples of underestimating the skills of the 8 year old. See reference: Hopkins and Smith (eds): Florey, L: Psychiatric disorders in childhood and adolescence.

150. (D) Regression. Regression involves a client's decreased responsibility, increased dependency, and disregard for others. Regression is a risk for client's who remain in treatment settings longer than necessary. Countertransferences are feelings that the therapist and client have about one another that are interfering with the process therapy. Continuity of care is a term that describes a range of services differing along treatment structure and intensity. Posttraumatic stress disorder is a psychiatric diagnosis versus a risk factor. See reference: Hopkins and Smith (eds): Richart, GZ, and Gibson, D: Practice settings.

151. (B) A physician's referral. Within acute care hospital settings, it is necessary to gain a physician referral to meet accrediting agency regulations and for third party reimbursement. Therefore, answers A, C, and D are incorrect. However, when in other settings, the occupational therapist may respond to a request for service and initiate services based on their own judgement. See reference: Reed and Sanderson: Referral or prescription?

152. (A) Reviewed and update annually. The JCAHO supports a long-term ongoing emphasis on quality and therefore recommends that policies and procedures be reviewed and updated annually. Facilities that attempt to update their manual specifically for JCAHO surveys will not be able to demonstrate a program of continual process assessment and improvement. Therefore, answers B and C are incorrect. Answer D is incorrect as well in that it does not allow for the manuals to be updated every year. See reference: Hopkins and Smith (eds): Perinchief, JM: Service management.

153. (B) With high risk. Because of the seriousness of high-risk areas, it is vital to continue monitoring secondary to the serious consequences. A consequence is a result of an occurrence within a specified monitor. An example would be a patient falling in the ADL shower. One incident could have serious consequences. Therefore, even if this area did not have any "incidents," it may continue to be monitored on an ongoing basis. However, when high volume/incidence or problem-prone areas achieve 100 percent, the quality issue is resolved. When this occurs, new monitors of quality care may be established. See reference: Hopkins and Smith (eds): Perinchief, JM: Service management.

154. (D) Occupational Safety and Health Administration (OSHA). The Occupational Health and Safety Administration is responsible for establishing and enforcing safe work place policies. As a part of this responsibility, OSHA established regulations regarding bloodborne pathogens in order to ensure employee safety. Their role was to develop standard requirements for employers to follow, which prevent and handle exposures. Therefore, answers A, B, and C are incorrect. Answer A is the Food and Drug Administration. Answer B is the Environmental Protection Agency. Answer D is the Joint Commission on Accreditation of Hospital Organizations. See reference: Hopp and Rogers: Bakland, LK, Burlew, SA, Clements, MJ, et al: Health care professional's role in the treatment of AIDS.

155. (A) Be aware of hazardous chemicals in the work environment, their side effects, and cleansing procedures for the chemicals. Facilities are required to meet the standard of the OSHA Hazard Communication Standard, which requires employee access to information on chemical handling, storage, spill response, and employee exposure. This information is contained in manuals that are referred to as Material Safety and Data Sheets or MSDS. Answers B, C, and D refer to other workplace information, which is not related to chemical handling. The most common chemicals that are handled in an occupational therapy department are related to splinting and serial casting. See reference: Federal Register: Rules and regulations.

156. (C) Frequent hand washing. Handwashing is the primary prevention against infection from bloodborne pathogens in the health care environment. Four workplace strategies aide in the prevention of exposure. Handwashing is considered an example of workplace practices. Other strategies include engineering controls, protective equipment, and universal precautions. Answers A, B, and D are examples of protective equipment. However, the primary prevention is handwashing. See reference: Hopp and Rogers: Elder, HA: Transmission of HIV and prevention of AIDS.

157. (C) Blood, semen, and saliva from dental procedures. OSHA has identified materials that require universal precautions to be blood, semen, vaginal secretions, cerebrospinal fluid, synovial fluid, pleural fluid, any body fluid with visible blood, any unidentifiable body fluid, and saliva from dental procedures. Answers A, B, and D all contain fluids that are not on this list. Items that OSHA identified as not needing universal precautions are feces, nasal secretions, sputum, sweat, tears, urine, and vomitus. See reference: Hopp and Rogers: Elder, HA: Transmission of HIV and prevention of AIDS.

158. (B) Rinse the eye with an eye wash or water immediately. It is necessary to immediately wash the eye because the "backwash" fluid in the I.V. is unidentifiable body fluid and universal precautions should be followed. It is recommended to flush an exposed area with warm water or normal saline immediately. Therefore, answers A, C, and D are incorrect. Following the cleansing of the eye, it is recommended to contact the immediate supervisor and report the exposure through the facility reporting system. See reference: Hopp and Rogers: Elder, HA: Transmission of HIV and prevention of AIDS.

159. (C) Contact with supervisor once a month. The description of general supervision given by the AOTA includes a minimum of monthly direct contact with supervision available as needed by phone or other forms of communication. Answer A describes close supervision with direct contact occurring daily. Answer B refers to routine supervision or direct contact occurring a minimum of every 2 weeks. Answer D is minimal supervision, which occurs on an as needed basis. See reference: AOTA: The Occupational Therapy Roles Task Force: Occupational Therapy Roles.

160. (A) Contact with supervisor once a day. *The Occupational Therapy Roles* document provides definitions for levels of supervision. Close supervision is defined as "daily, direct contact at the site of work." Other levels of supervision are routine, general, and minimal. Routine supervision is provided when direct contact is made every 2 weeks with "interim supervision occurring by other methods such as telephone or written communication." Under general supervision, contact is made monthly, answer C. Minimal supervision is provided on an "as

needed" basis as in answer D. It is possible that this may be less than once a month. See reference: AOTA: The Occupational Therapy Roles Task Force: Occupational Therapy Roles.

161. (A) An entry level. A therapist who is changing areas of practice within the profession of occupational therapy will return to the level of skill development. This level is referred to as entry level. At this level, the therapist will be regaining knowledge of the responsibilities and accountability in professional activities. Answers B and C involve the therapist being able to function independently with mastery of basic role functions. Answer D, educator, is a separate area of skills which is itself divided into proficiency levels of entry level, intermediate, and high proficiency. See reference: AOTA: The Occupational Therapy Roles Task Force: Occupational Therapy Roles.

162. (D) An intermediate therapist with routine or general supervision. Supervision is the oversight required of an occupational therapist and may be at any one of four levels based on the expertise of the professional. An intermediate therapist will have gained skill mastery and have the ability to function as a resource person. However, he or she has not yet gained the refinement of special skills to be considered advanced. Answers A, B, and C are incorrect in that they match the skill level of the therapist with inappropriate levels of supervision. See reference: AOTA: The Occupational Therapy Roles Task Force: Occupational Therapy Roles.

163. (C) Collaborative. The supervision of a certified occupational therapy assistant is intended to be collaborative. This term takes into account the sharing of information and utilization of each individual's skills in the process of working with patients. Answer A places the COTA in a role of not being able to provide information or have input into the treatment of the patient. Answer B is not appropriate in that it would have the COTA working independently without the supervision of an OTR. Answer D is incorrect in that open communication between the COTA and OTR is vital for a team approach. See reference: AOTA: The Occupational Therapy Roles Task Force: Occupational Therapy Roles.

164. (A) Complete the chart reviews. An identified role of the certified occupational therapy assistant is to complete data collection records such as a record review, general observation checklist, or behavior checklist. Answers B, C, and D indicate that the assistant is independently collecting nonstandardized data and interpreting the data. These roles are not appropriate for an assistant. See reference: Hopkins and Smith (eds): Entry Level Role Delineation Task Force for the Intercommission Council: Appendix F.

165. (B) Once service competency has been established. Service competency assures inter-rater reliability between the occupational therapist and the assistant. This concept indicates that two professionals working together in a collaborative relationship for patient treatment will obtain the same or equivalent results. Techniques for assuring service competency vary between facilities. Answers A, C, and D are inappropriate because they do not address the skill level required to administer a standardized test. See reference: Hopkins and Smith (eds): Entry Level Role Delineation Task Force for the Intercommission Council: Appendix F.

166. (B) An objective system for measuring appropriateness of patient care. Even though quality improvement programs are required by accrediting agencies, they do not represent the agencies' primary purpose; therefore, answer A is incorrect. Medical credentialing (answer C) is a process that is completed by the facility when hiring a medical professional to ensure that the individual is appropriately registered and licensed to practice in the state. Research projects to test validity and reliability of treatment approaches (answer D) are done on an individual basis and may not actually measure the appropriateness of patient care. See reference: Bair and Gray (eds): Shaw, KJ: Program evaluation.

167. (A) Advanced level with minimal supervision. Supervision is the oversight required of an occupational therapist and may be at any one of four levels based on the expertise of the professional. Advanced is the highest level of skill requiring only minimal supervision, which is defined as an on needed basis. These individuals have refined skills in their area of expertise and may have participated in research of providing continuing education. An intermediate therapist will have gained skill mastery and have the ability to function as a resource person. However, they have not yet gained the refinement of special skills to be considered advanced. Entry level therapists would be developing their skills and accepting responsibilities for relevant professional activities. See reference: AOTA: The Occupational Therapy Roles Task Force: Occupational Therapy Roles.

168. (A) Quality-improvement plan. Quality improvement plans should include the scope of services provided, indicators of quality, and the cost efficiency and effectiveness of the program. Results of program evaluations may also be included in quality improvement plans (i.e., *quality assurance plans*). Answer A reflects the policies that govern a department and the procedures to carry out tasks. Answer C covers safety information that may be pertinent to emergency resuscitation procedures, as well as fire and disaster plans. Answer D is a system of peer review that analyzes the appropriateness of services. See reference: Bair and Gray (eds): Joe, BE: Quality assurance.

169. (A) Quality improvement plan. Quality improvement programs have emerged from what was known as quality assurance programs. These programs look at the aspects of service, provision of care, identification of problems, and evaluation of the effectiveness of interventions. Quality improvement plans take this concept a step further to the continual evolution of identifying issues and working towards resolution. In these programs, once the issue is resolved, the team selects, monitors, and works toward resolution of another issue. Answer B, peer review, is the system of other service providers assessing the provision of care to assure appropriate interventions and documentation practices. Answer C, utilization review, is the process of analyzing the provision of services to promote the most economic delivery of service. Answer D, program evaluation, is a systematic collection and reporting of outcome data to document program effectiveness and cost efficiency. See reference: Hopkins and Smith (eds): Perinchief, JM: Service management.

170. (D) The standards with which outcomes are compared. Measures are the standards, which are established based on expertise and knowledge of the service intervention. Answer B, the results a program aims to achieve, are objectives. Answer C, characteristics according to severity or barriers to success, is referred to as descriptors. Answer D, the standards with which outcomes are compared, are thresholds. See reference: Hopkins and Smith (eds): Perinchief, JM: Service management.

171. (D) The Americans with Disabilities Act of 1990. Also referred to as the ADA, this act provides civil rights protection for disabled individuals in five specific areas. These areas include telecommunications, transportation, public accommodations, employment, and the activities of state and local government. Answer A, the Architectural Barriers Act of 1969, literally opened doors for changes to occur in gaining access for disabled individuals. Answer B, the Federal Rehabilitation Act of 1973, expanded service intervention for those individuals who were more severely disabled. Answer C, the Fair Housing Amendment Act of 1988, expanded the coverage of Title VIII. See reference: Hopkins and Smith (eds): Jacobs, K: Work assessments and programming.

172. (B) Protect consumers of occupational therapy. The purpose of licensure was to protect consumers of occupational therapy services, to improve the status of occupational therapy, and thereby to provide for increased coverage of service. Answer A is the delineation of roles between occupational therapists and certified occupational therapy assistants. Even though licensure guidelines will identify generalities of the roles of OTRs and COTAs, they do not go into depth and provide detail as to their roles. Answer C, ensuring the continued levels of competency of therapists, is not the primary purpose of licensure boards. Recently, many states have initiated requiring evidence of CEUs to maintain licensure. Answer D, justifying occupational therapy services for medicare and medicaid reimbursement, is also incorrect in that this may occur, but does so primarily from third-party payors. See reference: Hopkins and Smith (eds): Hopkins, HL: Scope of occupational therapy.

173. (A) Vary in each facility. Objectives are behavioral descriptors of the expectations the student will be required to achieve. Each fieldwork site is unique in the provision of occupational therapy and, therefore, the objective may vary from site to site. Therefore, answers B, C, and D are incorrect. See reference: Hopkins and Smith (eds): Cohn, ES: Fieldwork education: Professional socialization.

174. (A) A hypothesis. A hypothesis is a predicted outcome that the researcher defines prior to conducting research. The hypothesis is based on the current knowledge regarding the topic to be studied. The question, answer B, is the origin of any research. The qualities of a research question would be that the question is reasonable and has significance to the profession. The rational or theory base, answers C and D, are a foundation of knowledge from which a treatment approach may be selected (i.e., biomechanical, neurodevelopmental, behavioral). See reference: Bailey: Introduction.

175. (D) Reinforcement and enhancement of performance. The emphasis of occupational therapy since the early 1900s has been in performance. Performance is defined by *Webster*'s as the *execution of an action*. As occupational therapists, the focus has been on reinforcing and enhancing the execution of activities. Skill refers to ability and, therefore, answers A and C are incorrect. These areas focus on acquiring abilities and attaining abilities. See reference: Hopkins and Smith (eds): Hopkins, HL: Scope of occupational therapy.

176. (A) State licensure laws supersede NBCOT guidelines in the practice of occupational therapy. AOTA and the NBCOT recommend that therapists contact the state regulatory boards because each state has legal jurisdiction over the practice of therapists within the region. Therefore, answers B, C, and D are incorrect. See reference: Hopkins and Smith (eds): Hopkins, HL: Scope of occupational therapy.

177. (B) Expanding. Gerontologic occupational therapy is anticipated to expand, based on the fact that the number of older persons is expected to increase with individuals living longer. In addition, "baby boomers" will be reaching middle and older ages in the next two decades. Therefore answers A, C, and D are incorrect. See reference: Punwar: Current trends and future outlook.

178. (D) An increase in the amount of services available on an outpatient basis. Current trends in health care are reducing inpatient hospital stays and increasing the types and amounts of services that are available on an outpatient basis. Answers A and C are incorrect because it is projected that with the population getting older and patients moving out of hospitals faster, use of nursing homes and home health will increase. Answer B is incorrect because hospitalizations are anticipated to decrease, as only individuals with more serious illnesses and higher acuities of illness will be admitted. See reference: Punwar: Current trends and future outlook.

179. (B) A consultant. A consultant provides information based on his or her skill and knowledge base. Answer A is incorrect because a therapist provides services to remediate a disorder. Answer C is incorrect because a consumer actually uses goods or services. Answer D is also incorrect because a counselor generally gives advice, as well as has some sort of supervisory role. See reference: Jaffe and Epstein: Jaffe, EG: Theoretical concepts of consultation.

180. (B) Capitation. Capitation is a uniform payment or fee per diagnosis. This form of reimbursement has evolved with health care reform. Answer A, fee for service, is an outdated concept where health care providers were paid what they billed. This type of system allowed for various forms of abuse in the health care system. Answer C, cost shifting, actually occurs when a facility increases prices for all individuals who need service to cover the shortfalls in reimbursement by other carriers. Cost control is a general concept that focuses on keeping the expenses below the revenue generated. See reference: Bair and Gray (eds): Scott, SJ, and Somers, FP: Payment for occupational therapy services.

181. (C) Home care. Within the home care environment, the therapist needs to transport equipment to the home or use what is available for a therapeutic result. Therefore, the equipment resources are MOST limited within the home care setting, thus requiring the therapist to find creative alternatives for treatment. Acute care hospitals, nursing homes, and rehabilitation hospitals typically provide equipment resources from which the therapist may draw in treatment planning. Thus, answers A, B, and D are incorrect. See reference: Hopkins and Smith (eds): Levine, R, Corcoran, M, and Gitlin, L: Home care and private practice.

182. (A) Cerebrovascular accident. The diagnosis most frequently seen by occupational therapists is cerebrovascular accident at 28.2 percent. Answer B, cerebral palsy, is 11.2 percent. Answer C, developmental delay, is the second most frequent diagnosis seen by occupational therapists at 16.5 percent. Answer D, neuromuscular disorders, are seen by occupational therapists fairly infrequently at 0.6 percent. See reference: Punwar: The practice arena of occupational therapy.

183. (B) School systems. 16.3 percent of occupational therapists in the community settings are employed in the school system. Answer A is incorrect because 6 percent are employed in private practice. Answer C is incorrect because 4.5 percent are employed in home health agencies. Answer D is incorrect because 3.5 percent are in residential care facilities. See reference: Punwar: The practice arena of occupational therapy.

184. (A) The multiple baseline design. This type of design is the only design that requires three or more baselines, which may be taken across behaviors, across subjects, or across settings. In comparison, the withdrawal design consists of a baseline, treatment, and another baseline. This design requires a return to baseline. Answers C and D refer to the same form of design, which is an alternating treatment design. These designs are used to compare and contrast individuals who had treatment with individuals who did not. A baseline is taken and followed with an intervention, which is to cause an immediate change in behavior. See reference: Hopkins and Smith (eds): Deitz, JC: Research: A systematic process for answering questions.

185. (A) Refine the question and develop the background. Once the question has been identified, a review of the literature should occur. The next step in research is to refine the question and develop the background. Answer B is the next step of the process, which is deciding on the methodology. Answers C and D come later in the research, as the researcher establishes the boundaries and then collects and analyzes qualitative data. See reference: Bailey: Introduction.

186. (D) In collecting and analyzing qualitative data. The skills of a statistician may best be used in collecting and analyzing qualitative data. Even though the statistician may have knowledge in the other areas of research and research design, this is the area in which they may be of the MOST assistance. See reference: Hopkins and Smith (eds): Deitz, JC: Research: A systematic process for answering questions.

187. (B) Writing qualitative and quantitative facts in the results section. The results section should only contain measurable results. Conclusions, interpretive, and analytical information appear in the summary or conclusion of the research. Subjective information is not typically included into research. See reference: Bailey: Reporting results and drawing conclusions.

188. (A) Medicare. Medicare is a federal program for health coverage for individuals 65 years or older, disabled individuals, or people in the end stages of renal disease. Answer A, Medicaid, is a joint federal and state program which varies widely from state to state. Third party reimbursement is provided through insurance companies. Private pay is the individual receiving services taking full responsibility for payment of those services. See reference: Bair and Gray (eds): Scott, SJ, and Somers, FP: Payment for occupational therapy services.

189. (A) DRGs. Diagnostic categories were defined in order to establish the level of payment per diagnosis. The intent of government was to impose constraints on health care spending for the beneficiaries of Medicare. PROs were established to numerically assess unnecessary procedures, client/patient deaths, and substandard care. UB-82s are forms that must be completed on each patient listing his or her diagnosis, and co-morbidity information for the purpose of reimbursement. Cost shifting is what occurs when a hospital increases its prices to all customers in order to make up for the shortfall of reimbursement by a few providers. See reference: Bair and Gray (eds): Scott, SJ, and Somers, FP: Payment for occupational therapy services.

190. (C) Assist with stock and inventory control. Volunteer interaction within an occupational therapy department should be limited so that it is in the direct line of vision of an occupational therapist. In addition, it is not appropriate for a volunteer to treat a patient in that he or she lacks the skill and expertise of an occupational therapist. Answer D is incorrect because it violates the confidentiality of the patient. See reference: Reed and Sanderson: Direct service functions.

191. (C) Ascertain facts and impressions. Similar to the assessment process for treating a patient is the process for approaching an ethical dilemma. The Savage model outlines 14 steps of ethical contemplation. The first four steps were the answers to this questions. Initially, facts and impressions need to be gathered. Once this is done, information needs to be verified with key players. The third step is to identify problems to be solved and finally to sort the decisions to be made. Answers A, B, and D therefore are not the first response. See reference: Bair and Gray (eds): Opacich, K, and Welles, C: Ethical dimensions in occupational therapy.

192. (C) An ethical dilemma. Ethical situations are clearly defined by Opacich and Wells in the *Occupational Therapy Manager*. They define an ethical dilemma as "two or more equally unpleasant alternatives that are mutually exclusive." Ethical uncertainty is described as "uncertainty of what moral principles apply or if a problem is indeed a moral problem." Ethical distress is "knowing the right course of action but feeling constrained to act by institutional rules." Unethical behavior is behavior that is in conflict with the *Occupational Therapy Code of Ethics*. See reference: Bair and Gray (eds): Opacich, K, and Welles, C: Ethical dimensions in occupational therapy.

193. (A) A reprimand. A reprimand is a formal written expression of disapproval against a therapist's conduct that is retained in the NBCOT's file. This information is also communicated privately with the individual. Answer B, a censure, is a formal written expression of disapproval which is made public. Answer C, probation, is the period of time a therapist is given to retain the counseling or education required to remain certified. Answer D is permanent loss of NBCOT certification. See reference: Hopkins and Smith (eds): Hansen, RA: Ethics in occupational therapy.

194. (D) Revocation. Revocation is the permanent loss of certification from the National Board for Certification in Occupational Therapy (NBCOT). Answer A, a reprimand, is a formal written expression of disapproval against a therapist's conduct that is retained in the NBCOT's file. This information is also communicated privately with the individual. Answer B, a censure, is a formal written expression of disapproval which is made public. Answer C, probation, is the period of time a therapist is given to retain the counseling or education required to remain certified. See reference: Hopkins and Smith (eds): Hansen, RA: Ethics in occupational therapy.

195. (B) Competence. Principle 2 of the *Occupational Therapy Code of Ethics* is competence. This refers specifically to credentialing and the therapist functioning within the parameters of their skill level. Therapists are guided to refer patients to other service areas when the skills required do not fall within their expertise. Answer A, beneficence/autonomy, speaks to the concern that is to be demonstrated by a therapist towards patients. This includes provision of services without discrimination, providing appropriate information to patients regarding education/research, and involvement of the patient in treatment planning. Answer C, compliance with laws and regulations, is Principle 3. This principle refers to therapists following state, local, and federal in addition to facility-specific guidelines and requirements for accreditation. Answer D, public information, addresses the therapist accurately representing his or her expertise as well as not participating in any fraudulent statements or claims. See reference: Hopkins and Smith (eds): Hansen, RA: Ethics in occupational therapy.

196. (A) A guide to promote the highest standards of behavior. This answer is the purpose of the *Occupational Therapy Code of Ethics.* Answer B, "guidelines to assist the occupational therapist in the provision of services," is the answer that describes the purpose of the *Revision: Standards of Practice for Occupational Therapy.* Answer C, "a guide to assist the practitioner in identifying career options and developing career plans," is the purpose of the *Occupational Therapy Roles.* Answer D, "a document to assist therapist in applying uniform terminology," is the purpose of the *Uniform Terminology.* See reference: The American Occupational Therapy Association: Representative assembly.

197. (C) A guide to assist the practitioner in identifying career options and developing career plans. This answer is the purpose of the *Occupational Therapy Roles.* Answer A, "a guide to promote the highest standards of behavior," is the purpose of the *Occupational Therapy Code of Ethics.* Answer B, "guidelines to assist the occupational therapist in the provision of services," describes the purpose of the *Revision: Standards of Practice for Occupational Therapy.* Answer D, "a document to assist therapist in applying uniform terminology," is the purpose of the *Uniform Terminology.* See reference: AOTA: The Occupational Therapy Roles Task Force: Occupational Therapy Roles.

198. (D) To provide standard language for the description of occupational therapy services. This answer is the purpose of the *Uniform Terminology.* Answer A, "a guide to promote the highest standards of behavior," is a document referred to as the *Occupational Therapy Code of Ethics.* Answer B, "guidelines to assist the occupational therapist in the provision of services," describes the purpose of the *Revision: Standards of Practice for Occupational Therapy.* Answer C, the *Occupational Therapy Roles,* is "a guide to assist the practitioner in identifying career options and developing career plans." See reference: Hopkins and Smith (eds): Uniform Terminology Task Force: Appendix C.

199. (D) Health promotion. Health promotion is the advancement of healthy lifestyles, which may include education, behavioral change, and cultural support. Answer A, occupational behavior, is the developmental continuum of play to work. Answer B, synchrony, is actually the provision of treatment. Answer C, self efficacy, would be promoting the positive effects of occupational therapy services. See reference: Hopkins and Smith (eds): Levy, LL: The health care delivery system today.

200. (A) Efficacy studies. Efficacy studies demonstrate positive results in the ideal circumstances. Answer B, efficiency studies, compare outcomes of service compared with costs. Answer C, effectiveness studies, just look at the outcomes. Answer D, expenditure studies, just look at the cost of services. See reference: Punwar: Overview of occupational therapy.

SIMULATION EXAMINATION 3

Directions: Circle the correct answer to the following questions. When you have completed this examination, check your answers against the answer key that follows. As you will see, an explanation is given for each answer along with a reference for further study. The book author is listed as well as the chapter author. See the bibliography for complete references. Study the areas in which your comprehension was low, then test yourself again by taking Simulation Examination 4.

PEDIATRICS QUESTIONS

Assessment of Occupational Performance

1. A therapist evaluating a baby in the supine position observes that the infant is able to turn its head independently from the trunk to hear a sound. The therapist should conclude that the ability present in this child is:
   A. labyrinthine reaction.
   B. neck righting reaction.
   C. body righting on body reaction.
   D. optical righting reaction.

2. The asymmetrical tonic neck reflex pattern, when seen during the evaluation of a 1-year-old child, is considered to be:
   A. normal.
   B. abnormal.
   C. developmentally appropriate.
   D. developmentally inappropriate.

3. A 4-month-old infant being seen for an occupational therapy assessment shows a strong preference for the left hand when reaching for a rattle at midline. Considering the development of dominance in normal children, the therapist should conclude that:
   A. further observation of right body side for dysfunction is needed.
   B. development of hand dominance is proceeding in a typical manner.
   C. hand dominance will not develop until 1 year of age.
   D. unilaterality precedes bilaterality in typical development.

4. A 3-year-old child with spastic cerebral palsy uses "bunny-hopping" for functional mobility during the occupational therapy evaluation. This means that a primitive pattern is being used for mobility, specifically:
   A. symmetrical tonic neck reflex.
   B. asymmetrical tonic neck reflex.
   C. tonic labyrinthine reflex.
   D. neck righting reflex.

5. A 6-month-old child, when pulled into sitting with several trials, demonstrates a head lag. The therapist evaluating this child should conclude that head control is:
   A. developing in a typical manner.
   B. slightly delayed by 1 month.
   C. significantly delayed by several months.
   D. advanced.

6. A therapist is developing a treatment plan for an 18-month-old child with Down syndrome. The child needs to develop vertical righting reactions. Which of the following is a vertical righting reaction?
   A. neck righting reaction.
   B. body righting on body reaction.
   C. labyrinthine righting reaction.
   D. asymmetrical tonic neck reflex.

7. A 5-year-old child with Down syndrome and low muscle tone sits on the floor exclusively using a "W" sitting position (buttocks between heels). How should the therapist interpret this finding?
   A. Normal developmental skill, age appropriate
   B. Compensatory position to achieve stability
   C. Compensatory position to achieve mobility
   D. Normal developmental skill, but delayed

8. A child with athetoid cerebral palsy is able to reach and grasp a toy at "end ranges of shoulder and elbow control only." The therapist would interpret this finding, from a neurodevelopmental treatment frame of reference, as a problem with what area of concern?

A. Reciprocal innervation
B. Dissociation of movement
C. Stability and mobility
D. Delayed righting and equilibrium reactions

9. **A 6-month-old infant has begun to sit and is leaning forward onto his arms. The therapist assessing the child notes that this child is able to coactivate muscle groups around the shoulder and arm in order to bear weight on arms in sitting, or the child has developed:**
   A. protective reactions.
   B. equilibrium reactions.
   C. rotational righting reactions.
   D. support reactions.

Development of the Treatment Plan

10. **A child with a severe physical disability and no cognitive delays does not have a form of functional mobility. At what age should a powered wheelchair first be considered for this child?**
    A. 2 years
    B. 4 years
    C. 6 years
    D. 8 years

11. **When adapting a tricycle for a child with cerebral palsy, the child's tendency to flex forward increases when hip and lower extremities are positioned correctly. What further adaptation should solve this problem?**
    A. Raise the seat height.
    B. Raise the handle bars.
    C. Lower the seat height.
    D. Lower the handle bars.

12. **A 5-year-old child with spina bifida has developed daytime control of bowel and bladder, but not nighttime control. At what age for a typical child should the therapist consider lack of nighttime control as a delay and consider development of a therapeutic program?**
    A. 2 years
    B. 3 years
    C. 4 years
    D. 5 to 6 years

13. **A child with a physical handicap and poor postural stability is developmentally ready for toileting. Which of the following elements of a treatment plan should be considered first?**
    A. Training in management of fasteners
    B. Provision of foot support
    C. Provision of a seat belt
    D. Training in climbing onto the toilet

14. **A 3-year-old child with a disability of mental retardation is dependent in all areas of dressing skills. Which of the following abilities should** be addressed first by the therapist using a developmental approach?
    A. Correct arrangement of front and back of clothing
    B. Donning a t-shirt
    C. Doffing socks
    D. Buttoning and tying bows

15. **An ultralight wheelchair would be an appropriate wheelchair feature for a child with the following functional needs:**
    A. sliding transfers
    B. desk work
    C. wheeling efficiency
    D. work surface height adjustment

16. **Although the use of an adaptive device that supports the child for functional mobility in creeping may be helpful for the developmental and mobility experience, a disadvantage would be:**
    A. transitional movements to sitting are restricted.
    B. leg movements are restricted.
    C. arm movements are restricted.
    D. weight-bearing is restricted.

17. **In planning a therapeutic dressing program for a 5-year-old child who is mentally retarded, the therapist's first consideration should be the:**
    A. need for adaptive equipment.
    B. need for adaptive clothing.
    C. need for self-dressing adaptive techniques.
    D. need for adapted teaching techniques.

18. **The treatment plan for a child with a visual discrimination problem should include the following adaptation of visual material:**
    A. low contrast and defined borders.
    B. high contrast and defined borders.
    C. high contrast and unclear borders.
    D. low contrast and unclear borders.

19. **A child with visual perceptual problems may also have language problems which relate to spatial concepts. If a child can locate visually and understand directions about the "down" spatial concept, the appropriate next step in the therapeutic program would be development of:**
    A. behind.
    B. in.
    C. up.
    D. under.

20. **When planning a therapeutic program for a child who has visual discrimination problems, the first step would be to provide "matching" activities, which require discrimination in the areas of:**
    A. object function.
    B. object characteristics or details.
    C. object color, shape, and position.
    D. object recognition.

21. Using a visual perceptual frame of reference, the first step in planning a program for a child with visual perceptual problems would be to consider:
    A. visual memory skills.
    B. visual attention skills.
    C. general visual discrimination skills.
    D. specific visual discrimination skills.

22. The therapist is teaching a parent to change a diaper for a 2-year-old child who has spastic cerebral palsy. The child exhibits poor trunk balance and severe extensor and adductor patterns in the legs. The best method of inhibitory positioning to teach this parent is to have the child:
    A. supine, flex and abduct legs.
    B. prone over the parent's thighs; flex and abduct legs.
    C. in sitting with back supported and resting against parent's trunk, flex and adduct legs.
    D. prone over parent's thighs, extend and adduct legs.

23. When dressing a child with spastic cerebral palsy (predominantly extensor tone in lower extremities), which method, used before donning socks and shoes, would make the activity easier?
    A. Extend the hip and knee.
    B. Flex the hip and knee.
    C. Extend the shoulders.
    D. Dorsiflex the ankle.

24. A child with poor balance is unable to don and doff lower extremity clothing. Which of the following approaches would best deal with the functional problem?
    A. Child dresses in a sidelying position.
    B. Loops added to waistband of pants and skirts.
    C. Velcro fasteners applied instead of zippers.
    D. The child dresses while in a standing position.

25. The therapist is demonstrating how to bathe a child with hypertonic muscle tone to the parent. Which of the following approaches should be employed?
    A. Avoid using adaptive equipment.
    B. Provide few explanations of procedure.
    C. Handle the child slowly and gently.
    D. Stand and lean over the tub to support and wash child.

Implementation of the Treatment Plan

26. The sidelying position provides the infant the opportunity to work against gravity to develop:
    A. elongation on the nonweight-bearing side.
    B. extension on the nonweight-bearing side.
    C. elongation on the weight-bearing side.
    D. skilled arm movements on the weight bearing side.

27. The position that best provides the normal infant with the opportunity to develop the ability of trunk rotation is the:
    A. supine position.
    B. prone position.
    C. sidelying position.
    D. sitting position.

28. The standing position provides the normal infant with opportunities to develop the ability of:
    A. anterior pelvic tilt.
    B. posterior pelvic tilt.
    C. neutral pelvic position.
    D. flexor activity.

29. The therapist who teaches families therapeutic handling techniques, which can increase the opportunities for children with cerebral palsy to move with "more normal" patterns of movement, is using the following theoretical frame of reference:
    A. neurodevelopmental.
    B. sensory integrative.
    C. coping.
    D. biomechanical.

30. A child with a learning disability has difficulty attending to visual stimuli (i.e., as in textbook and chalkboard reading). The appropriate therapeutic approach would be to:
    A. provide visual tasks of low interest to the child.
    B. increase stimulation surrounding the visual task.
    C. provide visual tasks that lack novelty.
    D. prepare the child mentally and physically for visual tasks.

31. A child with a learning disability has significant problems with visual memory. The therapist may use the following approach to enhance visual memory:
    A. provide memory tasks which are of low interest to the child.
    B. decrease visual attention prior to memory tasks.
    C. combine task with additional sensory input (tactile, proprioceptive, and auditory).
    D. repeat the visual memory task one time.

32. After 6 months of therapy, a 5-year-old child with mild cerebral palsy is able to roll over to prone, rise to quadruped, and then push off of the floor to rise into standing. What would be the next developmental sequence in treatment for rising from supine to standing?
    A. The child will rise symmetrically to sitting, and then directly to standing with no rotation.
    B. The child will rise symmetrically to sitting, and then partially rotate to standing.
    C. The child partially rotates to sitting, and then partially rotates to standing.
    D. The child partially rotates to sitting, and then completely rotates toward prone, to then push on the floor in order to stand.

33. The therapist has been working with an 8-year-old child who has sensory-motor problems related to a learning disability. Objectives of treatment have included development of wrist extension, hand strength, and in-hand manipulation skills to improve pencil grasp and control. The child is now able to use a pencil for writing with a "dynamic tripod grasp." In terms of evaluating the treatment plan, this change means that:
    A. the child's pencil skills continue to be delayed.
    B. treatment for this problem may be discontinued.
    C. treatment for this problem should continue.
    D. other children his age have also just developed this pencil grasp.

34. A child with a learning disability has difficulty integrating visual, auditory, vestibular, and somatosensory stimuli, and responds to stimuli primarily with defensiveness. The area of the central nervous system which serves as a center for these functions would be the:
    A. reticular formation.
    B. superior and inferior colliculi.
    C. cerebral cortex.
    D. cerebellum.

35. A child with sensory-motor problems has difficulty performing a rapid alternating of forearm rotation (diadokinesis). This is a function of the:
    A. brain stem.
    B. cerebellum.
    C. thalamus.
    D. cerebral cortex.

Case Study

Megan is a 7-year-old girl with a diagnosis of spina bifida (myelomeningocele). A neurosurgical excision and closure surgery was completed soon after birth to repair the defect in the lumbosacral area. She also needed a shunt procedure (ventroperitoneal) due to presence of hydrocephalus, which developed after the repair of her back. Megan has had difficulty with recurring urinary infections. Her spine shows lumbosacral scoliosis, and equinovarus deformities are seen in the feet. She has fine motor coordination problems in the upper extremities. Megan wears long-leg braces when using a walker, but her primary mode of mobility is a wheelchair. Answer the following questions regarding this case study.

36. With Megan's condition of myelomeningocele, the major concern of medical treatment because it is the major cause of death is:
    A. respiratory infection.
    B. renal failure.
    C. spinal cord degeneration.
    D. hydrocephalus.

37. Megan's case study states that she has an equinovarus deformity of the foot. This means she has a/an:
    A. enlarged great toe.
    B. club foot.
    C. pronated foot.
    D. unstable heel.

38. Considering Megan's age, which of the following signs of shunt malfunction should be monitored by family and therapists?
    A. Increased head size
    B. Nausea and vomiting
    C. Back pain
    D. Intermittent headaches

39. Using an understanding of "neuroplasticity" as a guide, a therapist may focus therapeutic programming at their agency or school on the following population first:
    A. infants and toddlers.
    B. preschool aged children.
    C. elementary school-aged children.
    D. adolescents.

Evaluation of the Treatment Plan

40. The therapist has placed a child in prone on a wedge in order to develop vertical head righting. However, the child fatigues rapidly. What adjustment can the therapist make in the wedge that will make working in this position more successful for the child?
    A. Increase the height of the wedge (side A on diagram).
    B. Decrease the height of the wedge (side A on diagram).
    C. Shorten the length of the wedge (side B on diagram).
    D. Lengthen the wedge (side B on the diagram).

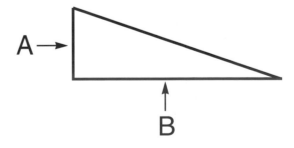

41. The therapist is positioning a child with poor muscle tone and postural stability in a prone stander to develop head righting. The child rapidly shows fatigue and associated reactions. How can the therapist best adjust the stander to decrease these reactions and yet work on the goal?

A. Place the child in prone on the floor.
B. Position the stander at 45 degrees from the floor.
C. Position the stander at 75 to 90 degrees from the floor.
D. Position the child upright in a prone or supine stander.

42. **A 10-year-old child with significantly low muscle tone due to Duchenne's muscular dystrophy is losing trunk control in sitting. Which of the following frames of references should the therapist consider when re-evaluating the treatment program?**
    A. Neurodevelopmental treatment
    B. Sensory integration
    C. Biomechanical
    D. Visual perceptual

43. **A young child with hypertonic muscle tone is unable to bring his hands to midline to reach for a toy while in the supine or sitting positions. The position that would be the best choice to incorporate next into the treatment plan, in order to reduce the effects of abnormal patterns and facilitate midline grasp, would be:**
    A. standing.
    B. prone.
    C. sidelying.
    D. quadruped.

44. **After many months of therapy, a 3-year-old child with Down syndrome has begun to demonstrate protective reactions when falling to either side. What type of arm movements have been facilitated?**
    A. Flexion
    B. Extension
    C. Internal rotation
    D. External rotation

45. **A child with sensory integration problems is demonstrating involvement of the limbic system. Which of the following answers describes the functions of this structure?**
    A. Regulator of several basic and vital functions of the CNS
    B. Smooth, orderly sequencing of the direction, extent, force time, and tone of movement
    C. Provides motivating force behind basic behaviors and personality traits
    D. Provides background movement patterns necessary for postural adaptation

Discharge Planning

46. **A therapist needs to explain to the parents of a child with cerebral palsy the importance of a correct sitting position for use of the hands in activity. Their child uses compensatory movements due to an inability to sit independently. What aspect of therapeutic positioning does the therapist need to emphasize as crucial for this child?**
    A. Stabilizing the trunk
    B. Weight on the arms
    C. Stabilizing the pelvis, hips, and legs
    D. Stabilizing the head and neck

47. **While making a discharge plan for a child with cerebral palsy, the therapist has decided that further modification must be made on the child's sidelyer. The therapist has observed increasing head extension and shoulder retraction when the child is positioned more than a few minutes. The technique that will improve this problem is:**
    A. increasing body flexion in general.
    B. rolling the child forward slightly.
    C. increasing lateral head flexion.
    D. extending both legs.

48. **A therapist is planning discharge for a child with paraplegic spina bifida who has just begun using a powered wheelchair. The community resource that will be most critical for this child is:**
    A. the local social service agency.
    B. a local wheelchair equipment vendor.
    C. the family physician.
    D. an early intervention program.

49. **A school-aged child with residual visual perceptual problems is being discharged from occupational therapy. Which compensatory technique would the therapist share with this child's teacher to assist with visual figure-ground problems?**
    A. Place a red line on the left side of the paper.
    B. Use a timer for certain activities.
    C. Teach the child to use lists and color coding of books and folders.
    D. Block out all areas of the page except important words.

50. **During discharge planning, a therapist is explaining how the wheelchair is adjusted to limit a child's hypertonic extension pattern. The adjustment which will fill this need is:**
    A. lengthening back support.
    B. use of a hip strap.
    C. use of a shoulder harness.
    D. increased angle of flexion at the hip.

PHYSICAL DISABILITY QUESTIONS

Assessment of Occupational Performance

51. **When the therapist is assessing the sense of proprioception at an individual's joint, movement within the range should be performed:**

A. until pain is elicited.
B. until the stretch reflex is elicited.
C. at the end ranges of the joint.
D. at the midrange of the joint.

52. **An individual who had a stroke is copying a picture of a clock. The drawing appears as a lopsided circle with a flat side on the left. The numbers one through eight are written in numerical order around the right side of the clock. The hands are correctly drawn on the clock to represent three o'clock. The individual's performance demonstrates:**
    A. right hemianopia.
    B. left unilateral neglect.
    C. cataracts in the left eye.
    D. bitemporal hemianopia.

53. **Which skills are necessary when completing the "Draw a Clock" test?**
    A. Visual memory, number sequencing, and constructional praxis
    B. Intact body image, visual sequencing, and 20/20 vision
    C. Auditory memory, visual closure, and proprioception
    D. Proprioception, body image, and visual memory

54. **An individual demonstrates normal range of motion in flexion of the elbow but hyperextends by 15 degrees when the elbow is straightened. The measurement should be recorded as:**
    A. −15 degrees to 140 degrees.
    B. 0.0 degrees to 140 degrees.
    C. 15 degrees to 140 degrees
    D. −15 degrees to 120 degrees.

55. **A therapist who has an individual repeat a list of random numbers 1 minute after hearing the list is evaluating:**
    A. short-term recall.
    B. attention.
    C. hearing.
    D. abstraction.

56. **An individual is sent to occupational therapy with a diagnosis of polymyositis and dermatomyositis. The individual is able to complete full range of shoulder flexion while in supine. However, against gravity, she is only able to achieve 50 percent of range for shoulder flexion. The grade for the muscle would be:**
    A. good (4).
    B. fair (3).
    C. fair minus (3−).
    D. poor plus (2+).

57. **The occupational therapist has assigned a level II fieldwork student to assess an individual with a closed-head injury and a fractured tibia (nonweight bearing). The student reports that the man answered his telephone when it was** not ringing in the room and frequently attempted to stand in spite of being restrained in the wheelchair with a seat belt. The man talked frequently about models of cars and coffee, and when questioned, invented a family. The man was able to comb his hair with verbal and physical cues and to brush his teeth impulsively after squirting the toothpaste in his mouth instead of on the toothbrush. The student would describe the man as functioning at which level on the Rancho Los Amigos Levels of Cognitive Functioning?
    A. Confused–Agitated (level IV)
    B. Confused–Inappropriate (level V)
    C. Confused–Appropriate (level VI)
    D. Automatic–Appropriate (level VII)

58. **A rating scale for head-injured individuals that uses a numerical scale to rate three types of response by the head-injured individual is the:**
    A. Rancho Los Amigos Levels of Cognitive Functioning.
    B. Claudia Allen Scale of Cognitive Functioning.
    C. Braintree Hospital Cognitive Continuum.
    D. Glasgow Coma Scale.

59. **Hypersensitivity training is graded from:**
    A. soft to hard to rough.
    B. tap to rub to touch.
    C. light to medium to heavy.
    D. rough to hard to soft.

60. **A person unable to name or demonstrate the use of common objects is exhibiting:**
    A. apraxia.
    B. stereognosis.
    C. visual agnosia.
    D. alexia.

61. **When performing sensation testing on an individual, the occupational therapist should do the following:**
    A. apply the stimuli distally to proximally.
    B. test the involved area first, then the uninvolved area.
    C. test stimuli should be presented in an organized pattern to improve reliability during retesting.
    D. apply the stimuli to the uninvolved area proximally to distally in a random pattern.

Development of the Treatment Plan

62. **Education of an individual with absent sensation should include:**
    A. training to inspect for pressure sores on bony prominences and affected areas.
    B. careful trimming of fingernails and toenails.
    C. providing padding to areas of a splint that cause redness on the individual.
    D. hypersensitivity training.

63. **Rood facilitation techniques include which of the following:**
    A. fast brushing, slow icing, and slow stroking.
    B. light stroking, fast brushing, and quick stretch.
    C. slow brushing and slow rolling.
    D. slow brushing, fast icing, and slow rolling.

64. **Teaching a task one step at a time and gradually adding more steps is called:**
    A. repetition.
    B. cuing.
    C. rehearsal.
    D. chaining.

65. **Which two tactile senses are the earliest to recover after a peripheral nerve injury?**
    A. Vibration and pain
    B. Temperature and pain
    C. Light touch and proprioception
    D. Tactile localization and proprioception

66. **An individual with an intravenous drug use problem has developed AIDS. The evaluation by occupational therapy determined the individual's major problems were with daily tasks (ADLs), self esteem, physical deconditioning, and anxiety. Which of the following approaches would be beneficial to the individual?**
    A. stress reduction using meditation and yoga, energy conservation, establishment of new leisure skills, and involvement with a support group
    B. re-establish former leisure skills, provide vocational training, and encourage participation in aerobic activities
    C. provide vocational training and video lectures on AIDs
    D. energy conservation, re-establish former leisure skills, and encourage participation in aerobic activities

67. **What type of feeding equipment would be MOST appropriate for an individual with a C5 spinal cord injury?**
    A. A wrist-driven flexor hinge splint
    B. A mobile arm support
    C. An electric self-feeder
    D. Built-up handled silverware

68. **The therapist is working with a confused individual who has difficulty placing his feet into his pants legs. A prefunctional treatment activity would be:**
    A. pulling up pants during toileting activities.
    B. teaching the individual to use a reacher to pull his pants up to knee level.
    C. doffing socks using a dressing stick.
    D. having him place his feet through loops of therapeutic band.

69. **Teaching a new method to perform an activity or skill is called:**
    A. problem solving.
    B. retraining.
    C. substitution.
    D. compensation.

70. **How quickly would sensation return in a hand that experienced an injury affecting both myelinated and unmyelinated fibers?**
    A. Myelinated and unmyelinated fibers recover at the same rate.
    B. Myelinated fibers would recover faster than unmyelinated fibers.
    C. Unmyelinated fibers would recover faster than myelinated fibers.
    D. Unmyelinated fibers would recover, but myelinated fibers would not recover.

71. **What hand position should an individual with quadriplegia as a result of a spinal cord injury maintain when performing weight-bearing activities?**
    A. Fingers extended and adducted
    B. Fingers flexed at all joints
    C. Fingers extended and abducted
    D. Fingers adducted and flexed only at the metacarpalphalangeal joints

72. **A continuous passive range of motion machine would be indicated for:**
    A. peripheral edema following an ulnar nerve reattachment.
    B. a fractured humerus and clavicle following an accident.
    C. finger flexion and extension in a person with ulnar drift from rheumatoid arthritis.
    D. peripheral edema following a cerebrovascular accident.

73. **When training an individual in meal preparation, the training would begin with:**
    A. a peanut butter and jelly sandwich.
    B. a hot cup of tea with sugar.
    C. a glass of orange juice.
    D. a grilled ham and cheese sandwich.

Implementation of the Treatment Plan

74. **When a person sees the relationship between cognitive or ADL training and daily life, carry-over is:**
    A. increased.
    B. decreased.
    C. unchanged.
    D. short term.

75. **An individual with which level of spinal cord injury would MOST benefit from using a wrist driven flexor hinge splint during functional activity?**
    A. C1
    B. C3
    C. C8
    D. T10

76. **An individual with Alzheimer's disease has difficulty following multiple step instructions. Which method will the therapist instruct the caregiver to use when presenting instructions?**
   A. One or two step instructions frequently repeated.
   B. Three step instructions with gestures for demonstration.
   C. Write instructions down that are over three steps for the individual.
   D. Have individual verbally repeat instructions after the therapist gives them.

77. **A swan neck deformity is:**
   A. hyperextension of the PIP and DIP joints.
   B. hyperextension of the PIP joint and flexion of the DIP joint.
   C. flexion of the PIP joint and hyperextension of the DIP joint.
   D. hyperextension of the MP joint and flexion of the PIP joint.

78. **An individual exhibits sensory changes only over the dorsum thumb and proximal phalanx of the index, long, and half of the ring finger. The therapist will MOST likely suspect involvement of the:**
   A. ulnar nerve.
   B. median nerve.
   C. radial nerve.
   D. brachial plexus.

79. **An individual demonstrates progressive weakness of the thumb, including atrophy of the thenar muscles as well as numbness and tingling in the index, long, and radial portion of the ring finger. The therapist will MOST likely suspect:**
   A. ulnar nerve.
   B. median nerve.
   C. radial nerve.
   D. brachial plexus.

80. **A power grip would MOST likely be used to hold:**
   A. a sewing needle while it is being threaded.
   B. a tall glass half filled with water.
   C. a heavy handbag held by the strap.
   D. a key while it is being placed in a lock.

81. **Inability to begin a task or activity may denote problems with:**
   A. attention.
   B. concentration.
   C. initiation.
   D. apraxia.

82. **An individual with a head injury is impulsive during self feeding. This is exemplified by placing too much food in her mouth at one time. What method may be used to control the rate of intake during self feeding?**
   A. Cut the food into smaller pieces.

   B. Have the individual count to 10 between bites of food.
   C. Have the individual set the utensil down until the mouth is cleared.
   D. Serve the food in separate containers on the meal tray.

83. **External memory devices include:**
   A. visual imagery and a diary.
   B. labeling and calendars.
   C. mnemonics and verbal cues.
   D. log and repetition.

84. **The therapist instructs the individual to pick up a cup with the left upper extremity, and place it in the sink to his right side while keeping the right upper extremity on the counter. The goals of this activity include weight shifting to the right side and weight bearing on the right upper extremity while incorporating trunk rotation to the right. Where should the cup be positioned initially in order to elicit the greatest amount of movement in the desired movement pattern?**
   A. The cup is placed at waist height and slightly left of midline.
   B. The cup is placed to the left and below waist line.
   C. The cup is placed to the right and below waist line.
   D. The cup is placed at waist height and slightly right of midline.

85. **The individual, who in the 1920s delineated principles for matching activities to individuals with specific diagnoses in order to achieve a therapeutic result, was:**
   A. Rood.
   B. Brunnstrom.
   C. Meyer.
   D. Dunton.

86. **During feeding training, what type of liquid is the most difficult to swallow?**
   A. Shake made with lime sorbet
   B. Tomato juice
   C. Coffee with nondairy creamer
   D. Lemonade

87. **An individual demonstrates internal rotation of the shoulder to 70 degrees. This range is:**
   A. within normal limits.
   B. within functional limits.
   C. hypermobile and needs further treatment.
   D. limited and needs further treatment.

88. **The first adaptive response to a disabling condition, which would normally pass in time without intervention, would be referred to as:**
   A. a dependency reaction.
   B. stress reactions.
   C. a grief response.
   D. a desire to set unrealistic goals.

89. An individual with joint changes that limit finger flexion would be more comfortable using utensils with:
   A. regular handles.
   B. weighted handles.
   C. a universal cuff attachment.
   D. built-up handles.

Evaluation of the Treatment Plan

90. During morning self care, an individual is able to place his dentures in his mouth, but has difficulty applying denture cream to the appropriate place on the dentures and attempts to place the cap on the tube backwards or on the wrong end of the tube. This individual most likely has:
   A. constructional apraxia.
   B. ideomotor apraxia.
   C. dressing apraxia.
   D. unilateral neglect.

91. While in occupational therapy, an individual with C6 quadriplegia complains of a headache, chills, and sweating. The therapist should immediately:
   A. tip the individual's chair backwards to increase his or her blood pressure.
   B. take the individual's heart rate and blood pressure.
   C. give the individual fruit juice to increase blood sugar levels.
   D. unclamp the individual's catheter and tap over the bladder.

92. An individual who is unable to see buttons on a printed fabric may be having difficulty with:
   A. spatial relations.
   B. figure-ground perception.
   C. body image.
   D. visual closure.

93. An alert, motivated individual who had a cerebrovascular accident affecting the parietal lobe is unable to learn compensation techniques for neglect after many ADL training sessions. This individual has a condition called:
   A. attentional deficit.
   B. apraxia.
   C. aphasia.
   D. anosognosia.

94. An individual stops after performing only one part of a self-care task and requires prompting to continue, although the individual is able to correctly list the next steps in the activity. This individual demonstrates difficulty with:
   A. impulsivity.
   B. initiation.
   C. memory.
   D. attention.

Discharge Planning

95. An individual who is being discharged home after participating in an inpatient pulmonary rehabilitation program for Chronic Obstructive Pulmonary Disease (COPD) is given a list of "tips" to use in the home to promote function. Which one of the following items is MOST likely to be on the list?
   A. Perform pursed lip breathing when doing activities.
   B. Use a long handled sponge while in the shower.
   C. Take hot showers to reduce congestion.
   D. Avoid air conditioned rooms during warm months.

96. Which of the following precautions should be included in a home program for an individual who had a total knee replacement?
   A. Avoid hip flexion past 80 degrees, and internal rotation.
   B. Avoid full knee extension.
   C. Limit weight bearing on the involved extremity.
   D. Limit full weight bearing on the uninvolved lower extremity.

97. An individual who has had a cerebrovascular accident with subsequent left hemiparesis is returning home to live with her husband and children after discharge. Prior to onset, the individual's primary role was a homemaker. To enable the individual to carry out her prior responsibility of meal preparation, what item would be recommended for stabilization when cutting a potato?
   A. A piece of nonskid backing under the cutting board
   B. A plate guard around the edge of the board
   C. A rocker knife
   D. A cutting board with two nails in it

98. The occupational therapist is training an individual in the principles of joint protection prior to discharge. These principles would include:
   A. using the strongest joint, avoiding positions of deformity, and ensuring correct patterns of movement.
   B. massaging a joint before exercise.
   C. practicing vivid imagery and relaxation exercises during difficult functional activities.
   D. application of heat before treatment and application of cold after range-of-motion treatment.

99. An individual with a high level spinal cord injury is returning home. What type of adaptive technology would the individual need to ensure safety?
   A. An environmental control unit.
   B. A call system for emergency and nonemergency use.

C. A remote control power door opener.

D. An electric page turner.

100. **Which piece of equipment would continue to be used at home by an individual with a total hip arthroplasty?**

A. A wire basket attached to a walker.

B. A padded foam toilet seat 1 inch in height.

C. A short handled bath sponge.

D. A long handled bath sponge.

PSYCHOSOCIAL QUESTIONS

Assessment of Occupational Performance

101. **In the review of an adolescent individual's chart, the DSM IV, Axis V diagnosis shows a score of 35. The BEST interpretation of functioning with this score is:**

A. slight impairment in social and school functioning (e.g., falls behind in schoolwork).

B. moderate difficulty in social or school functioning (e.g., few friends).

C. major impairment in several areas (e.g., defiant at home and failing at school).

D. serious impairment in communication or judgement (e.g., suicidal preoccupation).

102. **The following medication is considered to be an antipsychotic agent:**

A. Lithium carbonate.

B. Elavil.

C. Xanax.

D. Thorazine.

103. **According to OBRA (Omnibus Budget Reconciliation Act of 1987), the criteria that individuals with mental health problems must meet in order to be admitted to a nursing home is:**

A. the individual has Medicare.

B. the individual has Medicaid.

C. the individual's diagnosis is mental retardation.

D. the individual's diagnosis is mental illness or mental retardation with nursing care needs requiring active treatment.

104. **The therapist is working with an adult female whose admission to a psychiatric unit is related to her heavy drinking problem. The therapist should also expect that:**

A. her parents were substance abusers.

B. she has been asked whether she has been sexually or physically abused by other care givers.

C. she has received treatment for self-mutilating behaviors in the past.

D. she volunteered to someone on the treatment team that she has been abused in her past.

105. **The therapist reviews the 24-hour log of activities completed by a young Japanese-American man for the day before his admission to a mental health unit for depression. The therapist notices there are no leisure activities recorded on the log. The BEST interpretation for the therapist to make is:**

A. this individual has diminished involvement in leisure pursuits secondary to the onset of his depression.

B. this individual's absence of leisure involvement is an appropriate referral to the therapeutic recreation specialist.

C. that Asian-American's do not typically value leisure involvement.

D. this individual's satisfaction with the activities he listed on the log may not fit into work, leisure, and self-care categories.

106. **The occupational therapist is working in an eating disorders treatment program. The individuals that the therapist is MOST likely to treat in this program are:**

A. bulimics who weigh less than their normal body weight.

B. females over the age of 30.

C. males under the age of 30.

D. bulimics who are at or above their normal body weight.

107. **The following community vocational service that adults with mental retardation are most commonly referred to is:**

A. an adult activity center.

B. supported employment.

C. job coaching.

D. a sheltered workshop.

108. **The term that indicates a diagnosis from two mental diagnostic categories is:**

A. dual diagnosis.

B. multiply handicapped.

C. axis I and II duplicity.

D. primary and secondary diagnoses.

109. **Early stages of Dementia, Alzheimer's type, may be detected in behaviors such as:**

A. difficulty swallowing food.

B. forgetting to turn off the stove burner.

C. angry outbursts at close family members.

D. restless pacing around the house.

Development of the Treatment Plan

110. **An adolescent individual diagnosed with this disorder is most likely to engage in aggressive and violent behavior:**

A. Asperger's disorder

B. Attention deficit disorder

C. Conduct disorder

D. Oppositional defiant disorder

111. The approach that describes an occupational therapist's role when providing forensic psychiatry services is:
    A. helping individuals with criminal histories before they receive psychiatric medications and counseling.
    B. planning and implementing recreational and leisure activities in a prison setting.
    C. assessing and submitting reports for a competency hearing that determines an individual's ability to manage his or her own funds.
    D. providing treatment to individuals who are admitted to a locked psychiatric inpatient unit for individuals whose treatment is required by the court.

Questions 112–116 refer to this sample document

The Columbia-Madison Hospital

Section A. Individual is a 49-year-old WMM admitted to the unit with a diagnosis of major depression. Pt's self care, work, and leisure involvement were seriously impaired prior to admission as reported by his outpatient counselor at CMHC. Pt. referred to occupational therapy for evaluation and treatment.

Section B. Individual is unable to identify leisure interests.

Section C. Individual will identify two possible community locations offering leisure activities within 3 miles of individual's home prior to discharge. Individual will identify three new leisure interests that he wants to pursue at discharge.

Section D.   3-13-94; 4:00 PM
    "I really don't have any plans for myself once I go home."
    Individual identified 4 solitary and 2 leisure interests involving others at the casual interest level on the Interest Checklist Inventory. Individual's pattern and strength of leisure interests are inadequate to support leisure resource exploration in his community. Schedule individual to attend leisure group 3–4 times/week with focus on leisure interest exploration.
                                        Betty Smith, OTR/L

112. In section D of the sample document, the assessment and analysis statement is:
    A. "I really don't have any plans for myself once I go home."
    B. Individual identified 4 solitary and 2 leisure interests involving others at the casual interest level on the Interest Checklist Inventory.
    C. Individual's pattern and strength of leisure interests are inadequate to support leisure resource exploration in his community.
    D. Schedule individual to attend leisure group 3 to 4 times/week with focus on leisure interest exploration.

113. In section A of the sample document, CMHC stands for:
    A. Central Medical Health Care.
    B. Columbia-Madison Hospital Corporation.
    C. Community Mental Health Counselor.
    D. Community Mental Health Center.

114. In the sample document, the section containing the individual's goals is:
    A. section A.
    B. section B.
    C. section C.
    D. section D.

115. In the sample document, the section that contains the database is:
    A. section A.
    B. section B.
    C. section C.
    D. section D.

116. In the sample documentation, the section that contains a problem according to the Patient Oriented Medical Records (POMR) format is:
    A. section A.
    B. section B.
    C. section C.
    D. section D.

117. The therapist decides to use a woodworking kit with a client who has self concept deficits. The approach that is CONTRAINDICATED in this situation:
    A. Therapist presents woodworking kits that client could complete in one session.
    B. Therapist provides performance based praise during assembly of the kit.
    C. Therapist intervenes with a suggestion each time the client makes an assembly error.
    D. Therapist provides client with graded assembly instructions (1-step, 2-step, then 3-steps.)

118. The performance components found in the activity described in question 117 would be considered:
    A. sensory-perceptual components.
    B. cognitive components.
    C. social components.
    D. psychological components.

119. Directive group treatment is the MOST appropriate approach in acute care mental health for individuals with:
    A. substance abuse problems.
    B. eating disorders.
    C. adjustment disorders.
    D. disorganized psychosis.

120. The main purpose of a therapeutic group is to:
    A. decrease the sense of alienation among group members.
    B. bring about change among the members.
    C. enable members to experience several points of view.
    D. effectively manage the economic forces within the health care setting.

121. **The MOST important curative factor to regularly include in an assertiveness group is:**
    A. a leader who provides the group members with definitions of assertion, passive, and aggression.
    B. a group leader who allows and encourages all group members to physically and verbally release their aggressive feelings towards inanimate objects.
    C. a therapist who demonstrates common assertiveness techniques to the group members.
    D. a therapist who encourages group members to share similar situations and reactions with one another.

122. **The group leader observes that one member tends to monopolize the group. The intervention that would be best to implement LAST after other more conservative approaches were unsuccessful is to:**
    A. sit beside the person who is monopolizing and touch their hand or arm to remind them to not interrupt others who are talking.
    B. confront the individual's behavior: "Are you aware that your frequent interruptions prevent others from having a chance to contribute?"
    C. redirect the individual: "Now, let's hear what others have to say about this."
    D. restructure the task: select a group activity that requires sequential turn taking.

123. **The advantage of asking a closed question is that the question:**
    A. allows the therapist to obtain facts.
    B. avoids emphasizing feelings being expressed by the patient.
    C. can help the therapist who is in a hurry.
    D. forces the person to give the answer that the therapist needs.

124. **The occupational therapist is planning to demonstrate and then involve a group of individuals in practicing "broken record" behaviors. "Broken record" is part of:**
    A. music therapy activities.
    B. self-awareness activities.
    C. assertiveness training.
    D. psychodrama approaches.

125. **An example of a group norm is when:**
    A. one member contributes superficial comments.
    B. members role play.
    C. there is improved self-esteem among members.
    D. smoking during the group is prohibited.

Implementation of the Treatment Plan

126. **The therapist reviews an individual's chart as part of the screening process. The psychiatrist has written "observe for side effects with current anti-anxiety medications." The therapist is MOST likely to report about this side effect:**

A. Akathesia
B. Confusion
C. Extrapyramidal syndrome (EPS)
D. Tardive dyskinesia

127. **The OTR assessed an individual and developed a treatment plan that addresses functional deficits. The inpatient psychiatric services that may be billed as occupational therapy services for this individual are:**
    A. treatments from the therapist's plan provided by a COTA.
    B. treatments from the therapist's plan provided by a music therapist.
    C. treatments from the occupational therapist's plan provided by a recreational therapist.
    D. treatments from the occupational therapist's plan provided by an art therapist.

128. **The COTA describes an individual she is working with to her OTR supervisor. The COTA comments that the individual is "one of her favorites," and that she frequently allows this individual to spend extra time in the craft area after the group times. The supervisor is MOST likely to wonder if the COTA's comments may reflect:**
    A. self disclosure.
    B. over involvement.
    C. transference.
    D. burnout.

129. **In mental health treatment, the facility that offers the least restrictive level of care is:**
    A. a quarterway house.
    B. a halfway house.
    C. a supervised apartment.
    D. outpatient counseling.

130. **This is an example of a psycho-educational group:**
    A. stress management.
    B. directive group.
    C. group therapy.
    D. task group.

131. **The therapist is working with an elderly woman with a diagnosis of depression and dementia. During the clean-up portion of a cooking activity, the individual begins to dry the plates and utensils she has already dried. The therapist should:**
    A. tell the individual that she is redrying the utensils and dishes.
    B. put the dried dishes away and begin to hand the individual wet dishes.
    C. ask the individual to stop the activity because it seems too difficult.
    D. ask the individual to describe what she is doing.

Questions 132–134 refer to this group scenario:

Individual 1. "This is really stupid! Why are we doing this collage anyway?"

Occupational therapy group leader: "As I already told you before we started . . . this activity will help you to identify what is important or interesting to you."

Individual 2: "Should I tear from the magazine or use scissors?"

Occupational therapy group leader: "I want you to tear the pages out of the magazines and then use the scissors to cut out the pictures or words you want to use."

Individual 1: (tears out two whole pages from the magazine nearest to him and quickly glues the pages onto the paper provided) "O.K. I'm finished. I'm going back to my room now."

132. **Based on the previous scenario, the leadership style represented in the therapist's interactions is:**
    A. democratic leadership.
    B. laissez-faire leadership.
    C. bureaucratic leadership.
    D. autocratic leadership.

133. **In the scenario preceding question 132, the individual 1's last comment is MOST likely an indication of:**
    A. passivity.
    B. insecurity.
    C. hopelessness.
    D. indecision.

134. **The therapist uses AOTA Uniform Terminology to organize the subjective, objective, and assessment sections of SOAP notes. Based on the group scenario preceding question 132, the therapist should record individual 1's responses as:**
    A. "ineffective coping skills" in the objective section of the note.
    B. an example of individual 1's time management behaviors recorded in the subjective section of the note.
    C. "inappropriate social conduct" in the assessment section of the note.
    D. "self expression difficulties" in the objective section of the note.

135. **The item that is considered to be a positive symptom of schizophrenia:**
    A. Flat affect
    B. A lack of pleasure
    C. Hallucinations
    D. Withdrawal from others

136. **The term used to refer to individuals receiving mental health interventions through the psycho-educational approach is:**
    A. student.
    B. client.
    C. consumer.
    D. patient.

137. **The occupational therapist is visiting an individual in her home and working on a household budgeting activity. This individual is in her mid-60's and on anti-anxiety medication. As she stands up from the kitchen table to get her eyeglasses, she grabs onto the edge of the table and says "I'm having a dizzy spell." Later, when she sits down to work with the therapist, she has difficulty telling the difference between the phone bill and the utility bill. What is the first thing the therapist should do?**
    A. Advise the individual to discontinue taking her anti-anxiety medication until the physician can be reached.
    B. Look up the side effects of the medications in the *Physician's Desk Reference* upon return to the clinic.
    C. Ask the individual how often she has the "spells" and encourage her to sit back down until it passes and stop working on the budget activity for today.
    D. Teach the individual to get up slowly from seated and lying positions and to hold onto a stable surface until the dizzy feeling is over.

138. **The therapist is working with an individual in an inpatient psychiatric setting who is HIV positive. The individual has just started working on a copper tooling project. While placing the piece of copper over the template, the individual cuts his or her finger on the edge of the copper. The therapist should follow these precautions:**
    A. Suicidal precautions
    B. Universal precautions
    C. Escape from unit precautions
    D. Medical precautions

139. **Which complaints and behaviors are characteristic of geriatric individuals with major depression?**
    A. The individual has problems sleeping; difficulty with "thinking" or concentrating; describes oneself as "dumb" or "stupid;" and feels very hopeless that things will improve.
    B. The individual complains of feeling "blue" or sad; has lost interest in activities previously enjoyed; and reports decreased libido.
    C. The individual's complaints focus on physical concerns, denies feeling depressed but feels less energy, has lost weight, and complains of some concentration and memory problems.
    D. The individual cannot correctly identify the date or their present location; does not recall where he or she was earlier in the day; and has difficulty sleeping during the night.

Evaluation of the Treatment Plan

140. The occupational therapist wants to change the seating arrangement to facilitate communication among members of a group. The best arrangement is to:
A. provide enough chairs around a rectangle table.
B. provide enough chairs around a round table.
C. provide enough pillows to sit on the floor.
D. use the couches and chairs that are already in the room.

Questions 141–144 refer to the following scenario

Individual: "I'm so tired of coming to this group . . . It's a big waste of time!"

Occupational therapist: "Your coming to this group is a waste of your time."

Individual: (Looks down then changes position in the chair.) "Yes, it's pretty pointless . . . they won't give you a weekend pass even after going to groups all week."

Occupational therapist: "Seems like you might be feeling pretty discouraged and wondering about the whole point of groups and treatment."

Individual: "Discouraged isn't the word for it!"

Occupational therapist: "What is the word for it?"

Individual: (sighs deeply) "Hopeless."

Occupational therapist: "Roadblocks that are put in our way can stop most of us from wanting to continue with what we are doing. Maybe as a group, we can look at ways of getting around or over the roadblocks. I think it could help with the hopelessness."

141. In the preceding treatment scenario, the individual's first statement reflects this category of group interactions:
A. Giving a suggestion or possible direction
B. Showing tension, asking for help, or withdrawing from the process
C. Asking for information about the group's process
D. Giving information, clarifying, or confirming

142. In the preceeding group scenario, the therapist's statement that would be considered as clarifying is:
A. "Your coming to this group is a waste of your time."
B. "Seems like you might be feeling pretty discouraged and wondering about the whole point of groups and treatment."
C. "What is the word for it?"
D. "Roadblocks that are put in our way can stop most of us from wanting to continue with what we are doing. Maybe, as a group, we can look at ways of getting around or over the roadblocks. I think it could help with the hopelessness."

143. In the preceeding scenario, the therapist's statement that is an example of reflection:
A. "Your coming to this group is a waste of your time."
B. "Seems like you might be feeling pretty discouraged and wondering about the whole point of groups and treatment."
C. "What is the word for it?"
D. "Roadblocks that are put in our way can stop most of us from wanting to continue with what we are doing. Maybe, as a group, we can look at ways of getting around or over the roadblocks. I think it could help with the hopelessness."

144. In the preceding scenario, the therapist's statement that is an example of providing support:
A. "Your coming to this group is a waste of your time."
B. Seems like you might be feeling pretty discouraged and wondering about the whole point of groups and treatment."
C. "What is the word for it?"
D. "Roadblocks that are put in our way can stop most of us from wanting to continue with what we are doing. Maybe, as a group, we can look at ways of getting around or over the roadblocks. I think it could help with the hopelessness."

Discharge Planning

145. The therapist is considering possible topics for a discharge planning group for individuals treated in an inpatient psychiatric unit. The MOST important topic to address because of its significance in reducing re-hospitalization is:
A. managing family conflicts.
B. living skills needed for keeping aftercare appointments.
C. coping strategies for continuing medication compliance.
D. education about problems with alcohol and substance use.

146. The occupational therapist is conducting a predischarge interview with a female patient who has been treated on the psychiatric unit for schizophrenia. The therapist says "Are you ready to go home today?" The question is an example of a(n):
A. open question.
B. closed question.
C. directed or leading question
D. double question

147. The therapist is working with an individual who has identified his or her use of alcohol as a contributing factor to his or her depression. The therapist is discussing discharge plans with this individual. At discharge, the MOST appropriate type of group to refer this individual to is:
A. an advocacy group.
B. a self-help group.
C. a support group.
D. a psychotherapy group.

148. The individual described in question 147 asked the therapist for more information about self-help groups. The expectation for becoming a member in a self-help group for alcohol problems is:
    A. members are encouraged to tell the other members their name and where they live and work.
    B. members share their experiences and struggles with alcohol use.
    C. members are required to attend a set number of meetings.
    D. members are encouraged to give advice to others.

149. The group that is the MOST appropriate self-help group to recommend to the individual described in the previous two questions is:
    A. Mothers Against Drunk Drivers (MADD).
    B. Al-Anon.
    C. Alcoholics Anonymous (AA).
    D. Group therapy.

150. The therapist is working in an acute care inpatient psychiatric facility. The FIRST step in planning for the discharge of a socially isolated individual is:
    A. to provide community re-entry activities to introduce the individual to community resources to use after discharge.
    B. to evaluate the individual's occupational performance.
    C. to educate the family about the individual's ability to return home.
    D. to make a referral to an outpatient socialization program.

ADMINISTRATION AND MANAGEMENT QUESTIONS

Organize and Manage Services

151. OSHA has defined four strategies to help prevent workplace exposure to bloodborne pathogens. What is the strategy that teaches the concept of all blood and some body fluids being handled as if contaminated with HIV or HBV?
    A. Engineering controls
    B. Workpractice controls
    C. Personal protective controls
    D. Universal precautions

152. The occupational therapist worked for 6 years as a therapist and then took off work for 5 years to begin raising a family. As this therapist returns to work in a psychiatric setting, she would be entering the job with what level of skill? (Based on the *Occupational Therapy Roles*.)

A. Entry level
B. Intermediate level
C. Advanced level
D. Educator level

153. The manager of occupational therapy supervises an employee that demonstrates specialized skill in treatment and serves as an expert for her peers. This therapist has completed research, leadership training, and assisted in continuing education activities. The manager of the department is most likely to supervise this individual at what level?
    A. Close supervision
    B. Intermediate supervision
    C. Advanced supervision
    D. Educator supervision

154. The occupational therapist is working in a collaborative relationship with the certified occupational therapy assistant (COTA). The teamwork between the two professionals would be exemplified by:
    A. the occupational therapist completing the assessment and then telling the COTA what treatment to provide.
    B. the COTA updating the occupational therapist on improvements that the patient has made in the last week and both therapists providing information to update the goals.
    C. the COTA giving her progress note to the occupational therapist and the occupational therapist writing the discharge summary from the progress note.
    D. the occupational therapist telling the COTA what type of equipment to order from a durable medical equipment company.

Questions 155–157 refer to the following quality assurance plan

Section I	Compliance with facility documentation standards
Section II	Occupational therapy documentation in the patient's chart
Section III	Clinical findings are clearly documented according to the discipline's standards
Section IV	85%
Section V	25 patients
Section VI	Quarterly

155. Section III in the quality assurance plan represents:
    A. an indicator.
    B. a monitor.
    C. a threshold.
    D. the data source.

156. Section IV of the quality assurance plan represents:

A. the time frame.
B. the sample size.
C. the threshold.
D. the data source.

157. Section V of the quality assurance plan represents:
A. the time frame.
B. the sample size.
C. the threshold.
D. the data source.

158. Documentation has four major purposes. One of the MOST important purposes of documentation is to:
A. occupy the therapist's time between treatments.
B. satisfy accrediting agencies.
C. be used as a research tool.
D. facilitate effective treatment.

159. The manager of an occupational therapy department that provides services to pediatrics is reviewing the sterilization policy, which is based on universal precautions. The policy will MOST likely state:
A. all equipment is to be sterilized annually.
B. any equipment that has come into contact with body fluids will be sent to be sterilized prior to using the equipment again.
C. all equipment is to be sterilized at the end of each day.
D. all equipment is to be sterilized after each use.

160. The most common example of using the problem-oriented medical record would be:
A. completed patient checklists included in the medical record.
B. SOAP notes.
C. facility-specific documentation forms to be completed and placed into the patient chart.
D. narrative notes which do not follow a structured format.

161. In order for a school-aged child to receive services in the school system, which one of the following forms must be completed?
A. UB-82
B. FIM
C. IEP
D. I-9

162. The results of a service intervention and the status of the patient after care has been provided is referred to as:
A. process.
B. outcome.
C. program evaluation.
D. utilization review.

163. The interaction between the service provider and the manner in which care is provided for individuals is referred to as:

A. a process.
B. an outcome.
C. program evaluation.
D. utilization review.

164. Occupational therapy services should be discontinued when:
A. the goals have been met and the individual can no longer benefit from services.
B. the goals have not been met and the individual could benefit from continued services.
C. the goals have been met but the individual could benefit from continued services.
D. the individual feels that he or she has not made gains despite objective measures to the contrary.

165. Upon completion of the level II fieldwork, the student:
A. should be functioning slightly below entry level.
B. should be able to function at an intermediate skill level based on the *Occupational Therapy Roles*.
C. should be able to function at an advanced skill level based on the *Occupational Therapy Roles*.
D. should be able to function at an entry level or above the minimum entry level of competence.

166. In order to provide direct supervision for a level II fieldwork student, the supervisor MUST:
A. be a registered occupational therapist with 6 months of experience.
B. have at least 1 year of experience as a registered occupational therapist.
C. be certified by the NBCOT.
D. have previously supervised a level I student.

167. The concept of universal coverage is:
A. every American citizen having access to health care without financial or other barriers.
B. a guarantee that benefits will meet the full range of health care needs.
C. consumers having the opportunity to exercise choice regarding providers.
D. the health care system spreading the cost burden of care across the community.

168. The highest percentage of reimbursement paid for occupational therapy services is from:
A. Medicare.
B. Medicaid.
C. state and local programs.
D. Blue Cross.

169. The primary employment site of occupational therapist's is:
A. the school systems.
B. the general hospitals.
C. in rehabilitation centers.
D. in psychiatric hospitals.

170. The discharge disposition of an individual is: "The patient will return home upon discharge and receive services from the Bureau of Vocational Rehabilitation for vocational placement." This type of discharge plan demonstrates:
    A. a follow-up plan.
    B. aftercare.
    C. a home program.
    D. home health services.

171. One technique that is used to identify what should be billed for occupational therapy services is:

    A. $\dfrac{\text{present salary/earning potential} + \text{professional overhead}}{\text{billable hours}}$

    B. to set the rate at the equivalent of what physical therapy charges.
    C. to survey what other facilities charge and charge the same price.
    D. $\dfrac{\text{cost of equipment} + \text{building overhead}}{\text{billable hours}}$

172. The occupational therapist is working with a woman who recently experienced a stroke affecting the left side. Plans are to discharge the woman home to live independently. The therapist has worked with other individuals in similar situations and has developed a keen sense for all of the issues that may arise and need to be problem solved. The form of clinical reasoning that this therapist is MOST likely to use based on her past experience will be:
    A. procedural reasoning.
    B. conditional reasoning.
    C. interactive reasoning.
    D. narrative reasoning.

173. The occupational therapist is reviewing a patient's chart prior to evaluating the patient. Based on the physician's history and physical, the therapist is able to identify the patient's deficits and assessments that will best assess the problem areas. This form of clinical reasoning is an example of:
    A. procedural reasoning.
    B. conditional reasoning.
    C. interactive reasoning.
    D. narrative reasoning.

174. An example of resale equipment would be:
    A. a shoe horn.
    B. a dynamometer.
    C. a powder board.
    D. a desk chair.

175. An important criteria for medicare reimbursement of a patient referred to home care is that the patient:
    A. requires a wheelchair for mobility.
    B. is not able to drive to an outpatient treatment center.

C. is home-bound.
D. requires moderate assistance for ambulation.

Promote Professional Practice

176. The occupational therapist is passing a patient's room and witnesses another occupational therapist in an intimate position with a patient. Responding consistently with the Occupational Therapy Code of Ethics, the therapist will:
    A. notify AOTA.
    B. notify the state occupational therapy association.
    C. notify the state licensure board.
    D. discuss the situation privately with the therapist involved.

177. The principle that the individual be provided information regarding their own health status so that they may be involved with their own health care decisions, including collaboration in the treatment plan and goal setting, is:
    A. beneficence.
    B. therapeutic privilege.
    C. informed consent.
    D. competence.

178. The disciplinary action that designates a time frame in which the therapist is required to attain counseling or additional education in order to remain certified is referred to as:
    A. a reprimand.
    B. a censure.
    C. probation.
    D. revocation.

179. When completing research, the treatment variable, which is a condition that is manipulated by the researcher, is termed:
    A. a dependent variable.
    B. the independent variable.
    C. a sample.
    D. an interdependent variable.

180. The occupational therapist has completed research in which generalizations are made to the entire population. This research will have a condition of:
    A. internal validity.
    B. external validity.
    C. procedural agreement.
    D. reliability.

181. The occupational therapist is completing research on stroke patients and functional return of the upper extremities. This therapist has decided to get a random sample of patients. This means that the therapist will use:
    A. the entire population of the facilities stroke patients.
    B. all patients who have had a CVA with resulting deficits in the upper extremity function.
    C. a numbers table to select the population.

D. a small group of patients who are representative of the population with each individual meeting criteria, which validates that they are a representative subset of the population.

182. **The occupational therapist is supervising a level II student on an inpatient psychiatric unit. The student has led an awareness group on several occasions and is now comfortable with this activity. The fieldwork supervisor now asks the student to prepare for and lead an expression group. The fieldwork supervisor is using the basic educational principle of:**
A. meeting the learner at their current level.
B. moving from the familiar to the similar but unfamiliar.
C. involving the learner in the instruction.
D. proceeding from the simple to the complex.

183. **The occupational therapist is supervising a level II student in a rehabilitation center. The first patient on the students caseload was an individual who had a left hip replacement. The second patient assigned to the student's caseload was a patient with multiple fractures from an industrial injury. The third patient assigned to the student's caseload suffered a head injury from a car accident. The development of the student's caseload from lower acuity to higher acuity patients is an example of the educational principle of:**
A. meeting the learner at their current level.
B. moving from the familiar to the similar but unfamiliar.
C. involving the learner in the instruction.
D. proceeding from the simple to the complex.

184. **The term that mandates the confidentiality of patient information and holds the therapist to remain faithful to the patient's best interest is:**
A. informed consent.
B. fidelity.
C. beneficence.
D. nonmaleficence.

185. **The concept of always striving to bring about the best for other individuals through treatment and "doing good" is referred to as:**
A. informed consent.
B. fidelity.
C. beneficence.
D. nonmaleficence.

186. **The ADA set out regulations that include providing "reasonable accommodations." The term that BEST describes this is:**
A. making physical modifications to the environment to allow for wheelchair accessibility.
B. any modification to a job that will allow a disabled worker to perform the essential functions.

C. a standard job task that is fundamental to the position.
D. providing support personnel so that an employee may complete the essential functions with assistance.

187. **The section of the Occupational Therapy Code of Ethics that addresses the issue of a therapist complying with state, local, and institutional rules is:**
A. beneficence and autonomy.
B. competence.
C. compliance with laws and regulations.
D. public information.

188. **The *Revision: Standards of Practice for Occupational Therapy* was developed as:**
A. a guide to promote the highest standards of behavior.
B. guidelines to assist the occupational therapist in the provision of services.
C. a guide to assist the practitioner in identifying career options and developing career plans.
D. a document to assist therapists in applying uniform terminology.

189. **If a researcher chose a sample population for their research, they would use:**
A. the entire population of the facilities stroke patients.
B. all patients who have had a CVA with resulting deficits in the upper extremity function.
C. a numbers table to select the population.
D. a small group of patients who are representative of the population with each individual meeting criteria, which validates that they are a representative subset of the population.

190. **The obligation of health care providers to avoid doing harm to those they serve is referred to as:**
A. informed consent.
B. fidelity.
C. beneficence.
D. nonmaleficence.

191. **The role of the Commission on Education is to:**
A. promote coordination between academic programs and the fieldwork education centers.
B. collaborate with fieldwork coordinators to develop facility specific objectives that apply theoretical concepts.
C. provide fieldwork sites with the most current information on fieldwork education centers.
D. periodically review contractual agreements between the educational institutions and the fieldwork centers.

192. **The right of individuals to be provided information regarding their health care as well as to make choices about their own health care is:**

A. informed consent.
B. fidelity.
C. beneficence.
D. nonmaleficence.

193. **An outpatient treatment center that provides comprehensive rehabilitation services is most likely to be accredited by:**
    A. JCAHO and PSROs.
    B. CARF and JCAHO.
    C. JCAHO and CORF.
    D. CARF and CORF.

194. **The occupational therapist has assessed an individual and developed a treatment plan that addresses functional deficits. Which of the following inpatient services can be billed as occupational therapy services for the client whose hospitalization is covered by Medicare?**
    A. Treatments from the occupational therapy plan provided by a COTA.
    B. Treatments from the occupational therapy plan provided by a music therapist.
    C. Treatments from the occupational therapy plan provided by a recreational therapist.
    D. Treatments from the occupational therapy plan provided by an art therapist.

195. **The term given to the practice of an organization acting as an intermediary between an insurance agency and a hospital is:**
    A. managed care.
    B. utilization review
    C. peer review
    D. prospective payment

196. **When writing the results of a research project, the researcher should include:**
    A. writing conclusions in the results section.
    B. writing qualitative and quantitative facts in the results section.

C. writing subjective information in the results section.
D. interpretive and analytical information in the results section.

197. **An individual who is 70 years old is hospitalized after a cerebrovascular accident. The acute care stay for this individual will most likely be paid under:**
    A. a diagnostic related group (DRG).
    B. a functional rehabilitation group (FRG).
    C. Medicaid.
    D. third party reimbursement.

198. **Medicare will reimburse for equipment issued by an occupational therapist if it meets the criteria of:**
    A. increasing functional independence.
    B. medical necessity.
    C. maintaining patient function.
    D. reducing deformity.

199. **The concept of the federal government making a standard payment for health care services for individuals in diagnostic categories is known as:**
    A. DRGs
    B. PROs
    C. UB-82s
    D. Cost shifting

200. **The manager of an occupational therapy department is approached with an ethical dilemma by an occupational therapist. In using The Savage Model of Ethical Contemplation, her first response will be to:**
    A. identify problems to be solved.
    B. sort decisions to be made.
    C. ascertain facts and impressions.
    D. verify information with key players.

ANSWERS FOR SIMULATION EXAMINATION 3

1. (B) Neck righting reaction. Answer B is correct because the neck righting reaction allows the infant to turn the head independently from the trunk (rotational righting). Answer A is not correct because the labyrinthine righting reflex allows the child to lift and right the head against gravity when blindfolded (vertical righting). Answer C is not correct because the body righting on body reaction allows rotation between trunk segments (also a rotational righting reaction). Answer D is not correct because the optical righting reaction also allows the child to right the head against gravity with the assistance of vision (also a vertical righting reaction). See reference: Gilfoyle, Grady, and Moore: Strategies for developmental and purposeful sequences.

2. (C) Developmentally inappropriate. According to Dr. Milani, as referred to in a textbook by Rhoda Erhardt, OTR, many reflex patterns that exist beyond the age when they are normally integrated should be considered "developmentally inappropriate." Rather than considering these patterns "abnormal," because they existed and served a purpose in a child's life at one time, they should be considered "regressive" in terms of developmental progression. Answer A is incorrect because a pattern such as ATNR should be integrated by 6 months of age, and therefore its presence cannot be considered as normal. Answers B and D are incorrect because they both describe such patterns as abnormal, not considering their role in normal development. See reference: Erhardt: Patrick.

3. (A) Further observation of right body side for dysfunction is needed. Answer A is correct because infants usually use a bilateral approach at this age. Although unilaterality occurs several months later, most children will alternate hands in many activities until 6 years of age. This means that the infant should be observed for possible right-sided dysfunction. Answer B is incorrect because unilaterality at 4 months of age is not typical development. Answer C is incorrect because hand dominance begins to develop at 3 to 6 years of age. And answer D is incorrect because bilaterality precedes unilaterality in the course of infant development. See reference: Erhardt: Joanne.

4. (A) Symmetrical tonic neck reflex. The correct answer is A because the symmetrical tonic neck reflex when present provides the child with bilateral arm extension and hip flexion with the head raised (and bilateral arm flexion and hip extension with the head lowered), which can be used to move forward. Answers B, C, and D are not correct because these primitive patterns do not assist the child into a quadruped position, but primarily affect prone and supine positioning. See reference: Erhardt: Patrick.

5. (C) Significantly delayed by several months. Answer C is correct because at 6 months of age a child should initiate head flexion when pulled into a sitting position. The child assists with pulling of the arms and some trunk flexion or use of the abdominals at this age. Usually, by 2 months of age an infant is beginning to assist with being pulled to sit with some head flexion. Answers A, B, and D are not correct because they do not address the significance of the child's delay in head control. See reference: Erhardt: Kristy.

6. (C) Labyrinthine righting reaction. Vertical righting reactions "activate muscle groups that move the midline of the body into alignment with the center of gravity." Answer C is correct because it is the only reaction that aligns the body with the center of gravity. Gravity receptors are stimulated by movement and the infant lifts his or her head in order to vertically right himself or herself. Answers A and B are not correct because these are both rotational righting reactions; that is, the head or body are righted by turning the head or trunk segment on the central axis of the body. Answer D is not correct because the ATNR is a tonic reflex, not a righting reaction. See reference: Gilfoyle, Grady, and Moore: Strategies for developmental and purposeful sequences.

7. (B) Compensatory position to achieve stability. Answer B is correct because exclusive W-sitting by a child with low muscle tone indicates that the child is probably not using side-, ring-, or long-sitting positions (all of which are developmentally appropriate). The child is compensating for an inability to achieve stability in a variety of positions, which requires dynamic postural control, depending on skeletal rather than neuromuscular structures for stability. Answer A is not correct because exclusive W-sitting is not age-appropriate for a 5-year-old child, or a child at any age. Answer C is not correct because, although exclusive W-sitting is a compensatory position, it is used to achieve stability and in fact may limit mobility. Answer D is not correct because W-sitting is not a normal developmental skill. See reference: Kramer and Hinojosa (eds): Schoen, S, and Anderson, J: Neurodevelopmental treatment frame of reference.

8. (A) Reciprocal innervation. Answer A is correct because "reciprocal innervation" refers to the normal ability for interplay between agonists and antagonists in smooth, controlled movements. The child with athetosis who is reaching for a toy cannot control the midrange of the arm movements, and therefore uses excessive flexion and extension (poor grading of movement). Answer B is not correct because "dissociation of movement" refers to the normal ability to differentiate or separate one movement from another. Answer C is not correct because "stability and mobility" refer to the normal ability to hold stable positions or postures and move from one position to another. Answer D is not correct because poorly developed righting and equilibrium reactions limit positioning and posture capabilities, but not the gradation of arm movements (as in this example). See reference: Kramer and Hinojosa (eds): Schoen, S, and Anderson, J: Neurodevelopmental treatment frame of reference.

9. (D) Support reactions. Answer D is correct as the term "support reaction" refers to the ability to coactivate muscle groups of the appropriate extremity or about the midline in order to support the body weight or posture in a certain position. Answer A is incorrect because protective reactions follow the development of support reactions in the arms (which protect the child when falling) and require that the body is free from support. Answer B is not correct because equilibrium reactions are compensatory movements used to regain stability, not to maintain stability. Answer C is not correct because rotational righting reactions involve turning of the head or trunk in order to maintain body alignment. See reference: Gilfoyle, Grady, and Moore: Strategies for developmental and purposeful sequences.

10. (A) 2 years. Answer A is correct because, according to Colangelo, a powered wheelchair that provides rapid mobility to the nonambulatory child can be considered as early as 18 months. Because an 18-month-old child can direct his body through space safely, a nonambulatory child of the same age should also be able to direct a wheelchair. Answers B, C, and D are incorrect because the power wheelchair can first be considered at a much earlier age. See reference: Kramer and Hinojosa (eds): Colangelo, CA: Biomechanical frame of reference.

11. (B) Raise the handle bars. The correct answer is B because raising the handle bars demands that the arms are raised, which brings the child to the upright posture. Answers A and D are not correct because the hips and lower extremities are already positioned correctly and this positioning would be disrupted. Answer D is not correct because the arms would be lowered and trunk forward flexion would be increased. See reference: Kramer and Hinojosa (eds): Colangelo, CA: Biomechanical frame of reference.

12. (D) 5 to 6 years. Nighttime bowel and bladder control may not be accomplished until the child is 5 or 6 years of age. Other developmental trends in toilet training are that daytime control is usually attained by 30 months, and that girls may precede boys by 2.5 months. See reference: Case-Smith, Allen, and Pratt (eds): Shepherd, J, Procter, SA, and Coley, IL: Self-care and adaptations for independent living.

13. (B) Provision of foot support. This is probably the first concern of the therapist in order for the child to feel secure on the toilet and to be positioned for bowel control. Answer A is not correct as management of fasteners can be developed later, after positioning for stability has been achieved. Answer C is not correct because provision of a seat belt may not be necessary if foot support (or back support) is provided. Answer D is not correct because climbing onto the toilet independently may be developed later (as it in fact occurs with developmental progression). See reference: Case-Smith, Allen, and Pratt (eds): Shepherd, J, Procter, SA, and Coley, IL: Self-care and adaptations for independent living.

14. (C) Doffing socks. Answer C is correct because, according to most developmental scales, children first learn to remove garments, especially socks. Answer A is not correct because correct placement of front and back of garments, along with buttoning and tying bows (answer D) are later developing dressing skills. Answer B is not correct because children are able to remove garments before they are able to put them on. See reference: Case-Smith, Allen, and Pratt (eds): Shepherd, J, Procter, SA, and Coley, IL: Self-care and adaptations for independent living.

15. (C) Wheeling efficiency. Answer C is correct because the light weight of this type of wheelchair allows the child with weakness to be independent for longer periods of time. This type of chair is also easier for parents to handle when lifting in and out of a car. Answer A is not correct because the removable armrest wheelchair feature aides in sliding transfers. Answer B is not correct because the desk arm feature allows children to sit closer to tables for schoolwork and other table-top activities. Answer D is not correct because it is the adjustable arm rest feature that allows adjustment for varying heights of lap trays or work surfaces. See reference: Case-Smith, Allen, and Pratt (eds): Wright-Ott, C, and Egilson, S: Mobility.

16. (A) Transitional movements to sitting are restricted. Answer A is correct because children are unable to rotate onto their buttocks or sit back on lower legs when using such an adaptive device. Answers B, C, and D are incorrect because all of these movements are incorporated in the use of an adaptive device for support of creeping. See reference: Case-Smith, Allen, and Pratt (eds): Wright-Ott, C, and Egilson, S: Mobility.

17. (D) Need for adapted teaching techniques. Answer D is correct because the child with a mental retardation disability will characteristically have learning problems that require such teaching methods as "chain-

ing" or behavior modification. Answers A, B, and C would be of secondary importance as physical coordination may be impaired or other physical limitations such as abnormal muscle tone or significant problems with balance could also be present. These additional problems may require adaptive equipment, clothing, or techniques. However, the child's ability to learn procedures of dressing will still limit all aspects of dressing, and therefore there is the need to address task analysis and teaching approach first. See reference: Case-Smith, Allen, and Pratt (eds): Wright-Ott, C, and Egilson, S: Mobility.

18. (B) High contrast and defined borders. Answer B is correct because it provides the only combination of features when adapting visual material, which will assist the child with visual discrimination problems. High contrast of the stimuli (shape, letter, numbers, and so on) in relation to the background, and defining important areas of the stimuli with a border will attract the eye and provide clear input. Answer A is incorrect because low contrast of the stimuli, such as blue ditto lettering, is difficult to discriminate. Answer C is incorrect because undefined borders around the important stimuli make for less clear input. Answer D is incorrect because both features of the visual stimulus would make it difficulty to discriminate. See reference: Kramer and Hinojosa (eds): Todd, VR: Visual perceptual frame of reference: An information processing approach.

19. (A) Behind. According to Todd, the spatial concept of "down" develops around 4.6 to 5 years of age, and therefore the correct answer is A as the concept of "behind" follows this at about 5.0 to 5.6 years of age. Answer B is incorrect because the concept of "in" develops around 2.0 years of age (before the concept of down). Answer C is incorrect because the concept of "up" develops at 3.0 to 3.6 years of age (before down). Answer D is incorrect because the concept of "under" develops around 2.6 to 3.0 years of age. See reference: Kramer and Hinojosa (eds): Todd, VR: Visual perceptual frame of reference: An information processing approach.

20. (D) Object recognition. Answer D is correct because a child must first be able to recognize an object before dealing with its specific visual attributes. Answer A is incorrect because, in developmental order, matching object characteristics or details will be the last of the visual discrimination abilities to develop. Answer C is not correct because color, shape, and position are details of visual objects that also develop last in terms of visual discrimination or ability to match objects. See reference: Kramer and Hinojosa (eds): Todd, VR: Visual perceptual frame of reference: An information processing approach.

21. (B) Visual attention skills. According to Todd, Answer B is correct because development of visual attention skills should be worked on first because they prepare and provide foundation skills for other aspects of visual perception. Answer A is incorrect because visual memory skills can only be developed after visual attention skills are established. Answer C and D are incorrect because general and specific visual perceptual skills develop after visual memory. See reference: Kramer and Hinojosa (eds): Todd, VR: Visual perceptual frame of reference: An information processing approach.

22. (B) Prone over the parent's thighs; flex and abduct legs. Answer B is correct because it provides a position that is inhibitory to extensor patterns along with a reflex-inhibiting pattern (in opposition to abnormal pattern). Answer A is not the best position because extension can predominate in supine, making flexing of the hip and separation of the legs more difficult; however, the inhibitory pattern of flexion and abduction of the legs is correct. Answer A would be an appropriate choice if the child's neck were slightly flexed. Answer C is not the best position for a small child with undeveloped trunk balance but would be a good position as the child becomes larger and trunk balance develops; the inhibitory pattern is also incorrect (adduction is incorrect). Answer D is not correct because, although the positioning is optimal for decreasing extensor patterns, the pattern of movement at the hip (extension and adduction) is not inhibitory. See reference: Case-Smith, Allen, and Pratt (eds): Hunter, JG: The neonatal intensive care unit.

23. (B) Flex the hip and knee. Answer B is correct because flexing the hips and knees prior to donning socks and shoes provides inhibition of ankle plantar flexion (which makes the task very difficult) through the key point of the hip. Answer A is not correct because hip and knee extension is the position that already is contributing to the plantar flexion of the ankle; and, inhibition of plantar flexion could not occur. Answer C is not correct because the shoulder patterns may not influence the ankle patterns as significantly as hip and knee flexion; and, this is an extension pattern that could not be inhibitory to the abnormal ankle pattern interfering with dressing. Answer D is not correct primarily because the abnormal pattern at the ankle is usually influenced by inhibition from the key point of the hip. See reference: Case-Smith, Allen, and Pratt (eds): Hunter, JG: The neonatal intensive care unit.

24. (A) Child dresses in a sidelying position. Answer A is correct as the sidelying position eliminates the need for balance in order to dress the lower extremities. Answer B is not correct because loops will primarily help a child with limited grasp to pull in order to manage the clothing. Answer C is not correct because the addition of velcro instead of zippers also deals with limited grasp and pulling ability. See reference: Case-Smith, Allen, and Pratt (eds): Hunter, JG: The neonatal intensive care unit.

25. (C) Handle the child slowly and gently. Answer C is correct because the child with hypertonicity will be most relaxed, and easier to handle, if tone is inhibited by the therapist's slow and gentle handling of the body. Answer A is incorrect because adaptive equipment is frequently needed to provide a child with a sense of security during bathing. Answer B is not correct because an explanation of the procedures will also increase a child's sense of security during bathing. Answer D is not correct because it provides the parent with a poor model of good

body mechanics; rather, the therapist should kneel or sit on a stool. See reference: Case-Smith, Allen, and Pratt (eds): Hunter, JG: The neonatal intensive care unit.

26. (C) Elongation on the weight-bearing side. Answer C is correct because positioning of the child in side-lying position in normal development allows the weight-bearing side of the body to elongate, while flexion and skilled arm movements develop on the mobile or non-weight-bearing side of the body. Answers A and B are therefore incorrect because flexion is characteristic of the nonweight-bearing side in the sidelying position. Answer D is incorrect because stability or cocontraction develop on the weight-bearing side of the body, while skilled arm movements develop on the mobile, or nonweight-bearing side of the body. See reference: Kramer and Hinojosa (eds): Schoen, S, and Anderson, J: Neurodevelopmental treatment frame of reference.

27. (D) Sitting position. Answer D is correct because the upright sitting position provides the child with the opportunity not only to further control head movement (stability has developed in horizontal positions), weight bearing, and weight shifting, but to rotate the trunk as the child reaches toward the opposite side of the body. Answers A and B are not correct because head and neck stability have developed primarily in the prone and sidelying positions rather than trunk control because trunk rotation is limited to sidelying. See reference: Kramer and Hinojosa (eds): Schoen, S, and Anderson, J: Neurodevelopmental treatment frame of reference.

28. (C) Neutral pelvic position. Answer C is correct because the pelvis gradually changes from an anterior tilt caused by lordosis of the spine to a neutral (or slightly posterior) position as abdominal control develops. Therefore, Answers A and B are incorrect. Answer D is not correct because positioning in standing during normal development facilitates extensor activity throughout the child's posture. See reference: Kramer and Hinojosa (eds): Schoen, S, and Anderson, J: Neurodevelopmental treatment frame of reference.

29. (A) Neurodevelopmental. Answer A is correct because the neurodevelopmental treatment frame of reference has, as one of its postulates for change, increasing therapeutic handling opportunities in order to provide more normal experiences of posture and movement. Answer B is not correct because handling of the child is not a primary postulate for change; rather, the provision of situations requiring an adaptive response can promote growth and change. Answer C is not correct because the coping frame of reference is based on environmental modifications and expansion of the child's resources, rather than therapeutic handling. Answer D is not correct because the biomechanical frame of reference has as its most similar postulate for change increasing skill through practice (and use of adaptive equipment for positioning), and does not address managing tone and movement through therapeutic handling. See reference: Kramer and Hinojosa (eds): Schoen, S, and Anderson, J: Neurodevelopmental treatment frame of reference.

30. (D) Prepare the child mentally and physically for visual tasks. Answer D is correct because children with poor visual attention will find visual tasks facilitated by being prepared mentally and physically for the task. Answer A is not correct because concentration and task persistence are enhanced by motivation, comprehension, and intrinsic interest in the visual task. Answer B is not correct because stimulation surrounding the task should be minimized. Answer C is not correct because the novelty of the task increases visual attention. See reference: Kramer and Hinojosa (eds): Todd, VR: Visual perceptual frame of reference: An information processing approach.

31. (C) Combine task with additional sensory input (tactile, proprioceptive, and auditory). Answer C is correct because additional sensory input, when combined with a visual memory task, will facilitate memory. Answer A is not correct because interest in the task should be high in order to enhance visual memory. Answer B is not correct because visual attention is a prerequisite to visual memory. Answer D is incorrect because serial or varied repetition enhances visual memory. See reference: Kramer and Hinojosa (eds): Todd, VR: Visual perceptual frame of reference: An information processing approach.

32. (D) The child partially rotates to sitting, and then completely rotates toward prone, to then push on the floor in order to stand. Answer D is correct because the next sequence of rising to stand behavior, developmentally, modifies the complete rotation of rising to quadruped into a partial rotation into sitting. From sitting, the child will still need to completely rotate to prone to push to stand. The correct sequence developmentally (should the therapist choose to follow developmental sequence depending on the child's movement problem) would be answer D, answer C, answer B, and lastly, the most mature rising to stand behavior is answer A. See reference: Gilfoyle, Grady, and Moore: Strategies for developmental and purposeful sequences.

33. (B) Treatment for this problem may be discontinued. The correct answer is B because the child has developed the highest form of pencil grasp, which begins to appear at approximately 4 years of age. Answers A and C are incorrect because these answers imply that further development of grasp can be achieved. Answer D is incorrect because a dynamic tripod grasp of the pencil should be well established by this age. See reference: Erhardt: Joanne.

34. (B) Superior and inferior colliculi. The correct answer is B because the inferior and superior colliculi are "important centers concerned with integration of visual, auditory, vestibular, and somatosensory stimuli." They also respond to stimuli of a protopathic nature and play an important role in spatiotemporal orientation. Answer A is not correct because the brain stem reticular formation is responsible for regulation of reflex centers for eye movements, sleep-wake cycles, heart rate, respiration, perspiration, salivation, and vomiting. Answer C is not correct because the pathways of the dorsal medulla are an extension of the dorsal column (carrying kinesthetic informa-

tion). Answer D is not correct because the ventral aspect of the brain stem contains descending pathways responsible for voluntary control and coordination of skilled functions, relaying signals from cortical to subcortical structures, and modifying incoming sensory stimuli. See reference: Gilfoyle, Grady, and Moore: Highlights of nervous system development.

35. (B) Cerebellum. The correct answer is B because the cerebellum allows the nervous system to perform with synergy. The cerebellum provides smooth, orderly sequencing of direction, extent, force, timing, and tone involved in patterns of movement. See reference: Gilfoyle, Grady, and Moore: Highlights of nervous system development.

36. (B) Renal failure. Answer B is correct because the major cause of death in children with myelomeningocele is urinary infection with renal failure. Answers A, C, and D can contribute to the vulnerability of these children; however, respiratory infection, spinal cord degeneration, and hydrocephalus are usually not the major causes of death. See reference: Hopkins and Smith (eds): Atkins, J: Neural tube defect.

37. (B) Club foot. Equinovarus, or talipes equinovarus, is also called *club foot*. This deformity involves forefoot adduction and supination, heel varus, equinus through the ankle, and medial deviation of the foot in relationship to the knee, according to Schanzenbacher. See reference: Hopkins and Smith (eds): Atkins, J: Neural tube defect.

38. (D) Intermittent headaches. According to Atkins, the major signs of shunt malfunction in the older child are irritability, short attention span, increased paralysis, decreased upper extremity strength, decreased school performance, and intermittent headaches. Answers A and B (increased head size and nausea and vomiting) are major signs of shunt malfunction in very young children, and therefore are not correct answers. Answer D (back pain) is not among the symptoms given for this problem, and therefore is incorrect. See reference: Hopkins and Smith (eds): Atkins, J: Neural tube defect.

39. (A) Infants and toddlers. A is the correct answer because this is the youngest age group provided, and it is thought that the nervous system exhibits the greatest neuroplasticity at the earliest ages. However, neuroplasticity does exist throughout the life span. See reference: Gilfoyle, Grady, and Moore: Highlights of nervous system development.

40. (A) Increase the height of the wedge (side A on diagram). Answer A is correct because by increasing the height of the wedge from the floor, less weight is borne on the arms (which is a source of the heavy work involved in this position). Answer B is not correct because decreasing the height of the wedge from the floor will increase weight bearing and thus increase the postural work involved in the prone position. Answers C and D are not correct because shortening or lengthening the wedge will increase or decrease the lower back extension (lumbar curve or tilt) rather than weight bearing on the arms. See reference: Kramer and Hinojosa (eds): Colangelo, CA: Biomechanical frames of reference.

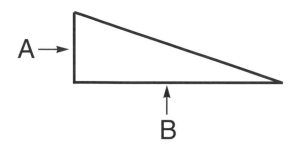

41. (C) Position stander at 75 to 90 degrees from the floor. Answer C is most correct because by adjusting the prone stander nearer to vertical (the least effect of gravity on the head or posture), the child will be able to tolerate work on head righting. Answer A is not correct because working on the floor in prone, the head and neck are doing the most work against gravity. Answer D is not correct because the head, neck, and postural work against gravity is the least in the standing position. See reference: Kramer and Hinojosa (eds): Colangelo, CA: Biomechanical frames of reference.

42. (C) Biomechanical. Answer C is correct because, according to Colangelo, "if postural reactions are delayed, weak, exaggerated, or performed by improper muscle groups, the biomechanical frame of reference should be considered." This child's physical status has changed with decreasing postural control. Adaptive support devices need to be considered, and a biomechanical frame of reference provides this approach. Answer A is not correct because the neurodevelopmental treatment (NDT) frame of reference is concerned with improving posture and movement, and supportive equipment is prescribed for that purpose. Answer B is not correct because the sensory integration (SI) frame of reference is concerned with sensory input in relation to posture and movement in children with SI disorders (specifically, Duchenne's disease is a neuromuscular disorder). Answer D is not correct because the visual perceptual frame of reference is concerned with guiding and compensating for visual perceptual problems, not postural delays. See reference: Kramer and Hinojosa (eds): Colangelo, CA: Biomechanical frames of reference.

43. (C) Sidelying. Answer C is correct because the sidelying position will reduce the influence of reflexes, extensor tone, and gravity, which make protraction of the shoulders and forward reach difficult. Answer A is incorrect because extensor tone will still predominate in standing, which encourages shoulder retraction and forward reaching of both arms to midline is more difficult. Answer B is wrong because the upper extremities are involved in weight bearing; however, this position may help facilitate forward reach by developing shoulder protraction. Answer D is not correct because the upper extremities are involved in weight bearing; however, if the position is attainable, shoulder protraction and forward reach may

be facilitated through this position. See reference: Kramer and Hinojosa (eds): Colangelo, CA: Biomechanical frames of reference.

44. (B) Extension. Protective arm reactions allow one to return to a support base or to protect the body when there are environmental changes. Answer B is the correct answer because the arms extend during this protective movement. Facilitation of protective reactions may be a beginning point for the development of arm extension in treatment. Answers A, C, and D are incorrect because these movements are not the major movement component of protective arm reactions. See reference: Gilfoyle, Grady, and Moore: Strategies for developmental and purposeful sequences.

45. (C) Provides motivating force behind basic behaviors and personality traits. Answer C is correct because the limbic system deals with behavior and personality. Answer A is not correct because it describes the functions of the brain stem reticular formation. Answer D is not correct because it describes functions of the cerebellum. Answer D is not correct because it describes the function of the basal ganglia. See reference: Gilfoyle, Grady, and Moore: Highlights of nervous system development.

46. (C) Stabilizing the pelvis, hips, and legs. The correct answer is C because compensatory movements can occur because of a poor central base of support provided by the pelvis, hips, or legs. Answer A is not correct because the pelvis is not stabilized, and arm movements may still be compromised. Answer B is not correct because use of a lapboard or chair arms for weight bearing of the upper extremities will compromise the use of the arms and hands to stabilize the body. Answer D is not correct because the pelvis continues to be unstable, and provides a poor base for arm movements. See reference: Kramer and Hinojosa (eds): Colangelo, CA: Biomechanical frames of reference.

47. (B) Rolling the child forward slightly. The correct answer is B because by rolling the child slightly forward, gravity can be used to increase shoulder protraction (the angle of the back support can be increased slightly). Answer A is not correct because the child's total body position in sidelying will become less stable. Answer C is not correct because increasing lateral head flexion will disrupt body symmetry in sidelying without improving head and shoulder retraction. Answer D is not correct because extending both legs would only increase head and shoulder retraction and extension, and body position in sidelying would be unstable. See reference: Kramer and Hinojosa (eds): Colangelo, CA: Biomechanical frames of reference.

48. (B) The nearest wheelchair equipment vendor. Although any community resource may be helpful to a child and family with a severe physical disability, answer B is correct because of the possible breakdown in this piece of equipment, which has already been purchased. The therapist needs to consider this possibility and provide local support for a problem solution. Therefore, although answers A, C, and D may serve as resources for other needs of the child, only a specialist in wheelchair equipment will be able to solve mechanical problems that arise. See reference: Case-Smith, Allen, and Pratt (eds): Wright-Ott, C, and Egilson, S: Mobility.

49. (D) Block out all areas of the page except important words. Answer D is correct because this compensatory technique represents methods for dealing with visual figure-ground or visual discrimination problems. The child needs to learn how to rule out extraneous stimuli and focus on an important area of a task, such as reading. Answer A is not correct because this is a technique used to orient the child with left-right visual tracking problems. Answer B is not correct because it is a technique used to deal with visual attention problems. Answer C is not correct because it is a technique used to help children deal with visual memory problems. See reference: Kramer and Hinojosa (eds): Todd, VR: Visual perceptual frame of reference: An information processing approach.

50. (D) Increased angle of flexion at the hip. The correct answer is D because increasing the angle of flexion at the hip will inhibit the extensor hypertonic pattern (or extensor reflex pattern). Answer A is not correct because lengthening the back support will primarily aide in head and neck support and stability. Answer B is not correct because a hip strap, although it may prevent thrusting out of the chair, will primarily stabilize the pelvis. Answer C is not correct because a shoulder harness primarily prevents the child from falling forward. See reference: Kramer and Hinojosa (eds): Colangelo, CA: Biomechanical frames of reference.

51. (D) At the midrange of the joint. Proprioception (or position sense) is demonstrated when the therapist passively positions the joint being tested and the individual is able to imitate the position with the opposite extremity. The joint should not be moved through range to an extent that would elicit a stretch or pain response, which would be at the end ranges of the joint. Movement should be at a rate of approximately 10 degrees per second to prevent the stretch reflex from being elicited. The end points of the range are used as the starting positions from which proprioception testing is started, for it is in these positions that the stretch or pain response would occur. See reference: Trombly (ed): Bentzel, K: Evaluation of sensation.

52. (B) Left unilateral neglect. This is the inability to respond or orient to perceptions from the left side of the body. Evidenced as left unilateral neglect, this deficit will also be apparent in the draw-a-man test, copy a flower test, house test, and completing a human figure or face puzzle. Unilateral neglect is contralateral to the side of a brain lesion; therefore, left unilateral neglect would result from right side brain damage. Left neglect occurs most commonly in right hemisphere lesions. A cataract would cause a visual impairment with detail on both sides of a page. Bitemporal hemianopia (hemianopia is also referred to as hemianopsia) is also known as "tunnel vision," with the individuals peripheral vision lost. The individual would

still be able to cross midline with cataracts or bitemporal hemianopsia. A right neglect would not see the right side, and would draw all the figures on the left side of the page. Visuospatial deficits are an important factor influencing functional independence outcomes. Visuospatial ability should be taken into account when establishing treatment goals as well as during discharge planning. See reference: Trombly (ed): Quintana, L: Evaluation of perception and cognition.

53. (A) Visual memory, number sequencing, and constructional praxis. Visual memory is the ability to recall a perception that was previously stored. Number sequencing is the ability to put numbers in the order of occurrence. Constructional praxis is the ability to produce a design in two or three dimensions. A person would not need an intact body image, visual sequencing, 20/20 vision, or auditory memory to complete a "draw-a-clock" test. Because these are skills that may not be used or may not be compensated for by the person in an appropriate manner, a person would need proprioception to grasp the writing utensil. Visual closure would not be used because an entire clock is the design from which the test is completed. See reference: Trombly (ed): Quintana, L: Evaluation of perception and cognition.

54. (A) −15 degrees to 140 degrees. Negative range of motion documentation may vary from one setting to another. However, this range may be written as a negative sign preceding the degree (−15 degrees) or as a positive number preceding the neutral position (15 degrees to 0 degrees to 140 degrees). Therefore, answers B, C, and D are incorrect. See reference: Pedretti: Evaluation of joint range of motion.

55. (A) Short-term recall. Short-term recall would be the ability to recall all information that has just been received and to hold it in temporary use from 1 to 5 minutes or more. Short-term recall is not just a selected part of the information. Attention, answer B, would allow the person to retrieve information from a long series and to single out a specific part of the information for use. A person who is being evaluated for hearing, Answer C, would be checked for the accuracy of sound at different pitches, not a specific sound. Abstraction, answer D, would be the ability to extrapolate information from an idea to generalize to another situation. See reference: Zoltan, Siev, and Freishtat: Cognitive deficits.

56. (C) Fair minus (3−). The definition of *fair minus (3−)* is that the part moves through incomplete range of motion (less than 50%) against gravity or through complete ROM with gravity eliminated against slight resistance. A grade of *good (4)*, answer A, indicates strength on the manual muscle test and ability to move through full range of motion against gravity and to take moderate resistance. A *fair (3)*, answer B, grade would be the ability to move through full range of motion and against gravity, but not take any additional resistance. A grade of *poor plus (2+)*, answer D, would move through full range of motion with gravity eliminated and take minimal resistance before suddenly relaxing. See reference: Trombly:

Evaluation of biomechanical and physiological aspects of motor performance.

57. (A) Confused–Agitated (level IV). Much of the physical behavior seen is impulsive with bizarre, random actions, and conversation is incoherent with confabulation noted when asked a direct question. The man has a very short attention span and is unable to follow commands but is able to demonstrate some automatic behaviors. A person functioning at the confused–inappropriate level has much of the same behavior and verbalizations; however, an increase in attention span is demonstrated by the individual responding more consistently to simple commands. A person functioning at the confused–appropriate level continues to follow simple directions consistently and has goal-directed behavior with external cues. An individual functioning at the automatic–appropriate level has appropriate behavior which is robotlike. This level also has minimal to no confusion noted, and the individual is able to initiate social or leisure activities within a structured setting. See reference: Trombly (ed): Scott, AD, and Dow, PW: Traumatic brain injury.

58. (D) Glasgow Coma Scale. The Glasgow Coma Scale rates the responses of the eye opening best motor response from 1 to 6 and verbal response from one to five. The score for each area is totaled and the scale developers consider any person with a score of eight or below to be in a coma and a score of nine or above to be out of the comatose state. The Claudia Allen Scale of Cognitive Function is a measurement, which uses task performance to evaluate a person's cognitive level of functioning. The Rancho Los Amigos Levels of Cognitive Functioning uses a scale of eight levels to describe a person's behavior as he or she emerges from a coma and progresses beyond the confused state to a more purposeful and appropriate behavior. The Braintree Hospital Cognitive Continuum rates a person in the five areas of arousal, attention, discrimination, organization, and higher level cognitive function. This scale demonstrates the neurological recovery neurologically from a diffuse head injury and the person may be at a different place on the continuum according to the environment. See reference: Trombly (ed): Scott, AD, and Dow, PW: Traumatic brain injury.

59. (A) Soft to hard to rough. Hypersensitivity stimuli is graded by texture and force. Texture begins with soft, progresses to hard, and finally to rough. The force begins with touch, progresses to rub, and then to tapping. The texture and force of the stimuli are graded together. Light, medium, and heavy do not specify what the texture and force of the stimuli would be during training. A person with hypersensitivity would be unable to tolerate training beginning with a rough texture. See reference: Trombly (ed): Bentzel, K: Remediating sensory impairment.

60. (C) Visual agnosia. Visual agnosia is the inability to recognize common objects and demonstrate their use in an activity. Apraxia is the inability to perform a purposeful movement on command. A person with alexia is unable to understand the written language. Stereognosis is the ability to identify an object by manipulating it with the fingers without seeing it. See reference: Trombly (ed): Quintana, L: Evaluation of perception and cognition.

61. (D) Apply the stimuli to the uninvolved area proximally to distally in a random pattern. The general guidelines for sensation testing are that the person's vision should be occluded, the stimuli should be randomly applied with false stimuli intermingled, a practice trial should be performed before the test, and the unaffected side or area should be tested before the affected side or area. Also, the amount of time a person has to respond should be established. See reference: Trombly (ed): Bentzel, K: Evaluation of sensation.

62. (A) Training to inspect for pressure sores on bony prominences and affected areas. Visual inspection of an area is important to prevent pressure sores, which may develop because there are no sensory cues to alert a person to the skin breakdown. It is recommended that an individual with absent sensation not trim his or her own nails due to safety issues. Another person may be able to assist by trimming the nails or the individual could file his or her own nails; however, the second option is often difficult and time consuming. Extra padding on a splint would cause increased pressure and redness to an area, which would lead to skin breakdown. Hypersensitivity training is performed with exaggerated sensation, not absent sensation. See reference: Trombly (ed): Bentzel, K: Remediating sensory impairment.

63. (B) Light stroking, fast brushing, and quick stretch. Facilitation techniques are used to stimulate the muscle to provide a specific response, such as to improve postural control or to evoke a movement. Some of the facilitory techniques are light stroking, fast brushing, and quick stretch. Any techniques that use slower movement or warmth act as inhibitory techniques in the Rood approach, such as slow stroking or rolling and neutral warmth. In addition, prolonged icing may act as an inhibitor. See reference: Trombly: Rood approach.

64. (D) Chaining. Chaining is frequently used when teaching a multiple step task, as it is easier to teach only one step at a time than a complete activity. Repetition and rehearsal involve repeating the whole activity over and over until the activity is learned. Cuing uses an external source to remind a person of the next step or part of that step. See reference: Zoltan, Siev, and Freishtat: Explanations for use of this manual.

65. (B) Temperature and pain. The sensations of pain and temperature are carried along small, unmyelinated nerve fibers, which recover more rapidly than senses carried by larger, myelinated fibers. The sensations of pain and temperature are also part of the "protective" or primary sensory systems, which are the receivers of simple information. More complex information is carried through the "discriminative or epicritic system." The senses carried on this system are vibration, light touch, proprioception, and tactile localization. See reference: Trombly (ed): Bentzel, K: Evaluation of sensation.

66. (A) Stress reduction using meditation and yoga, energy conservation, establishment of new leisure skills, and involvement with a support group. The individual with AIDS should implement a form of exercise to provide mobility and reduce stress without draining his or her physical resources, in addition to using energy conservation techniques during ADL. New leisure interests should be established within the individual's capabilities to promote satisfaction from completion and learning of a new task. A support group will assist the individual with coping with anxiety about AIDS. An individual with substance abuse needs new leisure interests to replace the former activities that the individual had involving drug use activities. New leisure interests may also need to be developed due to the individual's decreasing physical abilities. It would not be appropriate for an individual to participate in an aerobics program because of the high energy demands. Vocational training would also not be appropriate, as the individual may be unable to continue to work secondary to frequent hospitalizations and decreasing physical status. A lecture would provide information about AIDS but not support to reduce anxiety. See reference: Reed: Immunologic disorders.

67. (B) A mobile arm support. A C5 quadriplegic with fair shoulder flexors and abductors and at least poor minus biceps, upper trapezius, and external rotators will be able to operate a mobile arm support for self-feeding and facial hygiene activities. A wrist-driven flexor hinge splint would be used for a lower level spinal cord injury (C6-C8) in which the individual had functional use of the shoulder and arm muscles and has fair plus or better wrist extension strength. This splint is indicated for individuals who lack prehension power. An electric feeder is indicated for individuals with a higher level of involvement (C4) and who demonstrate poor plus or weaker shoulder strength. Built-up silverware may be indicated for individuals with C8 or T1 injuries because they may lack the strength to tightly grasp regular utensils. See reference: Trombly (ed): Hollar, L: Spinal cord injury.

68. (D) Having him place his feet through loops of therapeutic band. A prefunctional activity is when an individual is unable to perform a specific task, so an activity is used that practices the same movement as placing his feet into his pants legs. Activities that teach him to pull his pants up do not practice the same skill, and doffing socks is an activity that practices the opposite skill, removing feet from something. The other choices are also functional tasks that practice a specific skill. A prefunctional activity provides a base to improve a functional activity and may be practiced before or at the same time as a functional task. See reference: Kovich and Bermann (eds): Van Dam-Burke, A, and Kovich, K: Self-care and homemaking.

69. (C) Substitution. The use of a new method of response based on remaining skills to perform the same activity is substitution. An example would be to follow written directions when assembling a wood project versus using visual memory, which may be impaired after a cerebrovascular accident (CVA). Problem solving is the ability to organize information from several levels to generate a solution to a problem. Retraining teaches the same skills of an activity to the person who previously had mastery of those skills. For example, having a person with hand weakness practice tying knots. Compensation would be avoiding performance of the activity entirely by using an alternative piece of equipment or method. See reference: Zoltan, Siev, and Freishtat: Explanations for use of this manual.

70. (C) Unmyelinated fibers would recover faster than myelinated fibers. Unmyelinated fibers are thinner and recover more quickly than the large, myelinated fibers. Myelinated fibers also need to regenerate the sheath and the nerve fibers. The length of time it takes to recover will also vary according to the location, severity, and etiology of the disruption. See reference: Trombly (ed): Philips, C: Impairments of hand function.

71. (B) Fingers flexed at all joints. When weight bearing, the fingers should be flexed at all joints (the fisted position). This preserves the tenodesis function by protecting the finger flexors from over-stretching. Another reason for this position is to prevent claw-hand deformity by protecting the intrinsic hand muscles from overstretching. See reference: Hill: Farmer, A: Setting goals.

72. (D) Peripheral edema following a cerebrovascular accident. Continuous passive range of motion could not be used following laceration to an artery or nerve, because a stretch could cause sutures to separate following surgery. Also, an unstable joint (arthritis) or an unstable fracture (one healing poorly with multiple trauma sites or in an area unable to be casted) could have further trauma caused by constant movement. A CPM may be used as a secondary method for controlling edema in a hand following a CVA by using movement to flex and extend the fingers and thus act as a pump to push fluid out of the hand by the flexion and extension of the fingers. See reference: Trombly (ed): Philips, C: Impairments of hand function.

73. (C) A glass of orange juice. Meal preparation is graded from cold to hot foods or beverages, and from simple to multiple steps. An individual beginning practice in meal preparation would start with a cold item with the least number of steps possible, for example, pouring a glass of juice or other cold beverage. Cold sandwich preparation adds another step as each topping to the bread is added, as well as for each utensil used. After preparation of cold items have been mastered, training in hot food or beverage preparation would begin if appropriate. See reference: Kovich and Bermann (eds): Van Dam-Burke, A, and Kovich, K: Self-care and homemaking.

74. (A) Increased. When a person sees the relationship between treatment and daily life, it increases carryover of techniques. A person will only continue to perform activities or techniques after therapy when the importance is seen to the person and his or her family. Carryover of ADL and cognitive training is unchanged or short term after discharge if the person sees no value or relevance to his or her daily life and will therefore, soon be discarded after discharge. See reference: Trombly (ed): Versluys, H: Facilitating psychosocial adjustment to disability.

75. (C) C8. An individual with C8 quadriplegia will have some use of the abductor pollicis longus, extensor pollicis longus, extensor digitorum communis, and extensor carpi ulnaris. The extensor tone of the muscles in conjunction with the splint will operate the power for prehension force. Individuals with C1 or C3 injuries have higher level lesions and will lack the wrist extension strength needed to operate the wrist-driven flexor hinge splint. An individual with a T10 injury will be able to grasp and manipulate utensils without difficulty or need for assistance. See reference: Trombly (ed): Hollar, L: Spinal cord injury; and Hill: Farmer, A: Evaluation.

76. (A) One or two step instructions frequently repeated. The best method to use with an individual with Alzheimer's disease is short instructions of one to two steps keeping them to the point and repeating them frequently. Demonstration with multiple-step instructions can be confusing as it provides too much stimulation. Multiple-step written instructions are unlikely to be retained in the individual's short-term memory after reading, or remembered in order. Also, written instructions could be lost if the individual puts them down. Verbally repeating directions over and over, or rehearsal, does not enable a person with Alzheimer's to retain information in the memory, and he or she may not repeat the instructions properly. See reference: Glickstein: Working with dementia clients.

77. (B) Hyperextension of the PIP joint and flexion of the DIP joint. Answer B is the only answer provided that describes a swan neck deformity. The pattern of hyperextension of the PIP and DIP joints may be seen in lower motor neuron palsies. Flexion of the PIP joint and hyperextension of the DIP is descriptive of a boutonniere deformity. An individual who has overstretched the volar plates at the PIP and DIP joints would have hyperextension of the MP joint and flexion of the DIP joint. See reference: Hunter, Schneider, Macklin, and Bell (eds): Phillips, C: The management of patients with rheumatoid arthritis, and Swanson, A: Pathomechanics of deformities of the hand and wrist.

78. (C) Radial nerve. Injury to the radial nerve in the wrist area will cause sensory damage only. This damage will occur to the radial two thirds of the dorsum of the hand. Damage to the median nerve at the wrist will cause decreased thumb and prehensile strength and complete or partial loss of sensation in the distal portion of the second digit (index finger) and third digits (long finger) with some loss in the fourth digit (ring finger). Damage to the ulnar nerve at the wrist will cause decreased grip strength and complete or partial loss of sensation to half of the fourth digit (ring finger) and all of the fifth digit (little finger) as well as the proximal hypothenar region. The ulnar and median nerves are frequently entrapped together. A brachial plexus injury causes peripheral nerve damage to

any or all of the fibers from C5 to T1. See reference: Kisner and Colby: The elbow and forearm complex.

79. (B) Median nerve. The median nerve passes through the carpal tunnel at the wrist. Impingement in this region will cause sensory changes in the thumb, index, and long fingers. Prolonged impingement in the carpal tunnel will result in atrophy of the thenar eminence and weakness of the opponens pollicis. Injury to the radial nerve in the wrist area will cause sensory damage only. Damage to the ulnar nerve at the wrist will cause decreased grip strength and complete or partial loss of sensation over half of the fourth digit (ring finger) and all of the fifth digit (little finger) plus the proximal hypothenar region. A brachial plexus injury causes peripheral nerve damage to either the C5-6 or C8-T10 levels. This will cause motor and sensory impairments. See reference: Kisner and Colby: The elbow and forearm complex.

80. (C) A heavy handbag held by the strap. The power grip is strongly based on the ulnar nerve and flexion of the ulnar fingers. The wrist is in a slightly extended position, which allows the object to be pressed firmly into the palm of the hand with the thumb in opposition. A needle would be held with two-point pinch while being threaded. A glass would be held with a cylindrical grasp. Finally, a key being placed in a lock would be held by a lateral pinch. See reference: Fess, Ewing, and Philips: Strickland, JW: Anatomy and kinesiology of the hand.

81. (C) Initiation. Initiation, or the ability to begin a task, affects a person's spontaneity in performing activities and how much he or she is able to perform. An individual with initiation problems may be able to plan or carry out activities, but unable to begin until prompted by another person. Problems with attention, concentration, or apraxia is evidenced as the incomplete or incorrect completion of an activity, but no difficulty is noted with beginning the activity. See reference: Zoltan, Siev, and Freishtat: Cognitive deficits.

82. (C) Have the individual set the utensil down until the mouth is cleared. The individual needs to the establish a routine to pace him or herself during feeding. This skill may then be used after discharge from therapy. An individual with problems relating to the rate of intake will put too much food in the mouth in spite of the size of the pieces. An impulsive person who eats too fast will also have difficulty counting slowly enough to have the mouth cleared by the time the count of 10 is reached. Food in separate containers would slow the meal down if they were presented one at a time, but would not slow the rate of food intake. See reference: Kovich and Bermann (eds): Van Dam-Burke, A, and Kovich, K: Self-care and homemaking.

83. (B) Labeling and calendars. An external memory device uses environmental adaptations or structure to assist the person in remembering specific information. Examples include setting an alarm clock to wake up in the morning, labeling drawers according to contents, and using a log or calendar to keep track of events and activities. An internal memory device would be the use of internalized memory techniques to structure information. Examples would be rehearsal, visual imagery, mnemonics, or elaborating on the information. See reference: Zoltan, Siev, and Freishtat: Cognitive deficits.

84. (C) The cup is placed to the right and below waist line. Reaching for objects placed on the left side would use little trunk rotation and no weight shift to the right side. It also decreases weight bearing to the right upper extremity. Reaching for an object on the right side increases trunk rotation, weight shift to the right, and weight bearing on the right arm, but the greatest amount of shift is needed when reaching for objects below waist level. See reference: Trombly: Proprioceptive neuromuscular facilitation (PNF) approach.

85. (D) Dunton. William Rush Dunton, Jr. wrote the first textbook on occupational therapy in 1915, *Occupational Therapy–A Manual for Nurses.* He wrote that the primary purpose of occupation is to "divert the individual's attention from unpleasant subjects to keep the individual's train of thought in more healthy channels." His primary work was to analyze activities and categorize individual's needs. He then worked to match the activity to the individual to achieve a therapeutic result. Rood and Brunnstrom are both therapists who developed treatment approaches to the brain-injured population. Adolf Meyer was a psychiatrist who promoted health through the use of activities. See reference: Hopkins and Smith: Hopkins, H: Scope of occupational therapy.

86. (D) Lemonade. Lemonade would be the most difficult to control since it is a thin liquid and a tart citrus product that would stimulate thin saliva flow with its sweet, citrus taste. Products that contain milk-thicken secretions making them easier to control. Tomato juice, although a citrus product, has much pulp in the juice to thicken it, which allows easier control. A shake with lime sorbet would still contain milk to counteract the effects of the lime (citrus) flavoring, plus the firmer consistency is easier to control with the tongue. The nondairy creamer would have little noticeable effect on the consistency of the coffee when swallowing. Coffee also contains caffeine, which is dehydrating and would leave a drier taste in the mouth, because less saliva is produced. See reference: Kovich and Bermann (eds): Van Dam-Burke, A, and Kovich, K: Self-care and homemaking.

87. (A) Within normal limits. The normal range of motion for both internal and external rotation is 70 degrees. Rotation may be assessed with the humerus adducted against the trunk or with the shoulder abducted at 90 degrees. If the humeral movements for internal or external rotation were observed during the performance of activities and were found to be adequate for the performance of any functional activities, the range of motion may be noted as within functional limits (WFL). A formal joint measurement may not be performed if the joint is WFL, even though the end of the range may be lacking a few degrees, since the loss of movement may not be seen as significant by the individual. Hypermobility at a joint is

motion past the average range of motion, which at the shoulder would be past 80 degrees of internal rotation. If hypermobility is a deformity caused by an unstable joint, as might occur after a surgical repair or a disease process, then splinting or another form of stabilization or immobilization may be used to correct the problem. If hypermobility is seen during range of motion, it may be compared with the individual's opposite side to assess normal range. A limitation of internal rotation at the shoulder would be less than 80 degrees of motion. If a limitation is seen, it may only be treated if it interferes with the function of the upper extremity. See reference: Trombly: Evaluation of biomechanical and physiological aspects of motor performance.

88. (C) A grief response. Grief is an adaptive mechanism used for dealing with a disabling condition, since a loss of function has occurred. Dependency, stress reactions, and unrealistic goals are responses that would not normally pass with time. They also interfere with the recovery process when in the extreme, as with grief. See reference: Trombly (ed): Versluys, H: Evaluation of emotional adjustment to disabilities.

89. (D) Built-up handles. Built-up handles would allow a comfortable grasp that regular utensils would not provide without adding extra weight. A weighted handle would cause more rapid fatigue and strain to the joints. An arthritic person would have adequate grasp and release with a built-up handle, making it easier to use than a universal cuff. See reference: Trombly (ed): Feinberg, J, and Trombly, C: Arthritis.

90. (A) Constructional apraxia. An individual with constructional apraxia may have full sensory awareness of the affected side of the body, but still may be unable to perform the construction of one or more objects onto each other to carry out a verbal command or don clothing in the proper sequence or position. Unilateral neglect occurs as the individual neglects the affected side of the body and performs activities toward or with the unaffected side. An example would be an individual only combing one side of his hair or shaving one side of his face. See reference: Trombly (ed): Quintana, L: Remediating cognitive impairment.

91. (D) Unclamp the individual's catheter and tap over the bladder. The individual is suffering a condition, which is termed autonomic dysreflexia. If not promptly addressed, death may result. This condition may be caused by a bowel impaction, plugged catheter, or suppository insertion. Do not recline the individual in that this may result in a higher cerebral blood pressure. The condition must be treated promptly so taking a heart rate and blood pressure postpone action on the condition. A drop in blood sugar is usually associated with diabetes, which is counteracted by having the individual consume fruit juice to raise the blood sugar level. Autonomic dysreflexia causes the blood pressure to increase to dangerous levels, so no action should be performed to the individual that would cause the blood pressure to rise. See reference: Trombly (ed): Hollar, L: Spinal cord injury.

92. (B) Figure-ground perception. Figure ground perception is the ability to visually separate an object from the surrounding background. An example of this would be an individual having the ability to find a button on a plaid shirt. A problem with spatial relations is seen in dressing by a person over or underreaching for buttons. The person is unable to judge the relationship between the object and the body. Body image is a mental picture of the person's body that includes how the person feels about the body. Visual closure is the ability to recognize an object although only part of it is seen, for example, recognizing a partially covered button. See reference: Zoltan, Siev, and Freishtat: Spatial relations syndrome.

93. (D) Anosognosia. Anosognosia is a form of neglect in which the individual denies any deficits. Compensation techniques can not be taught to someone who has no awareness of his or her deficits. A person with a visual field cut has a loss of a specific area of vision related to an area of the visual system that has been damaged. When there is an awareness of the loss, compensatory techniques can be taught. A person who has apraxia is unable to perform a purposeful movement on command, but is able to understand a loss of ability, and can perform activities spontaneously or follow some cues. Aphasia is an impairment of receptive or expressive communication verbally, but a person with this is able to comprehend gestures or pictures and use them as a compensatory technique. See reference: Trombly (ed): Quintana, L: Evaluation of perception and cognition.

94. (B) Initiation. Initiation problems are often seen when an individual is unable to perform the first step of an activity without requiring prompting. A problem with impulsiveness during self care would be seen by attempting to complete many steps of an activity rapidly, requiring slowing the rate for safety reasons. Memory or attention problems are seen by skipping the steps of an activity either because he or she does not remember the steps or is distracted by internal or external stimuli. Memory deficits are also evidenced as steps of a task not performed in sequence. The lack of initiation (the ability to begin a task) will affect a person's spontaneity in performing activities. The individual with initiation problems may be able to plan or carry out activities, but may be unable to begin until prompted by someone else. An individual who has difficulty with impulsivity, memory, or attention would have no difficulty with beginning the activity, but would have difficulty listing the steps. See reference: Kovich and Bermann (eds): Bermann, D: Treatment of sensory-perceptual and cognitive deficits.

95. (A) Perform pursed lip breathing when doing activities. Pursed lip breathing is a technique that narrows the passage of air during expiration. This technique helps individuals with chronic obstructive pulmonary disease (COPD) to keep the airway open and improve breathing efficiency. The overall effect is improved endurance and tolerance for activities. Taking hot showers and avoiding air conditioning during the warm weather are incorrect in that both activities are contraindicated for individuals with COPD. Using a long handled bath sponge may be helpful but is not the MOST likely tip to be on a home program for an individual with COPD. See reference: Kisner and Colby: Management of obstructive and restrictive pulmonary conditions.

96. (C) Limit weight bearing on the involved extremity. Precautions for following a total knee replacement would include graded lower extremity weight bearing determined by the surgeon. These precautions may range from nonweight bearing, toe touch, and partial or full weight bearing. The level usually changes between the day of surgery and discharge, according to the person's rate of healing as seen in radiographs. The individual usually has a course of physical therapy to practice the appropriate level of weight bearing during gait and may or may not be seen by an occupational therapist to receive self care or home management training. Following the knee surgery, a person is allowed full hip movement and is allowed full weight bearing on the uninvolved lower extremity. Full knee extension is encouraged, and flexion exercises for the knee are part of the individual's physical therapy. See reference: Trombly (ed): Bear-Lehman, J: Orthopaedic conditions.

97. (D) A cutting board with two nails in it. The potato is placed on the nails to hold it in place while working. The dycem would only hold the cutting board in place, not the potato being cut. A plate guard would not be secured tightly enough to the plate to withstand the force of cutting the potato. A rocker knife would be unable to both stabilize the potato and be used for cutting. See reference: Trombly (ed): Stewart, C: Retraining housekeeping and child care skills.

98. (A) Using the strongest joint, avoiding positions of deformity, and ensuring correct patterns of movement. These principles of joint protection are beneficial for all individuals. The significance of using these principles for individuals with pre-existing joint deformities and adverse musculoskeletal changes may help to restore function as well as prevent further impairments. Answers B, C, and D involve muscle relaxation and stress management. See reference: Trombly (ed): Bear-Lehman, J: Orthopaedic conditions.

99. (B) A call system for emergency and nonemergency use. A call system is necessary for a person with a high level spinal cord injury to allow the caretaker to leave the room, but remain available to answer the person's call for assistance for daily needs or an emergency. This is frequently the first opportunity that a person with a spinal cord injury would have to control some part of his or her life, giving some feeling of independence or choice. An environmental control unit does allow independence in operating appliances, lights, and so on through the use of switches or voice control, but would not be a necessity for safety. A remote control power door opener that would allow a caretaker to enter would be useless if the person is unable to call for assistance. An electric page turner is useless without the ability to call for someone to position or replace reading material. See reference: Hill, Intagliata, and Allen (eds): Jones, R: Home environmental control.

100. (D) A long handled bath sponge. A person with a total hip arthroplasty needs to avoid hip flexion of 80 degrees or more, hip adduction with internal rotation at the knee or ankle, or to lift the knee higher than the hip during self care or home management activities. A wire basket attached to the walker would not allow the person to come close to a counter without having to step sideways, which causes hip adduction to either move toward or away from the counter. A padded toilet seat of 1 inch height or a short handled sponge would cause the person to flex the hip past 80 degrees during the performance of self care activities. See reference: Trombly (ed): Bear-Lehman, J: Orthopaedic conditions.

101. (C) Major impairment in several areas (e.g., defiant at home and failing at school). Axis V indicates a person's Global Assessment of Functioning score. GAF is a numerical scale ranging from persistent danger of hurting self (1) to superior functioning (100). Major impairments are scored between 31 and 40. Answer A would be a score between 71 and 80. Answer B would be score between 51 and 60. Answer D would be scored between 21 and 30. See reference: American Psychiatric Association: Multiaxial assessment.

102. (D) Thorazine. Thorazine is an antipsychotic medication. Lithium, answer A, and elavil, answer B, are used to treat mood disorders. Answer C, is an anti-anxiety medication. See reference: Hopkins and Smith (eds): Gibson, D, and Richert, GZ: The therapeutic process.

103. (D) The individual's diagnosis is mental illness or mental retardation with nursing care needs requiring active treatment. As of October 1990, all individuals admitted to long-term nursing homes must have a clear need for skilled nursing care. If mental health problems also exist that require active treatment in addition to the identified nursing care needs, the mental health treatment must also be provided. See reference: Eichmann, MA, Griffin, BP, Lyons, JS, Larson, DB, and Finkel, S: An estimation of the impact of OBRA-87 on nursing home care in the United States. *Hosp Community Psychiatry*, 43, 781–788, 1992.

104. (A) Her parents were substance abusers. Adult children of alcoholics are at much greater risk for abusing substances themselves. Unfortunately, individuals rarely volunteer and are rarely asked about a history of physical or sexual abuse. The incidence of abuse is quite high with individuals who grow up with alcoholic caretakers. Even when abusive histories and self-mutilating behaviors are known to the treatment team, they are often inadequately addressed. See reference: Rose, SM, Peabody, CG, and Stratigeas, B: Undetected abuse among intensive case management clients. *Hosp Community Psychiatry*, 42, 499–503, 1991.

105. (D) This individual's satisfaction with the activities he listed on the log may not fit into work, leisure, and self-care categories. It is important to find out how each individual categorizes his or her daily activities, especially when the individual comes from a culture that is different from the therapist's. Answer A is incorrect because the occupational therapist does not know if there is a change or reduction of interests. Answer B is premature because the occupational therapist does not know if the absence of leisure activities is a problem. Answer C is incorrect because it involves the use of stereotypes to explain individual behavior. See reference: Christiansen and Baum (eds): Krefting, LM, and Krefting, DV: Cultural influence on performance.

106. (D) Bulimics who are at or above their normal body weight. Ninety percent of all eating disorders occur in women. Most women with eating disorders, bulimics and anorexics, are between adolescence and adulthood. Only one third of all bulimics weigh less than their normal body weight. See reference: Hopkins and Smith (eds): Beck, NL: Eating disorders: Anorexia nervosa and bulimia nervosa.

107. (D) A sheltered workshop. This is the most available type of vocational service for adults with mental retardation. Although two alternatives (answers B and C) that incorporate an actual job and may be preferred, these are not as commonly available. See reference: Hopkins and Smith (eds): Humphrey, R, and Jacobs, K: Mental retardation.

108. (A) Dual diagnosis. Examples of dual diagnostic categories are mental health and mental retardation and mental health and substance abuse. Multiply handicapped refers to the coexistence of physical and mental health types of problems. Answers C and D are not terms commonly used in health care. See reference: Hopkins and Smith (eds): Humphrey, R, and Jacobs, K: Mental retardation.

109. (B) Forgetting to turn off the stove burner. The progression of dementia of the Alzheimer's type is often described by its phases of impairment in functioning. Behaviors linked to memory impairments usually occur in the early stages, whereas social and motor impairments occur later. See reference: Bonder: Delerium and dementia.

110. (C) Conduct disorder. Conduct disorders often involve aggression to people or animals and property destruction. Individuals with Asperger's disorder, answer A, demonstrate restricted or limited social behaviors. Answer B, attention deficit disorders, involve impulsive but not typically violent behaviors. Answer D, oppositional defiant disorders, involve similar but less severe behaviors as conduct disorders. See reference: American Psychiatric Association: Disorders usually first diagnosed in infancy, childhood, or adolescence.

111. (C) Assessing and submitting reports for a competency hearing that determines an individual's ability to manage his or her own funds. Forensics is a specialty area dealing with problems linking psychiatry and the law. Answer C is the situation that clearly links psychiatry and the law and is a common role for occupational therapists. Answer A does not describe the type of "help" provided, so the occupational therapy role is not addressed. Answer B is typically the role of therapeutic recreation or activity therapy. Answer D does not specify if patients with legal involvement are being treated by the occupational therapist. See reference: Hopkins and Smith (eds): Gibson, D, and Richert, GZ: The therapeutic process.

112. (C) Individual's pattern and strength of leisure interests are inadequate to support leisure resource exploration in his community. This statement represents an analysis of the objective findings about the individual's responses during the interest checklist inventory using the SOAP note format. Answer A is the "subjective" component of the progress note. Answer B is the "objective" findings and answer D is the "plan" section of the note. See reference: Hopkins and Smith (eds): Perinchief, JM: Service management.

113. (D) Community Mental Health Center. CMHC is an abbreviation for Community Mental Health Center. Individuals are often recommended for hospitalization from outpatient care such as that provided by community mental health centers. See reference: Hopkins and Smith (cds): Richert, GZ: Program planning, development, and implementation.

114. (C) Section C. Statement's that identify the direction and the criterion that the individual will achieve are goals. Section A contains demographics. Section B contains the problem. Section D contains a SOAP progress note. See reference: Hopkins and Smith (eds): Perinchief, JM: Service management.

115. (A) Section A. The database of a problem-oriented medical record includes demographics such as age, marital status, and diagnosis. This section should also contain an overall statement of the individual's chief complaint. See reference: Christiansen and Baum (eds): Bruce and Borg: Assessing psychological performance factors.

116. (B) Section B. In the POMR format, problems are numbered descriptions of the individual's problems. Progress should be linked to the problem list (see section D). See reference: Hopkins and Smith (eds): Perinchief, JM: Service management.

117. (C) Therapist intervenes with a suggestion each time the client makes an assembly error. Self concept deficits are addressed through feedback from the therapist and through the activity. Answers A, B, and D are appropriate approaches for self-concept deficits. Intervening to prevent errors, answer C, can elicit frustration and can emphasize incompetence with the client. This approach should be avoided. See reference: Denton: Treatment planning and treatment intervention.

118. (D) Psychological components. Psychological properties of activities include delayed gratification and predictability of results that enhance success experiences.

Social components involve interactions with others. Sensory–perceptual and cognitive components involve an awareness and processing of incoming information. See reference: Hopkins and Smith (eds): Simon, CJ: Use of activity and activity analysis.

119. (D) Disorganized psychosis. Directive group treatment is a highly structured approach that is used in acute care psychiatry for minimally functioning individuals. This approach is useful for disorganized and disturbed functioning with psychoses and other neurologic disorders. Task groups are more appropriate for substance abuse. Psychoeducation groups are appropriate for eating disorders and adjustment disorders. See reference: Hopkins and Smith (eds): Beck, NL: Substance abuse: Drug addiction and alcoholism.

120. (B) Bring about change among the members. Change is the overall purpose of therapeutic groups. Both answers A and C are methods by which members may change. Answer D is an advantage of groups but is not a main purpose. See reference: Posthuma: The small group counseling and therapy.

121. (D) A therapist who encourages group members to share similar situations and reactions with one another. Answer D is an approach designed to develop cohesiveness and universality among members. Seeing others as similar has been identified by individuals as a curative factor. Answers A and C are approaches designed to impart information. Answer B is an example of catharsis, which may not be helpful to all members and requires the therapist to understand precautions for the use of catharsis. See reference: Posthuma: The small group counseling and therapy.

122. (B) Confront the individual's behavior: "Are you aware that your frequent interruptions prevent others from having a chance to contribute?" In general, the group leader should try A, C, or D before trying confrontation of the individual's monopolizing. Confrontation within a group setting is difficult for many individuals to accept. See reference: Posthuma: What to do if . . .

123. (A) Allows the therapist to obtain facts. Fact gathering is the primary advantage to closed questions. The occupational therapist should be aware that posing mostly closed questions can lead to biased information gathering, as with answers B and D. Although you can generally ask more closed questions in a short amount of time, this is generally not a patient-focused goal. See reference: Denton: Effective communications.

124. (C) Assertiveness training. Broken record is a specific assertiveness skill concerned with repeating your position without losing control. Music therapy is a creative arts discipline. Psychodrama is a group technique for expressing catharsis. Self-awareness groups tend to focus on feeling identification and expression versus skill building. See reference: Posthuma: Appendix A—Small group programs.

125. (D) Smoking during the group is prohibited. Norms are guidelines for behavior in groups, whether stated explicitly or shared implicitly by the members. Answer A is an individual's behavior versus the group's guidelines. Answer B is a group activity. Answer C is a general group goal. See reference: Posthuma: Goals and norms.

126. (B) Confusion. Medication side effects are observed and reported by occupational therapists. Anti-anxiety medications often cause confusion. Akithesia, EPS, and tardive dyskinesia (answers A, C, and D, respectively), are adverse effects commonly linked to antipsychotic medications. See reference: Hopkins and Smith (eds): Gibson, D, and Richert, GZ: The therapeutic process.

127. (A) Treatment from the occupational therapist's plan provided by a COTA. It is fraudulent to bill any other services as occupational therapy services. Billings are limited to charges for services rendered by the occupational therapist's and assistant's for the evaluation and treatment of functional deficits. See reference: Novak: Improving payent for occupational therapists, in mental health through effective documentation strategies.

128. (B) Over involvement. The conscious use of self is an area that should be addressed in supervision. There are some therapist-patient interactions that can stall or interfere with treatment goals. One of these problematic interactions is over involvement. Behaviors that can signal this are making extra time for an individual at the expense of others. Transference, answer C, is a reaction that the individual has toward the therapist. Long-term over involvement can lead to burnout, answer D. Self disclosure, answer A, is the comments the therapist makes to an individual to emphasize a point made by the individual. See reference: Hopkins and Smith (eds): Schwartzberg, SL: Tools of practice—Therapeutic use of self.

129. (D) Outpatient counseling. Transitional programs after hospitalization offer a range or continuum of support to mental health consumers. Outpatient counseling is the least restrictive situation as it provides support through counseling but does not require any residential treatment. Answers A, B, and C are all residential programs with varying amounts of supervision. See reference: Hopkins and Smith (eds): Richert, GZ, and Gibson, D: Practice settings.

130. (A) Stress management. Psychoeducational groups focus on specific content areas such as stress management or assertiveness. These groups focus on education of individuals about the specific content areas and are appropriate for short-term treatment facilities. The use of directive groups and task groups are described for question 119. Group therapy focuses on verbal psychotherapy and is conducted by other disciplines. See reference: Hopkins and Smith (eds): Niestadt, ME: Stress management.

131. (B) Put the dried dishes away and begin to hand the individual wet dishes. Compensating for mistakes is helpful for increasing the self worth and integrity of individuals with dementia. This approach is recommended

over drawing attention to errors, especially in situations where safety is not an issue. Answers A, C, and D all draw attention to the individual's errors. See reference: Trace, S, and Howell, T: Occupational therapy in geriatric mental health. *Am J Occup Ther*, 45:833–838, 1991.

132. (D) Autocratic leadership. Autocratic leadership styles focus on directing and dominating the group and its tasks. A democratic style offers suggestions, but leaves most decisions up to the members. Laissez-faire leadership provides minimal to no task direction. Bureaucratic leadership is rule focused. See reference: Posthuma: Leadership.

133. (B) Insecurity. Feelings of insecurity are often covered up by projecting difficulties onto other objects (the collage) or other people. Hopelessness involves negative statements about oneself or about changing. Individual 2's comments reflect indecision. Passivity is often only "heard" through nonverbal communication. See reference: Posthuma: Observation and analysis.

134. (B) An example of individual 1's time management behaviors recorded in the subjective section of the note. The time management component involves planning and participating in activities that promote satisfaction. Individual 1's behaviors indicate difficulty with planning, participation, and satisfaction aspects. An individual's statements are appropriate for recording subjective information. The sample interaction does not provide the occupational therapist with enough information about individual 1 to determine if the behavior is ineffective coping or self expression difficulties (answers A and D). There is no information about personal space, eye contact, and so on to determine if individual 1 has inappropriate social conduct (answer C). See reference: Bonder: Appendix B—Uniform terminology for reporting occupational therapy services.

135. (C) Hallucinations. The symptoms of schizophrenia are generally classified as either negative or positive. Negative symptoms tend to persist after the positive or "acute" symptoms are treated with medications. Negative symptoms greatly impact an individual's level of function. A, B, and C are all negative symptoms. See reference: Hopkins and Smith (eds): Richert GZ: Program planning, development, and implementation.

136. (A) Student. The roles of the care givers and service recipients vary according to the general approach being used. Labels and language reflect these varied roles. *Patient* is terminology connected to a biomedical approach. *Client* is often linked to outpatient or community approaches. *Consumer* is often linked to activist and advocacy approaches. *Student* is the term linked to a psychoeducational approach. See reference: Crist: Community living skills: A psychoeducational community-based program.

137. (C) Ask the individual how often she has these "spells" and encourage her to sit back down until it passes and stop working on the budget activity for today. Advising the discontinuation of prescribed medications is outside the domain of occupational therapy. The occupational therapist should have a general understanding of possible adverse reactions to common antianxiety medications. Frequent adverse reactions are dizziness and confusion. Although ultimate responsibility of the therapist is to report the individual's reactions to the treatment team as soon as possible, additional information from the individual as well as recommending immediate safety precautions is necessary. Answer D is the safety precaution for orthostatic hypotension, not dizziness. See reference: Hopkins and Smith (eds): Gibson, D, and Richert, GZ: The therapeutic process.

138. (B) Universal precautions. Health care personnel are to follow universal precautions when blood or body fluids are present. Suicidal, escape, and medical precautions are guidelines developed for individuals identified with those risks that are not noted in this question. See reference: Hopkins and Smith (eds): Pizzi, M: HIV infection and AIDS.

139. (C) The individual's complaints focus on physical concerns, denies feeling depressed but feels less energy, has lost weight, and complains of some concentration and memory problems. The general presentation of depression varies somewhat with an individual's age group. Answer A is more descriptive of adolescent depression and answer C is descriptive of middle adult depression. Depression and dementia are also important for care givers to distinguish between in working with geriatric patients. Answer D is a description of complaints consistent with dementia. See reference: Hopkins and Smith (eds): Rogers, JC: Geriatric psychiatry.

140. (B) Provide enough chairs around a round table. Circular seating arrangements generally facilitate the most communication among members. Rectangle-shaped tables can lead to unbalanced communications. Difficulties in maintaining comfort and attention are problems related to floor seating arrangements. Using available chairs and couches frequently provide different seating heights and rectangular or square arrangements. See reference: Posthuma: Group dimensions.

141. (B) Showing tension, asking for help, or withdrawing from the process. Answer B is a category that describes the underlying emotional impact on the process with this group. The individual's first statement is about withdrawing or discontinuing effort within this group. The other categories are concerned with communication and control concerns within a group. See reference: Posthuma: Observation and analysis.

142. (C) "What is the word for it?" Clarifying is designed to facilitate understanding of an individual's comments or the process within a group. Answer C is an example of asking to clarify the client's meaning. See answers for 139 and 140 to identify other response types. See reference: Posthuma: Leadership techniques.

143. (B) "Seems like you might be feeling pretty discouraged and wondering about the whole point of groups and treatment." Reflection conveys that you

have heard and understood, particularly the feelings behind the statement. Reflection is deeper than restatement of what the person said as is shown in answer A. See reference: Posthuma: Leadership techniques.

144. (D) "Roadblocks that are put in our way can stop most of us from wanting to continue with what we are doing. Maybe, as a group, we can look at ways of getting around or over the roadblocks. I think it could help with the hopelessness." Support is an approach that can be helpful when an individual is pulling back or away from difficult, intense feelings or a situation. Support should be encouraging the individual or the group to work on the difficulties. See reference: Posthuma: Leadership techniques.

145. (C) Coping strategies for continuing medication compliance. Studies designed to determine the factors related to frequent readmissions for psychiatric individuals have found medication noncompliance to be the major reason for readmission. The other strategies listed may be important issues for specific individuals, however, they are not the primary issue. See reference: Green, JH: Frequent hospitalization and noncompliance with treatment. Hosp Community Psychiatry, 39:963–964, 1988.

146. (B) Closed question. Closed questions can be answered with one word responses such as "yes" or "no." Open questions, answer A, are very broad and can be answered many different ways. Leading questions, answer C, suggest the desired response. A double question, answer D, asks two questions at once or forces a choice. See reference: Denton: Effective communications.

147. (B) A self-help group. Self-help groups are supportive and educational and focus on personal growth around a single major life disrupting problem. Support groups, answer C, focus on assisting members who are in crises until the crisis is past. Advocacy groups, answer A, focus on changing others or changing the system versus changing one's self. Psychotherapy groups, answer D, focuses on understanding the influence of past experiences on present conflicts. See reference: Posthuma: Self-help groups.

148. (B) Members share their experiences and struggles with alcohol use. Shared experiences can build feelings of understanding, hope, and acceptance among the members of a self-help group. Answers A, C, and D are all examples of member roles that are NOT encouraged in self-help groups. See reference: Posthuma: Self-help groups.

149. (C) Alcoholics Anonymous (AA). Self-help groups focus on personal growth in which leadership comes from the membership. AA is an example of such a group. MADD is an example of an advocacy group that focuses on changing the legal system. Group therapy involves leadership and expertise from outside of the membership itself. Al-Anon is a combination of support group and self-help group for the family members of the alcoholic. See reference: Posthuma: Self-help groups.

150. (B) To evaluate the individual's occupational performance. Discharge planning in short term hospitalizations should begin at admission. The therapist's evaluation of occupational performance is the first step in the occupational therapy discharge planning. Answers A, C, and D would all occur later in the treatment pro-cess. See reference: Sederer (ed): Schwartzberg, SL, and Abeles, J: Occupational therapy.

151. (D) Universal precautions. Treating blood and body substances as though they are contaminated is the concept of universal precautions. There are four strategies to protect an employee from potential exposure. Engineering controls modify the work environment to reduce risk of exposure. An example would be using sharps containers, eye wash stations, and biohazard waste containers. Work practice controls are policies that require a procedure be done a certain way so that potential for exposure may be reduced. An example of such would be the *technique* for disposal of sharps using only one hand or frequent handwashing during and after patient contact. Personal protective equipment would include wearing the appropriate gear to prevent contact with blood or identified body substances. Equipment may include goggles, masks, and gowns. See reference: Hopp and Rogers: Elder, HA: Transmission of HIV and prevention of AIDS.

152. (A) Entry level. As this therapist re-enters the profession of occupational therapy, he or she will be striving to regain previous skills and become accountable in relevant professional activities. Therefore, this individual will be functioning at entry level. Intermediate and advanced levels require specialization in an area along with increased responsibility and participation in relevant professional activities. Educator levels are separate from practitioner levels and they themselves go into entry-level, intermediate, and high proficiency. See reference: AOTA: The Occupational Therapy Roles Task Force: Occupational Therapy Roles.

153. (C) Advanced supervision. Advanced levels of supervision occur on an as needed basis. Individuals being supervised at this level have demonstrated skill and expertise in the area of occupational therapy in which they are working. They may also serve as a resource person and assist in continuing education or research as it relates to their expertise. Answer A describes close supervision, which is direct daily contact between the supervisor and the employee. This form of supervision is recommended for entry level therapists or therapists re-entering the profession of occupational therapy. Answers B and D describe routine supervision and general supervision. These forms of supervision are for the therapist who can function independently and have mastered basic role functions of occupational therapy. See reference: AOTA: The Occupational Therapy Roles Task Force: Occupational Therapy Roles.

154. (B) The COTA updating the occupational therapist on improvements that the patient has made in the last week and both therapists providing information to up-date the goals. A collaborative relationship between an occupational therapist and the assistant supports sharing of information and utilization of each professional's skills. In this type of relationship, communication is two-way and both individuals work as a team to the benefit of the patient. Answers A and D demonstrate one-way communication with the therapist telling the assistant what to do. Answer C is incorrect in that the therapist only takes information off of the progress note and does not allow for feedback or input from the COTA into the patients discharge status or discharge disposition and recommendations. See reference: AOTA: The Occupational Therapy Roles Task Force: Occupational Therapy Roles.

155. (B) A monitor. A monitor, is a specific area that will be systematically checked for compliance to the established standard measured. Answer A, an indicator, is an overall aspect of care, which has set criteria that are established. Answer C, a threshold, is a numerical measure of the level at which quality services are provided. Answer D, the data source, is the area or way in which information will be gathered. See reference: Jacobs and Logigian: Quality assurance.

156. (C) The threshold. The threshold is a numerical measure of the level at which quality services are provided. The threshold serves as a "breaking point" in that areas that fall on the negative side of the threshold are monitored and actions are taken to improve the service. Answer A, the time frame, indicates the period in which the sample of subjects who will be studied are taken. Answer B, a sample size, is the number of subjects or items that will be included in a study. Answer D, the data source, is the area or way in which information will be gathered. An example would be a concurrent or retrospective chart review to analyze the appropriateness of documentation. See reference: Jacobs and Logigian: Quality assurance.

157. (B) The sample size. A sample size is the number of subjects or items that will be included in a study. This may be represented by a number or a percentage. An example would be studying "10 percent of the patient charts for the first quarter." A numerical sample size could be "25 charts will be reviewed each quarter." Answer A, the time frame, indicates the period in which the sample of subjects who will be studied are taken. Answer C, the threshold, is the minimum acceptable level of performance. Answer D, the data source, is the area or way in which information will be gathered. An example would be a concurrent or retrospective chart review to analyze the appropriateness of documentation. See reference: Hopkins and Smith (eds): Perinchief, JM: Service management.

158. (D) Facilitate effective treatment. The primary purpose of documentation is to facilitate the treatment process. By defining the problem, goals and objectives, and a treatment plan, the therapist's thoughts are organized in order to carry out goal-directed services. Additional purposes of documentation are to serve as legal documentation, report services provided for reimbursement, and provide communication among the team, patient, or family. Answers A, B, and C, are incorrect in that they are not part of the primary reasons for documentation. However, some forms of documentation may be necessary to meet accrediting agencies guidelines or be used in research. See reference: Hopkins and Smith (eds): Perinchief, JM: Service management.

159. (B) Any equipment that has come into contact with body fluids will be sent to be sterilized prior to using the equipment again. OSHA has set out strategies to protect individuals from potential exposure to HIV or HVB. This situation would be an example of an engineering control. These controls are to modify the work environment to reduce risk of exposure. Other examples would be using sharps containers, eye wash stations, and biohazard waste containers. Answers A, C, and D would not meet guidelines set forth by OSHA. See reference: Hopp and Rogers: Elder, HA: Transmission of HIV and prevention of AIDS.

160. (B) SOAP notes. The problem oriented medical record is based on assessing an individual's limitations and listing problem areas. A SOAP note is a structured format of documentation that consists of four sections: subjective, objective, assessment, and plan. This format may be used in initial, progress, and discharge notes as well as consultation documentation. Answer A is incorrect because most checklists are not designed to assess and list problem areas. Answer C is incorrect because the answer is vague and does not indicate whether the format is structured or assesses and documents problem areas. Answer D is incorrect in that a structured format is not followed. See reference: Hopkins and Smith (eds): Perinchief, JM: Service management.

161. (C) IEP. The individual education plan is a form that must be completed for children receiving services in the school system. This documentation standard was defined in The Education of the Handicapped Children Act (1975 and 1986). Answer A, UB-82, is incorrect in that this form is used to process insurance claims. Answer B is incorrect in that FIM stands for "functional independence measure," which is used on rehabilitation units to measure patient's levels of independence. Answer D is incorrect in that the I-9 is a form used by employers to verify citizenship in the employment process. See reference: Hopkins and Smith (eds): Perinchief, JM: Service management.

162. (B) Outcome. Outcomes are the results of service intervention that an individual receives. These measures are taken at the completion of service intervention. Answer A, the process, is the manner in which services are rendered. Each process has an order in which activities occur. An example of the process of interaction between the consumer and therapist may progress from initial interview, to evaluation, to treatment, to family training, to discharge intervention. Answer C, program evaluation, is the compilation of the intervention results for a population of individuals. One of the most frequently used program evaluation systems is the FIM (Functional Independence

Measure). FIM scores may be compiled and compared with regional and national norms. Answer D, utilization review, reviews the care that is provided to ensure that services were appropriate and not over or under utilized. Overall, utilization review analyzes the services to ensure that the interventions were provided in an economical manner. See reference: Hopkins and Smith (eds): Perinchief, JM: Service management.

163. (A) A process. The process is the manner in which services are rendered. Each process has an order in which activities occur. An example of the process of interaction between the consumer and therapist may progress from initial interview, to evaluation, to treatment, to family training, to discharge intervention. Answer B, outcome, is the results of service intervention that an individual receives. These measures are taken at the completion of service intervention. Answer C, program evaluation, is the compilation of the intervention results for a population of individuals. One of the most frequently used program evaluation systems is the FIM. FIM scores may be compiled and compared with regional and national norms. Answer D, utilization review, reviews the care that is provided to ensure that services were appropriate and not over or under utilized. Overall, utilization review analyzes the services to ensure that the interventions were provided in an economical manner. See reference: Hopkins and Smith (eds): Perinchief, JM: Service management.

164. (A) The goals have been met and the individual can no longer benefit from occupational therapy services. Discontinuation of occupational therapy should occur when an individual has met the goals and further progress is not anticipated within the therapeutic environment. Answer C is incorrect in that often times, individuals may achieve their goals and new goals are established because it is anticipated that further progress may be made. Answer B is incorrect in that if the therapist does not anticipate progress and the goals have not been met, it is necessary for the therapist to discharge the individual. Depending on an individual's status at discharge, recommendations may be made for community services, outpatient care, day care, or home health services. A vital role of the occupational therapist is to provide appropriate linkages to the community for those individuals served. The preparation for discharge planning should include the patient's support system, discharge environment, and possible need for continued health care services. Answer D is incorrect in that discharge of an individual should be made on objective information. If an individual does not "feel" that he or she is making progress, the therapist should be able to clarify with the individual his or her status based on objective measurements and observations. See reference: Hopkins and Smith (eds): Perinchief, JM: Service function.

165. (D) Should be able to function at an entry level or above the minimum entry level of competence. According to the *Guide to Fieldwork Education*, it is recommended that entry-level therapists practice in settings where they may be supervised by an experienced occupational therapist. Entry-level therapists are more likely to be able to receive coaching and mentoring in development of clinical skills while in settings that provide the opportunity to be supervised by an experienced therapist. See reference: AOTA: Commission on Education: Guide to Fieldwork Education.

166. (B) Have at least 1 year of experience as a registered occupational therapist. Based on the *Essentials* for level II fieldwork, an occupational therapist supervising a level II occupational therapy student is required to have a minimum of 1 year of experience. Occupational therapy with 6 months of experience may supervise level I or II COTA students. See reference: AOTA: Commission on Education: Guide to Fieldwork Education.

167. (A) Every American citizen having access to health care without financial or other barriers. Universal coverage was a term put forth in the health care reform platforms in 1994. This term related to the provision of health care for all legal United States citizens. The level of coverage for services would vary based on additional contributions by employees and/or employers. Answers B, C, and D are incorrect in that this term does not refer to the types of services covered or choice in selecting a provider or reimbursement for services. No reference available.

168. (C) State and local programs. State and local programs represent the largest source of reimbursement for occupational therapists. In this system, occupational therapists are most likely paid based on grant programs, which have broad goals regarding the provision of services. Stricter forms of reimbursement include insurance companies. These payment systems may regulate to what extent occupational therapy services are provided. This includes the type of occupational therapy that will be paid for as well as a frequency of services that may be covered. Answer A, Medicare, is the second highest source of reimbursement. Answer B, Medicaid, represents 12 percent, and Answer D, Blue Cross, represents 8 percent. See reference: Punwar: Current trends in the field.

169. (B) The general hospitals. The primary employment site of occupational therapists is in general hospitals with a percentage of 22.5. The next largest area of concentration of occupational therapists is in the school systems with a percentage of 16.3. Rehabilitation hospitals have 11.6 percent and psychiatric hospitals have 6.6 percent. See reference: Punwar: Current trends in the field.

170. (B) Aftercare. Aftercare is the arrangement for postdischarge services, which may be needed by the individual once he or she is discharged from an occupational therapy program. For individuals having received services in a rehabilitation unit, this may include linkages with the Bureau of Vocational Rehabilitation in order to prepare for gainful employment. Another example would be a psychiatric patient being referred to a community center to continue the program that has been established on an inpatient unit. Answer A is a follow-up plan. This is different in that these services are provided by the same program. An example of this would be when an individual on

a rehabilitation unit is asked to return for a visit 1 month after discharge. This is generally done to verify that issues or problems have not arisen and that the individual's health status is not declining. Answer C is a treatment program that may be prescribed to an individual to do during treatment or after discharge so that the health status may be maintained or progress will be enhanced. Home health services, answer D, is the provision of health care in the patient's home. These services are provided for those who are physically unable to commute to an outpatient center for treatment. See reference: Reed and Sanderson: Practice with the elderly populations.

171. (A) $\dfrac{\text{Present salary/earning potential} + \text{professional overhead}}{\text{billable hours}}$

This is the only correct answer in that it takes into account all overhead related to the provision of services. This includes overhead and salaries. See reference: Hopkins and Smith (eds): Perinchief, JM: Service function.

172. (B) Conditional reasoning. Conditional reasoning is a form of clinical reasoning that takes into account various systems and dynamics involved with the patient and his or her illness or injury. This approach is more "holistic" in that takes into account the "whole patient" as he or she functions and interacts within his or her environment. Reasoning based on corresponding an individual's deficits and physical symptoms with a procedure that may benefit the area is referred to as procedural reasoning. Interactive reasoning is a process by which the therapist and patient collaborate so that the therapist may better understand the patient's environment or situation. Narrative reasoning is a form of "story telling" in which therapists share similar experiences, allowing for problem solving to occur. See reference: Mattingly and Fleming: Fleming, MH: The therapist with the three-track mind.

173. (A) Procedural reasoning. Reasoning based on corresponding an individual's deficits and physical symptoms with a procedure that may benefit the area is referred to as procedural reasoning. Procedural reasoning is the process of identifying a particular treatment or procedure. Conditional reasoning is a form of clinical reasoning that takes into account various systems and dynamics involved with the patient and his or her illness or injury. This approach is more holistic in that takes into account the whole patient as he or she functions and interacts within his or her environment. Interactive reasoning is a process by which the therapist and patient collaborate so that the therapist may better understand the patient's environment and situation. Narrative reasoning is a form of story telling in which therapists share similar experiences, allowing for problem solving to occur. See reference: Mattingly and Fleming: Fleming, MH: The therapist with the three-track mind.

174. (A) A shoe horn. Resale items and adaptive equipment may be frequently turned-over. This is due to the nature of a patient population needing specific pieces of adaptive equipment to promote independence. Departments that have resale items should also have stock and inventory procedures for purchase and billing of equipment. Answers B and C are incorrect in that a dynamometer and a powder board are used in treatment and are categorized as having an operational life of 2 years and therefore are considered expendable equipment. Answer D is incorrect because a desk chair would be considered office equipment or capital equipment. See reference: Bair, Jeanette, and Gray (eds): Scammahorn, G: Program planning.

175. (C) Is home-bound. The definition of home-bound involves the ability of the patient to physically leave his or her home, with or without assistance. Answers A and D are incorrect in that even if a patient requires a wheelchair or assistance for mobility, home care services would not be covered if he or she could leave his or her home. Answer B is incorrect in that if a patient is unable to drive to an outpatient center, community transportation services may be arranged. See reference: Hopkins and Smith (eds): Levine, RE, Corcoran, MA, and Gitlin, LN: Home care and private practice.

176. (C) Notify the state licensure board. Licensure is regulatory legislation, which is established to protect the consumer. Therefore, any occurrence of unprofessional conduct involving a consumer should be reported to the licensure board. Answers A and B are incorrect in that AOTA and the state occupational therapy association do not have regulatory jurisdiction over therapists. Answer D, discuss the situation with the therapist, is partially correct, however, this answer does not include the responsibility of the therapist to protect the consumer. See reference: Hopkins and Smith (eds): Hopkins, HL: Scope of occupational therapy.

177. (C) Informed consent. One of the fundamental components of the *Occupational Therapy Code of Ethics* is informed consent. The basis of informed consent is that the patient be given relevant medical information so that he or she may be an active participant in the decision making process. Therapeutic privilege or the withholding of medical information is no longer acceptable in reference to the provision of services; therefore, answer B is incorrect. Beneficence is a charitable or kindly act, and even though we would like to offer these to our patients, answer A is not the correct answer. Competence is a quality of expertise that is expected from occupational therapists but does not refer to the involvement of the patient in the treatment plan; therefore, Answer D is incorrect. See reference: Hopkins and Smith (eds): Hansen, R: Ethics in occupational therapy.

178. (B) A censure. A censure is formal disapproval of the conduct of an occupational therapist that is made public. It is used for conduct that is more serious and differs from a reprimand in that it is public. Answer A, a reprimand, is a formal written expression of disapproval against a therapist's conduct, which is retained in the NBCOT's file. This information is also communicated privately with the individual. Answer C, probation, is the period of time a therapist is given to retain the counseling

or education required to remain certified. Answer D is permanent loss of NBCOT certification. See reference: Hopkins and Smith (eds): Hansen, R: Ethics in occupational therapy.

179. (B) The independent variable. The independent variable is one that may be manipulated so that the researcher may see the effects on a dependent variable. An example would be in that actual treatment of edema may be referred to as the "independent variable," and the edemitous hand would be considered the "dependent variable." Various treatments may be attempted to identify a treatment that has a positive effect on the dependent variable. It is this ability to manipulate and modify a variable to observe the effects on another variable which is termed "independent." Answer A, a dependent variable, is the variable that is used to measure the effect of a treatment. In this way, the dependent variable acts as a yardstick for assessing the effectiveness of an independent variable. Answer C, a sample, is incorrect in that it is the number of subjects or items to be studied. Answer D is incorrect in that "interdependent variable" is not a commonly recognized term in research. See reference: Hopkins and Smith (eds): Deitz, J: Research: A systematic process for answering questions.

180. (B) External validity. In this case, the occupational therapist studied the effects of utilizing proper body mechanics in an industrial plant in which the employees handled 10 to 20 pound boxes frequently. Because the information gained from the study could be generalized to the entire population, a condition of external validity existed. Answer A, "internal validity," would be represented by the incidence of back and neck injuries (dependent variable) being positively impacted by the implementation of body mechanics (independent variable). Answer C is the process in which the independent variables are applied. Answer D is the level to which the stability of the study can be measured. See reference: Hopkins and Smith (eds): Deitz, J: Research: A systematic process for answering questions.

181. (C) A numbers table to select the population. Numbers tables are utilized to select members of a population at random. An example would be an occupational therapy department choosing to study the charts of patients who had rehabilitation services to identify the typical occupational therapy charges that these patients are most likely to incurr. Within 1 year, the occupational therapy department treated over 170 individuals with the diagnosis of cerebrovascular accident. Instead of reviewing all of the cases, the department may choose to review 10 percent of the cases and employ a numbers table to identify which charts should be reviewed. Answers A and B represent studies of an entire population. Answer D is an example of a sample population. See reference: Jacobs and Logigian: Quality assurance.

182. (B) Moving from the familiar to the similar but unfamiliar. This is the only answer that represents the student moving from the familiar activity of leading an awareness group to leading an expression group, which is similar but unfamiliar. This principle is one of six educational principles utilized by fieldwork supervisors to facilitate adult education. The other principles include; meeting the learner at their current level, involving the learner in the instruction, proceeding from the simple to the complex, utilizing spaced learning intervals, and facilitating generalization or transference of learning. See reference: Jacobs and Logigian: Designing fieldwork programs.

183. (D) Proceeding from the simple to the complex. In this example, the acuity of the student's caseload was increased. Typically, patients who have had a hip replacement require a fairly straightforward plan-of-care. As the student progressed, she also worked with patients who were likely to have more complicated cases as a result of multiple injuries or comorbidity. This is an example of one of the basic principles of education in "proceeding from the simple to the complex." There are six basic principles of working with adults in an educational environment. These six principles relate to the educational process a fieldwork supervisor may employ as he or she works with fieldwork students. See reference: Jacobs and Logigian: Designing fieldwork programs.

184. (B) Fidelity. Fidelity is defined as "remaining faithful to the patient's best interest." This includes statements regarding the confidentiality of patient information. Answer A, informed consent, is in reference to the rights of individuals to be provided information regarding their health care as well as to make choices about their own health care. Answer C, beneficence, is the concept of striving to bring about the best possible outcome for patients served through treatment modalities. Answer D, nonmaleficence, is defined as the obligation of the therapist to deliberately create a situation or cause harm or injury to a patient. See reference: Jacobs and Logigian (eds): Bloom, G: Ethics.

185. (C) Beneficence. Beneficence is the concept of striving to bring about the best possible outcome for patients served through treatment modalities. Answer A, informed consent, is in reference to the rights of individuals to be provided information regarding their health care as well as to make choices about their own health care. Answer B, fidelity, is defined as "remaining faithful to the patient's best interest." This includes statements regarding the confidentiality of patient information. Answer D, nonmaleficence, is defined as the obligation of the therapist to deliberately create a situation or cause harm or injury to a patient. See reference: Hopkins and Smith (eds): Hansen, R: Ethics in occupational therapy.

186. (B) Any modification to a job that will allow a disabled worker to perform the essential functions. "Reasonable accommodation" refers to the modification of an environment so that it is realistic and fiscally responsible. An example would be that if the offices of a small company were on the second floor of a building and could only be accessed by stairs, it might be impossible to complete the accommodation due to the expense of putting in an elevator. However, other options such as a stair lift, may be considered for an employee in a wheelchair. See reference: Hopkins and Smith (eds): Reed, K: The beginnings of occupational therapy.

187. (C) Compliance with the laws and regulations. Compliance with laws and regulations is the third principle of the Code of Ethics. This principle refers to therapists following state, local, federal, and facility-specific guidelines and requirements for accreditation. Answer A, beneficence and autonomy, speaks to the concern that is to be demonstrated by therapists towards patients. This includes provision of services without discrimination, providing appropriate information to patients regarding education and research, and involvement of the patient in treatment planning. Answer B, principle two of the Occupational Therapy Code of Ethics, is competence. This refers specifically to credentialing and to the therapist functioning within the parameters of his or her skill level. Therapists are guided to refer patients to other service areas when the skills required do not fall within their expertise. Answer D addresses the therapist accurately representing his or her expertise as well as not participating in any fraudulent statements or claims. See reference: Hopkins and Smith (eds): Representative Assembly: Occupational Therapy Code of Ethics.

188. (B) Guidelines to assist the occupational therapist in the provision of services. This answer describes the purpose of the *Revision: Standards of Practice for Occupational Therapy*. Answer A, "a guide to promote the highest standards of behavior," is the purpose of the *Occupational Therapy Code of Ethics*. Answer C, "a guide to assist the practitioner in identifying career options and developing career plans," is the purpose of the *Occupational Therapy Roles*. Answer D, "a document to assist the therapist in applying uniform terminology," is the purpose of the *Uniform Terminology*. See reference: Hopkins and Smith (eds): AOTA Commission on Practice: Standards of Practice for Occupational Therapy.

189. (D) A small group of patients who are representative of the population with each individual meeting criteria, which validates that they are a representative subset of the population. Answer D is the MOST correct answer because the question asks for a sample (subset) population (defined group of people). Answers A and B are representative of an entire population versus a subset. In research, a sample is a small subset of a group or population. The sample is to be representative of the entire population. Answer C is an example of a system used to identify members of a population to utilize for a random sampling. See reference: Hopkins and Smith (eds): Deitz, J: Research: A systematic process for answering questions; and Jacobs and Logigian: Quality assurance.

190. (D) Nonmaleficence. Nonmaleficence, is defined as "the obligation of the therapist to deliberately create a situation or cause harm or injury to a patient." Answer A, informed consent, is in reference to the rights of individuals to be provided information regarding their health care as well as to make choices about their own health care. Answer B, fidelity, is defined as "remaining faithful to the patient's best interest." This includes statements regarding the confidentiality of patient information. Answer C, beneficence, is the concept of striving to bring about the best possible outcome for patients served through treatment modalities. See reference: Hopkins and Smith (eds): Hansen, R: Ethics in occupational therapy.

191. (C) Provide fieldwork sites with the most current information on fieldwork education centers. As defined in the *Guide to Fieldwork Education*, the Commission on Education is responsible for developing and reviewing educational standards, consulting with developing and existing occupational therapy programs, reviewing and revising educational documents, developing and implementing continuing education opportunities, and reporting to the representative assembly. It is also stated in the *Guide to Fieldwork Education* that each facility has its own unique philosophy of care in addition to roles of each discipline. It is for this reason that each individual facility establishes their own objectives for students. See reference: AOTA: Commission on Education: Guide to Fieldwork Education.

192. (A) Informed consent. Informed consent, is in reference to the rights of individuals to be provided information regarding their health care as well as to make choices about their own health care. Answer B, fidelity, is defined as "remaining faithful to the patient's best interest." This includes statements regarding the confidentiality of patient information. Answer C, beneficence, is the concept of striving to bring about the best possible outcome for patients served through treatment modalities. Answer D, nonmaleficence, is defined as the obligation of the therapist to deliberately create a situation or cause harm or injury to a patient. See reference: Hopkins and Smith (eds): Hansen, R: Ethics in occupational therapy.

193. (B) CARF and JCAHO. The Commission on Accreditation of Rehabilitation Facilities and the Joint Commission on Accreditation of Hospital Organizations are the agencies most likely to accredit a comprehensive outpatient rehabilitation program. CARF defines its mission as serving as "the preeminent standards-setting and accrediting body promoting quality services to people with disabilities." JCAHO certifies hospital organizations including ambulatory services, which may include an outpatient rehabilitation. PSROs are peer standards review organizations, which review quality of care. Therefore, answer A is incorrect. Answers C and D are incorrect in that a CORF is an institution (public or private), which provides comprehensive rehabilitative services on an outpatient basis. It is NOT an organization that accredits outpatient facilities. See reference: Bair and Gray (eds): Scott, SJ, and Somers, FP: Payment for occupational therapy services; and Hopkins and Smith (eds): Levy, LL: The health care delivery system today.

194. (A) Treatments for the occupational therapy plan provided by a COTA. Based on the Occupational Therapy Code of Ethics second principle (competence), occupational therapy may only be done by "those individuals

holding appropriate credentials for providing services." These credentials are certification from NBCOT and, when appropriate, state licensure as an occupational therapist or occupational therapy assistant. Therefore, answers B, C, and D are incorrect because recreational, music, or art therapists do not hold these credentials. See reference: Hopkins and Smith (eds): Representative Assembly: Occupational Therapy Code of Ethics.

195. (A) Managed care. These companies serve as the link between hospitals and insurance companies. Managed care providers identify the need for medical care of an individual by referring to the patient's medical information as it relates to pre-established criteria for services. Utilization review, Answer B, compares the length of stay or duration of services provided with the cost to ensure efficiency. Peer review, answer C, is a form of quality improvement in which charts are reviewed for indicators that represent the level of quality of a service. Prospective payment, Answer D, is a system for payment of services based on DRGs (Diagnostic Related Groups). See reference: Hopkins and Smith (eds): Gibson, D, and Levy, LL: The health care delivery system today.

196. (B) Writing qualitative and quantitative facts in the results section. The results section should only contain measurable results. Conclusions and interpretive and analytical information appear in the summary or conclusion of the research. Subjective information is not typically included into research. See reference: Hopkins and Smith (eds): Deitz, J: Research: A systematic process for answering questions.

197. (A) A diagnostic related group (DRG). DRGs are a part of the prospective payment system established by Medicare. In that this patient is over 65, she would qualify under Medicare. An FRG, or Functional Related Group, is not in effect as of the printing of this guide. However, this term relates to groups of diagnoses, which are admitted to rehabilitation facilities. Medicaid, Answer C, is incorrect in that this population is poor or indigent. Answer D is partially correct in that if the woman involved did have insurance, it would be used. However, it would be considered the secondary insurance and Medicare would be the primary provider. See reference: Bair and Gray (eds): Scott, SJ, and Somers, FP: Payment for occupational therapy services.

198. (B) Medical necessity. Medicare defines medical necessity as "necessary and reasonable to treat an illness or an injury or to improve the functioning of a malformed body member." Answer B is the MOST correct answer. Answers A, C, and D are correct but are a part of the broader statement of medical necessity. See reference: Bair and Gray (eds): Scott, SJ, and Somers, FP: Payment for occupational therapy services.

199. (A) DRGs. Diagnostic categories were defined in order to establish the level of payment per diagnosis. The intent of government was to impose constraints on health care spending for the beneficiaries of Medicare. PROs were established to numerically assess unnecessary procedures, client and patient deaths, and substandard care. UB-82s are forms that must be completed on each patient, listing their diagnosis and comorbidity information for the purpose of reimbursement. Cost shifting is what occurs when a hospital increases its prices to all customers in order to make up for the shortfall of reimbursement by a few providers. See reference: Bair and Gray (eds): Scott, SJ, and Somers, FP: Payment for occupational therapy services.

200. (C) Ascertain facts and impressions. Similar to the assessment process for treating a patient is the process for approaching an ethical dilemma. The Savage model outlines 14 steps of ethical contemplation. The first four steps were the answers to this question. Initially, facts and impressions need to be gathered. Once this is done, information needs to be verified with key players. The third step is to identify problems to be solved, and finally to sort the decisions to be made. Answers A, B, and D therefore are not the first response. See reference: Hopkins and Smith (eds): Hopkins, HL: Scope of occupational therapy; and Bair and Gray (eds): Opacich, KJ, and Welles, C: Ethical dimensions in occupational therapy.

SIMULATION EXAMINATION 4

> **Directions:** Circle the correct answer to the following questions. When you have completed this examination, check your answers against the answer key that follows. As you will see, an explanation is given for each answer along with a reference for further study. The book author is listed as well as the chapter author. See the bibliography for complete references. Study the areas in which your comprehension was low, then test yourself again by taking Simulation Examination 5.

PEDIATRIC QUESTIONS

Assessment of Occupational Performance

1. A 7-year-old girl with a visual perceptual problem is lacing a series of geometric beads from a stimulus card. She is unable to identify a triangle shape when the lacing bead is turned sideways on the table. This is called a problem with:
   A. figure-ground perception.
   B. form constancy perception.
   C. visual memory.
   D. visual sequencing.

2. A 7-year-old child with a learning disability is unable to focus on a blackboard 20 feet away from him, and refocus on his paper in order to copy a mathematics problem. The therapist also observes the same problem during clinical observations requiring the child to focus on a pencil at 12 inches and refocus on the wall clock at 20 feet. The therapist should conclude that the child has a visual problem with:
   A. ocular motility.
   B. binocular vision.
   C. convergence.
   D. accommodation.

3. A 10-year-old girl with a behavior disorder is being evaluated by an occupational therapist for the development of play skills. The child has considerable difficulty with problem solving during any play activity. She becomes frustrated and gives up easily. In terms of development of play skills, the therapist can conclude that this child's major play problem is in the area of:
   A. sensorimotor.
   B. imaginary.
   C. constructional.
   D. game.

4. When a child with a behavior disorder demonstrates problems with innate temperament, the therapist should consider the following treatment approach:
   A. help care providers get tough with the child during activities.
   B. help the child develop cognitive strategies for anxiety-producing activities.
   C. help care providers develop an unpredictable routine for activities that disorganize the child.
   D. provide a play environment where the parent and child can demonstrate conflicts.

5. A therapist planning a program for a 10-year-old child with multiple handicaps needs to develop self-feeding skills at a low cognitive level. Of the following approaches, which would provide the most support to learning this skill?
   A. Physical guidance
   B. Verbal cues
   C. Visual cues
   D. Forward chaining

6. A 12-year-old girl with behavior problems has difficulty with peer interactions. The therapist needs to develop a plan that:
   A. provides activities in an authoritarian environment.
   B. allows the children the opportunity to develop basic social skills on their own.
   C. provides enjoyable activities in a safe and accepting environment.
   D. establishes rules for group play.

7. An elementary-aged boy is being observed for diagnosis in an outpatient psychiatric clinic. He was unable to listen to directions for a constructional play activity. He had difficulty sequencing steps and became very frustrated, appearing to be angry with himself. He appears to be in constant motion while attempting to sit

and work on the project. He grabs tools and materials away from other children and constantly interferes with their work. The occupational therapist observes and reports to the team that this child is demonstrating symptoms of the following disorder:
A. attention-deficit hyperactivity.
B. mood disorder-manic episode.
C. conduct.
D. anxiety.

8. A child diagnosed with arthrogryposis has been referred for an occupational therapy evaluation. In preparation for this evaluation, the therapist needs to focus on ADLs because these children have the following problem from birth:
A. obstetric paralysis.
B. hip dislocation.
C. joint inflammation.
D. joint contracture.

9. The occupational therapist evaluating a 4-year-old child notices a bruise on the child's shoulder, which looks like an adult hand and finger print. Based on this observation, the therapist should:
A. discuss this with family members who pick up the child.
B. wait until more injuries can be observed.
C. make a report to appropriate authorities.
D. not become involved in personal family members.

10. Promoting good parenting skills is often a therapy objective for children and families where child abuse and neglect exist. What characteristic of these families makes this an important objective?
A. Teenage parents
B. High socioeconomic status
C. Older parents
D. Low socioeconomic status

Development of the Treatment Plan

11. The therapist working in an acute care hospital receives an occupational therapy referral for a 1-year-old child with congenital hip dislocation. The child has recently been hospitalized for traction prior to body casting. The initial concern of the therapist when developing a treatment plan should be:
A. upper extremity strengthening.
B. developmental stimulation.
C. preacademic skill development.
D. activities of daily living.

12. A child with sensory integration problems demonstrates hypersensitivity to movement activities by becoming nauseated and dizzy. Which of the following activities would be the most appropriate use of the large therapy ball for this child?

A. Movement in any position or direction.
B. No movement.
C. Slow and predictable movement.
D. Quick and unpredictable movement.

13. The therapist is carrying out a sensory integration program using activities to improve sensory processing. If she is working with a child who has underreactive sensory processing, the activities should have the following facilitatory characteristics:
A. arrhythmic and unexpected.
B. arrhythmic and slow.
C. sustained and slow.
D. unexpected and rhythmic.

14. A therapist considering the use of classical sensory integration therapy for a child with a learning disability would carry out the therapy in the following way:
A. include the child in a group of children using a program of sensory stimulation activities.
B. encourage the child to participate in activities that are passive and do not require adaptive responses.
C. design an individualized program that requires advanced training.
D. promote the development of specific motor skills such as standing balance.

15. The therapist's goal is to develop reach and voluntary release of grasp in a child with flexor spasticity in the upper extremities. Using a neurodevelopmental treatment frame of reference, the therapist would begin the treatment sequence with the following procedure:
A. apply a quick stretch to flexor groups of muscles at the shoulder, elbow, and wrist.
B. facilitate cocontraction at the shoulder, elbow, and wrist joints using compression.
C. strengthen shoulder, elbow, and wrist flexors using resisted bilateral sanding.
D. decrease abnormal muscle tone by positioning and moving shoulder, arm, and wrist in a reflex-inhibiting pattern.

16. According to a neurodevelopmental frame of reference, a therapist working with a child in an effort to inhibit hypertonus, should grade treatment in the following order:
A. begin with assistive movement (support).
B. begin with passive movement (placing and holding).
C. begin with active movement (independent).
D. ignore abnormal patterns.

17. The therapist, when working with a child who has a learning disability, observes an unusually tight grip and frequent breaking of the pencil from too much pressure on the paper. This type of problem would most likely be caused by inadequate sensory information from the:

A. vestibular system.
B. auditory system.
C. somatosensory system.
D. visual system.

18. The therapist is working with a 6-year-old girl who has Down syndrome and demonstrates a 3-year delay in fine motor skills. The child has just developed the stability and strength in her right hand to hold scissors properly, hold paper in the nondominant hand, and make snips or single cuts in the paper. Which of the following would be the next scissors skill to develop?
A. Cut cardboard and cloth.
B. Cut along curved lines to cut out a circle.
C. Cut along straight lines to cut a triangle.
D. Cut the paper in two following a straight line.

19. An 8-year-old girl receiving occupational therapy has low muscle tone, which results in problems in the following print and handwriting subskill areas: (1) postural stability, (2) shoulder stability, and (3) immature grasp of the pencil. Treatment of her problems should proceed in the following order if the therapist follows a central to peripheral approach to development:
A. 1-2-3.
B. 2-1-3.
C. 3-1-2.
D. 2-1-3.

20. The therapist who is assisting a child in developing reach and pointing skills, needed to point to a picture on a picture board, is training the child in the following type of augmentative communication system:
A. scanning mode.
B. encoding mode.
C. direct selection mode.
D. output mode.

Case Study

Jason is a 1-year-old boy who was born prematurely (31 weeks of gestation), weighing 6 pounds. Labor was induced when ultrasonography showed an insufficiency of amniotic fluid. There was a long labor of 28 hours with no apparent distress as measured by fetal monitors. Following the birth, Jason had a collapsed lung and a spirated meconium. He was transferred to a neonatal intensive care unit (NICU) for 15 days, experienced several seizures, and was put on a respirator. A computed tomography (CT) scan showed that there was brain damage from anoxia. He was fed by gavage method for 1 month, and the seizures continued to be successfully treated with phenobarbital. Jason's mother is a single parent with two other children (both girls) whose ages are 6 and 8 years. Jason has been referred to an early intervention program for evaluation and programming. Jason's presenting problems are: (1) sensitivity to sound and changes in position; (2) dislike of baths and undressing; (3) mild-to-moderate hypertonicity in the trunk, shoulders, and legs

(extensor patterns) and mild to moderate hypertonicity in arms and hands (flexor pattern); (4) weak sucking; (5) strong Moro reflex; and (6) poor head control.

21. Through an early intervention program, Jason is eligible to have the following type of program plan developed by an interdisciplinary team:
A. Individual Education Plan (IEP).
B. Least Restrictive Environment Plan (LREP).
C. Individual Family Service Plan (IFSP).
D. Early Intervention Program Plan (EIPP).

22. From the following list, select the most appropriate assessment for the occupational therapist to give to Jason according to his age.
A. Southern California Sensory Integration and Praxis Tests
B. Bruininks-Oseretsky Test of Motor Proficiency
C. Motor-Free Visual Perception Test
D. Peabody Scale of Motor Development

23. Considering Jason's postural patterns, the following positioning would best suit his need for feeding:
A. hips and legs flexed, shoulders protracted.
B. hips and legs extended, shoulders protracted.
C. hips and legs flexed, shoulders retracted.
D. hips and legs extended, shoulders retracted.

24. From the following list, select the piece of adaptive equipment that would best meet Jason's positioning needs during eating and feeding:
A. prone stander with lateral trunk supports.
B. corner chair with head support and padded abductor post.
C. supine on a wedge with hips flexed 15 degrees.
D. bolster chair without back support.

25. The therapist is developing Jason's treatment plan. What aspect of postural control should first be developed to improve success of eating and feeding goals?
A. Shoulder
B. Head
C. Trunk
D. Hand

Implementation of the Treatment Plan

26. The therapist has recommended that Jason's mother use a shallow spoon when feeding Jason. This will help develop:
A. jaw opening.
B. jaw closing.
C. lower lip control.
D. upper lip control.

27. If a child such as Jason has been fed by the gavage method, he may have developed some resistance to introducing oral foods. What symptom from use of gavage could produce this negative response?

A. Nose and throat irritation
B. Stomach soreness
C. Infection
D. Skin breakdown

28. **The therapist, when treating Jason's tactile defensive reactions, should instruct the parents to handle him in the following manner:**
    A. tickle him during playtimes.
    B. play loud music when undressing him.
    C. lightly stroke his arms and legs during bath time.
    D. hold him firmly when picking him up.

29. **From the following list, select the best treatment activity for development of Jason's head control:**
    A. standing in a standing frame with knee and hip support.
    B. quadruped with chest supported in a sling.
    C. prone over a wedge.
    D. sitting on a therapy ball with hips supported by the therapist.

30. **Considering all of Jason's needs, select the most important referral to be made at the time of discharge or transition:**
    A. psychologist.
    B. social worker.
    C. orthotist or prosthetist.
    D. teacher.

33. **When planning for discharge, Janet's therapist would like to focus on the most important information to share with Janet's classroom teacher. This would be the:**
    A. child's level of visual perceptual skills.
    B. information on juvenile rheumatoid arthritis.
    C. degrees of range of motion in involved joints.
    D. occupational therapy treatment plan in general.

34. **Janet's therapist is designing a splint for Janet's right wrist. Considering her problems, what would be the most appropriate goal for her splint?**
    A. Inhibition of hypertonus
    B. Increase range of motion
    C. Prevent deformity
    D. Correct deformity

35. **Janet is being discharged from occupational therapy in an outpatient clinic. Although the active nature of her condition is gone, there is remaining hand strength weakness. Which of the following pieces of adaptive equipment would be most important to prevent hand fatigue in Janet's situation?**
    A. Reacher
    B. Jar opener
    C. Pencil gripper
    D. Plate guard

Case Study

Janet is a 12-year-old girl with a diagnosis of juvenile rheumatoid arthritis. She has normal intelligence and, although she misses school occasionally, is able to maintain her age group grade level. Onset was sudden and she has periodic episodes of acute inflammation, which primarily affect her knees, hips, elbows, and hands. Also, there is a slight loss of range of motion in these joints. Besides a low grade fever, she is frequently listless and irritable. There is neither lymph node nor spleen involvement. Hand strength has become weaker in the past year, and her right dominant hand now shows 1 to 2 pounds of grasp strength. Answer the following questions regarding this child:

31. **Which type of juvenile rheumatoid arthritis (JRA) is described by Janet's symptoms:**
    A. polyarticular.
    B. systemic.
    C. pauciarticular.
    D. Still's disease.

32. **Janet's therapist is planning for discharge and needs to consider the possibility of permanent disability. What percentage of children with juvenile rheumatoid arthritis will not recover completely from this condition?**
    A. 100 percent
    B. 75 percent
    C. 50 percent
    D. 15 percent

Case Study

Megan is a 7-year-old girl with a diagnosis of spina bifida (myelomeningocele). A neurosurgical excision and closure surgery were completed soon after birth to repair the defect in the lumbosacral area. She also needed a shunt procedure (ventroperintoneal) because of the presence of hydrocephalus developing after the repair of her back. Megan has had difficulty with recurring urinary infections. Her spine shows lumbosacral scoliosis, and equinovarus deformities are seen in the feet. She has fine motor coordination problems in the upper extremities. Megan wears long-leg braces when using a walker, but her primary mode of mobility is a wheelchair. Answer the following questions regarding this case study:

36. **Megan's case study states that she has an equinovarus deformity of the foot. This means she has a/an:**
    A. enlarged great toe.
    B. club foot.
    C. pronated foot.
    D. unstable heel.

37. **Considering Megan's age, which of the following signs of shunt malfunction should be monitored by family and therapists?**
    A. Increased head size
    B. Nausea and vomiting
    C. Back pain
    D. Intermittent headaches

38. **Knowing the problems that are part of Megan's diagnosis, select the most appropriate areas of occupational therapy testing from the list below:**
    A. development and ADL.
    B. ADL and sensory integration.
    C. development, ADL, and vocational.
    D. development, ADL, and sensory integration.

39. **With Megan's condition of myelomeningocele, the major concern of medical treatment, because it is the major cause of death, is:**
    A. respiratory infection.
    B. renal failure.
    C. spinal cord degeneration.
    D. hydrocephalus.

40. **Considering her condition, which of the following precautions should be stressed with Megan and her family at the time of discharge?**
    A. Practice regular skin inspections.
    B. Avoid chewy foods which may cause choking.
    C. Monitor apnea episodes.
    D. Avoid tactile defensive situations.

Evaluation of the Treatment Plan

Case Study

Michael is a 4-year-old boy with a diagnosis of developmental delay following interdisciplinary assessment. Medical testing showed a high level of lead in blood samples, from continuing exposure to materials in the family home. Michael received an intelligence quotient of 65 when tested on the Wechsler Intelligence Scales for Children (WISC). Initially, he was referred to a speech clinician about 6 months ago due to language delays caused by oral dyspraxia. His developmental milestones have been delayed, as evidenced by sitting at 10 months of age and walking at 18 months. Clinical observations of posture and movement show below average muscle tone, with instability in quadruped and kneeling positions. Balance is delayed in sitting, kneeling, and standing. He also avoids playing with toys or on playground equipment where his feet are off the ground. When introduced to the occupational therapy environment, it took several minutes for him to figure out how to mount a rocking horse, and play on a scooter board. His developmental test scores using the Peabody Scales of Motor Development are 36 months for gross motor skills, and 28 months for fine motor skills. Answer the following questions regarding the case study of Michael:

41. **When re-evaluating Michael's low muscle tone and joint stability, the therapist could use the following sensory integration clinical observation:**
    A. arm extension test.
    B. joint hyperextensibility observation.
    C. Adiadokinesis test.
    D. thumb-finger touching.

42. **The cause of Michael's developmental delays or mental retardation would be classified under the following category:**
    A. birth complications.

B. congenital infection.
C. genetic.
D. environmental.

43. **When writing up Michael's initial evaluation report, the therapist should describe his avoidance of play equipment where his feet would be off the ground using the following sensory integration terminology:**
    A. tactile defensiveness.
    B. developmental dyspraxia.
    C. gravitational insecurity.
    D. intolerance for motion.

44. **When selecting a treatment activity for Michael's problem with management of the rocking horse and scooterboard, the therapist would search for activities that meet the following goal:**
    A. improve fine motor skills.
    B. improve gross motor skills.
    C. improve reflex integration.
    D. improve motor planning.

Case Study

Martha is an 8-year-old girl who has recently been identified as having a learning disability. She had been referred to occupational therapy by an educational psychologist in the school system. Besides academic difficulties in reading and writing, she was distractible, frustrated, and easily discouraged in many of her school and home activities. Martha was given the Southern California Sensory Integration and Praxis Tests (SIPT) and the SIPT Clinical Observations of postural control and other neuromuscular responses. The results of the evaluation indicate the presence of a bilateral sequencing disorder, with vestibular processing dysfunction (underreactivity). Martha showed depressed postrotary nystagmus, low muscle tone, inadequate equilibrium reactions, poor balance, difficulty with assumption of the prone extension posture, and irregular eye pursuits. There was also evidence of tactile defensiveness, and depressed visual perception scores. The school system provided sensory integration therapy through a private clinic, since her sensory integration dysfunction appeared to have a direct influence on her academic performance. Answer the following questions regarding this case study:

45. **Considering Martha's presenting sensory integration problems, which of the following goals should be considered first when developing her treatment plan?**
    A. Improve eye pursuit skills
    B. Improve vestibular processing
    C. Improve muscle tone
    D. Increase postrotary nystagmus

46. **Which of the following activities would be the most appropriate initial activity for Martha in the treatment of her tactile defensiveness?**
    A. Therapist brushes her neck and face
    B. Balancing on a therapy ball
    C. Rolling in a carpeted barrel
    D. Swinging in a hammock swing

Discharge Planning

47. **When planning discharge for Martha, the therapist should inform parents of precautions if use of a hammock swing is an appropriate activity. Which of the following observations would indicate autonomic responses indicating sensory overload during this activity?**
    A. Suddenly scratching oneself.
    B. Spinning oneself very fast.
    C. Hitting one's head on the floor.
    D. Flushing, blanching, or perspiration.

48. **Which of the following tests would best measure progress for discharge planning in the specific area of visual perceptual dysfunction for Martha?**
    A. Purdue Perceptual Motor Survey (Kephart)
    B. Denver II
    C. Test of Visual-Motor Integration (Beery)
    D. Test of Visual Perceptual Skills (Gardner)

49. **When making discharge plans, the therapist should recommend the following activity to the classroom teacher as best meeting Martha's goal "to improve bilateral coordination?"**
    A. Walk sideways on a rope taped to the floor (in stocking feet).
    B. Crawl on top of a rope taped to the floor.
    C. Kick a ball when sitting on a T-stool.
    D. Follow an obstacle course.

50. **At the time of discharge the therapist could expect Martha's sensory integration problem to have responded to therapy (compared with other types of sensory integration dysfunction) in the following way:**
    A. Best responder
    B. Worst responder
    C. Neither best nor worst responder
    D. Unresponsive

PHYSICAL DISABILITY QUESTIONS

Assessment of Occupational Performance

51. **An example of a nonstandardized test used by occupational therapists in a physical disabilities setting would be the:**
    A. Motor Free Visual Perceptual Test.
    B. Minnesota Rate of Manipulation.
    C. Manual Muscle Test.
    D. Purdue Pegboard.

52. **The name of the standardized test that uses seven tasks of daily living to assess hand function is called the:**
    A. Purdue Pegboard Evaluation.
    B. Jebson-Taylor Hand Function Test.
    C. Minnesota Rate of Manipulation.
    D. Crawford Small Parts Dexterity Test.

53. **According to Signe Brunnstrom, a person who demonstrates developing spasticity on the hemiplegic side of the body with weak, associated movements in synergy and little active finger flexion would be in which stage of recovery?**
    A. One
    B. Two
    C. Three
    D. Four

54. **A person may be diagnosed with chronic pain from cervical disk disease when the symptoms of acute pain with impairment and disability have lasted longer than the acute stage of pain had disappeared by how many weeks?**
    A. 1 week
    B. 3 weeks
    C. 6 weeks
    D. 9 weeks

55. **To measure gross hand grasp (strength), the instrument used is called:**
    A. a goniometer.
    B. a dynamometer.
    C. a pinch meter.
    D. an aesthesiometer.

56. **Which hand function test includes seven subtests and may be easily constructed by a hospital therapy department?**
    A. Minnesota Rate of Manipulation Test
    B. Purdue Pegboard Test
    C. Jebsen-Taylor Hand Function Test
    D. Valpar Upper Extremity Range of Motion Work Sample

57. **What instrument is used to measure edema in the hand?**
    A. Goniometer
    B. Aesthesiometer
    C. Volumeter
    D. Dynamometer

58. **The part of the evaluation process in which the methods are selected to approach the problems and specific needs of a person would be the:**
    A. initial interview.
    B. performance of assessments.
    C. analysis of data.
    D. development of a treatment plan.

Development of the Treatment Plan

59. **A work hardening program plan would include:**
    A. recreational activities.
    B. pain management techniques.
    C. driver re-education.
    D. joint protection techniques.

60. The second level of use in an augmentative communication hierarchy after understanding picture symbols and their use would be:
    A. sequencing of picture symbols.
    B. recognizing letters of the alphabet.
    C. recognizing whole words.
    D. spelling letter by letter.

61. When an occupational therapist decides to use a neurophysiologic approach to treat a person with a cerebrovascular accident, the therapist has selected:
    A. a treatment technique.
    B. an exercise.
    C. a treatment plan.
    D. a frame of reference.

62. A woman who had a cerebrovascular accident (CVA) has random movements in all four extremities. What is the most appropriate switch to use on the controls for her wheelchair?
    A. Infrared switch
    B. Sip and Puff switch
    C. P-switch
    D. Rocking lever switch

63. After a transient ischemic attack (TIA), a man has demonstrated some impairments with proprioception, which has caused uneven letter formation during writing activities. What activity would best improve his letter formation?
    A. The therapist verbally describes to him how to make a letter as he writes.
    B. The man is encouraged to watch his grip during writing with a pen.
    C. The man works with putty to strengthen his hand.
    D. The therapist has the man trace letters through a pan of rice with his fingers.

64. The part of a treatment objective that describes the performance of an individual to be changed is the:
    A. terminal behavior.
    B. condition.
    C. criterion.
    D. plan.

65. What is the criteria in the treatment objective "the individual will dress himself with moderate assistance of one person using a reacher, long shoe horn and a sock aid?"
    A. A reacher, a long shoe horn, and a sock aid
    B. The individual
    C. Moderate assistance of one person
    D. Dress himself

Case Study

A hospital volunteer has brought a 70-year-old man to occupational therapy. This man has had a right cerebrovascular accident resulting in left hemiplegia. The man uses his right unaffected upper extremity to push himself to the left, because "I feel like I am going to fall out of my chair." His left upper extremity dangles over the armrest of the chair and his hips are extended, placing him in a posterior pelvic tilt.

66. After the man's hips have been realigned in the wheelchair to place him in hip flexion, where should the line of pull at a 45 degree angle be placed from the seat belt to provide maximal pelvic stability?
    A. Inferior to the ischial tuberosity.
    B. Superior to the iliac crest.
    C. Inferior to the anterior superior iliac spine.
    D. Superior to the posterior superior iliac spine.

67. The best positioning device used to support the man's flaccid arm as described in the previous question would be:
    A. a half lap tray.
    B. the wheelchair armrest.
    C. an arm sling.
    D. an arm trough.

68. A type of wheelchair adaptation used to stabilize the man's upper body in a midline position would be:
    A. a reclining wheelchair.
    B. an arm trough.
    C. a lateral trunk support.
    D. a lateral pelvic support.

69. The occupational therapist would recommend which one of the following items for a person with fine motor incoordination who frequently drops small objects?
    A. A shirt with contrasting buttons.
    B. A spray deodorant.
    C. A toothpaste container with a flip-open cap.
    D. Pants with a drawstring waist.

70. An example of a prevocational activity, used with a woman who had worked as a cashier in a clothing store, would be having the woman:
    A. make a grocery list while sitting.
    B. fold laundry and place in a basket.
    C. wash dishes while standing.
    D. add a column of numbers by hand while sitting.

71. An activity may be effectively used when the adaptation:
    A. is complicated.
    B. needs to be adjusted frequently.
    C. is performed in a comfortable position.
    D. is monotonous.

72. An activity that may be graded to improve a person's arm strength and endurance would be:
    A. passive range of motion.
    B. Codman exercises.
    C. popping a balloon.
    D. batting a balloon.

73. The therapist will need this information before a work hardening program may begin:
    A. evaluation of the individual's job site.
    B. physician's written consent and medical precautions.
    C. insurance information.
    D. individual's work history.

Implementation of the Treatment Plan

74. The temperature range in which paraffin may be used comfortably without developing a film on top is:
    A. 108 degrees F to 116 degrees F.
    B. 118 degrees F to 126 degrees F.
    C. 128 degrees F to 136 degrees F.
    D. 138 degrees F to 146 degrees F.

75. A man who has a fractured radial head has his elbow immobilized by a cast. He wants to maintain his strength in the affected arm and has asked his therapist for some exercises. The therapist instructs him in performing:
    A. isometric exercises.
    B. isotonic exercises.
    C. progressive resistive exercises.
    D. passive exercises.

76. A person with a spinal cord injury at the C8 level would be able to perform self-feeding:
    A. not at all.
    B. while using a mobile arm support.
    C. while using a universal cuff independently.
    D. independently without using equipment.

77. One form of shoulder exercise to reduce adhesions is referred to as the Codman exercises. These exercises are performed with the person leaning forward at the waist with the involved arm dangled in a vertical position. The involved arm is then moved:
    A. actively by the shoulder muscles.
    B. actively by the body.
    C. passively by the shoulder muscles.
    D. passively by active motion of the body.

78. The occupational therapist is working on weight shift using the proprioceptive neuromuscular facilitation (PNF) method to the affected left side of a person in a standing position. The therapist is using the activity of putting groceries away to facilitate weight shift. If the grocery bag is sitting on the floor to the right side, where should the groceries be placed (using the right hand) to stimulate the left arm and leg?
    A. On the counter directly in front.
    B. On the counter to the left side.
    C. In the upper cabinet to the right side.
    D. In the upper cabinet to the left side.

79. The combined movements of the upper extremities of the person in the previous question would be described as:
    A. bilateral reciprocal.
    B. ipsilateral.
    C. bilateral symmetric.
    D. bilateral asymmetric.

80. An occupational therapist working in a satellite outpatient clinic would like to find the information about the use of dynamic splints after tendon repair surgery. A computer access to the main hospital's library provides journal information through a program called:
    A. The *Index Medicus*.
    B. Medline.
    C. The *American Journal of Occupational Therapy*.
    D. Dissertation Abstracts.

81. An occupational therapist uses a program involving specific exercises to improve a patient's strength in the shoulders. This treatment approach would be considered:
    A. neurophysiologic.
    B. neurodevelopmental.
    C. biomechanic.
    D. rehabilitative.

82. The most common usage of the computer in most occupational therapy departments would be for:
    A. administrative functions.
    B. treatment planning activities.
    C. patient evaluation functions.
    D. patient and family education activities.

83. The two carpometacarpal (CMC) joints, which provide a fixed axis for the other CMC joints to move around to form the palmer arches, would be the:
    A. first and second CMC joints.
    B. second and third CMC joints.
    C. third and fourth CMC joints.
    D. fourth and fifth CMC joints.

84. Excessive anterior pelvic tilt over an extended period of time will increase what curves of the vertebral column in an individual with normal muscle tone?
    A. Lordosis and scoliosis
    B. Scoliosis and kyphosis
    C. Lordosis and kyphosis
    D. Lordosis only

85. The adult spine has curves in the following areas:
    A. cervical, lumbar, and sacral.
    B. thoracic, lumbar.
    C. cervical, lumbar.
    D. cervical thoracic, lumbar, sacral.

86. **Precision handling of an object involves:**
    A. a static grip of the hand.
    B. the stabilization of an object between the fingers and the palm.
    C. the placement of an object between the fingers and the thumb.
    D. a power grip.

87. **A set of norms to provide moral guidance to a professional group is called a:**
    A. policy or procedure.
    B. regulation.
    C. code of ethics.
    D. protocol.

88. **A promotional photograph of an occupational therapist treating a man who has had a cerebrovascular accident is planned. The photographer wishes to include the photograph in a marketing brochure for the hospital since the man is a prominent community leader. What information would need to be obtained prior to the photography session?**
    A. The correct spelling of the therapist's and man's name for the photograph caption.
    B. The man's written consent to take the photograph.
    C. The therapist's written consent to take the photograph.
    D. The correct spelling of the man's diagnosis and name for the photograph caption.

Evaluation of the Treatment Plan

89. **A nonspeaking person in a wheelchair is suddenly making many errors on the augmentative communication device, but experienced no difficulty the previous day. The first step the occupational therapist would need to do to correct this problem is:**
    A. refer the person to contact a physician for a physical.
    B. reposition the person in the wheelchair to allow an optimal range of motion.
    C. reassess the person's communication abilities.
    D. replace the communication device.

90. **A woman is trying to improve shoulder flexion endurance by performing towel pushes with both hands up on an incline board set at a 30 degree angle. The woman is able to accomplish 25 repetitions easily, so the occupational therapist upgrades the task. What change in the activity would improve the endurance of the shoulder flexors?**
    A. Change the angle of the incline board to 15 degrees.
    B. Increase the number of repetitions to 40.
    C. Turn the incline board around so the woman is pushing down the incline.
    D. Add 1 pound of weight to each arm.

91. **An occupational therapy student has completed a manual muscle test on a person and asks her supervisor to retest the person to check her results. This is an example of:**
    A. split-half reliability.
    B. test-retest reliability.
    C. interrater reliability.
    D. intrarater reliability.

92. **During home management activities with a woman who has a pelvic fracture, the occupational therapist notices that the woman is unable to hold her left arm in 90 degrees of shoulder abduction against gravity for more than a few seconds and has shoulder pain in that position. The woman most likely also has:**
    A. carpal tunnel syndrome.
    B. deltoid weakness.
    C. a dislocated clavicle.
    D. a rotator cuff tear.

Discharge Planning

93. **A person who uses a mouthstick on a home computer would benefit from what device to keep the mouthstick from striking other keys accidentally?**
    A. A moisture guard
    B. A key guard
    C. An auto-repeat defeat
    D. One-finger access software

94. **Which features are necessary when ordering a wheelchair for an individual who will be performing a sliding board transfer with assistance of the family upon discharge?**
    A. One arm drive, low back rest
    B. Reclining back rest, elevating leg rests
    C. Swing away leg rests, removable arm rests
    D. Elevating leg rests, removable arm rests

Case Study

A 38-year-old woman newly diagnosed with multiple sclerosis will return home in approximately 1 month. The woman's goal is to perform activities independently from a wheelchair level within the home to conserve her energy. The woman plans to perform some walking in the home for short distances (10 to 15 feet) and is only able to do 2 to 3 steps with assistance. The woman and her husband are in the process of having a house built. The husband has filled out a home assessment form for the occupational therapist to review and make suggestions for adaptations prior to the home visit. The form reveals a two-story home with a walk-in basement. The front door opens inward with an outward opening storm door and has two steps in with a platform that is flanked by two bushes. The basement is unfinished at present with plans to finish part into a recreation room with a half bath. The unfinished area will contain a storage area, laundry room, and a place for the family's dog, an Irish Setter. The first floor contains areas for the kitchen, formal dining room, breakfast nook, entry way, informal and formal living areas, office or library, and a half bath. There is also a door to the back yard with an area planned for a spa, and a changing area that is part of the garage. The second floor has four bedrooms and two full baths, with a sitting area at the top of the stairs.

The woman's 62-year-old mother, who is widowed, will be living with the family to assist her daughter as needed and to supervise the 8-year-old twin boys after school when the father and 18-year-old daughter are at work. The grandmother has arthritis in her knees, and had her right knee replaced 2 months previously, however, she still uses a cane when walking. The grandmother would like to have her own separate living area to entertain her own friends.

95. **The husband would like to know what minimum width the doorways should be for adequate accessibility from either a wheelchair or walker. The distance would be:**
    A. 46 cm.
    B. 58 cm.
    C. 70 cm.
    D. 82 cm.

96. **Where should the family place the bedrooms for the mother and the grandmother?**
    A. The mother and the grandmother on the second floor.
    B. The mother on the first floor and the grandmother on the second floor.
    C. The mother on the first floor and the grandmother in the basement.
    D. The mother and the grandmother in the basement.

97. **How much space is needed around the front door to allow easy access by a wheelchair?**
    A. 3 feet by 5 feet
    B. 4 feet by 4 feet
    C. 4.5 feet by 3 feet
    D. 5 feet by 5 feet

98. **The family would like to place grab bars around the toilets in the house for easy access during transfers by the mother. At what height should they be placed?**
    A. 28 to 32 inches
    B. 33 to 36 inches
    C. 38 to 41 inches
    D. 43 to 46 inches

99. **After the occupational therapist has completed the home visit, the therapist should include in the report of the visit the:**
    A. outpatient therapy recommendations.
    B. status of the woman at the time of discharge.
    C. changes necessary for furniture arrangement.
    D. appropriate method of transportation.

100. **It should be recommended to the family prior to an individual's discharge home in a wheelchair that the:**
    A. toilet paper dispenser should not be used as a grab bar.
    B. the bathroom mirror should be placed with the bottom 48 inches from the floor.
    C. carpeting should not be short pile.
    D. stove controls should be place on the back.

PSYCHOSOCIAL QUESTIONS

Assessment of Occupational Performance

101. **The occupational therapist has organized a group of individuals to evaluate their group interpersonal skills in an activity-based group. Six clients have been told about the evaluation group. The therapist is asked to add two additional clients to the group. These individuals are new admissions to the unit. The therapist would:**
    A. ask one or two of the original six members to wait until later and include the two new admissions to the group.
    B. add the two new admissions and then divide the members into two groups of four.
    C. interview the two new admissions separately and continue with the original evaluation group of six.
    D. agree to include one of the new admissions to the group, interview the other new admission separately.

102. **In the above activity-based evaluation group, the best activity to select is:**
    A. clients make individual collages and share a set of magazines to complete the activity.
    B. all group members construct one tower that incorporates all of the pieces provided in a set of constructional materials (e.g., Legos, Tinkertoys, or Erector set).
    C. all group members work together to make pizza and salad for their lunch that day.
    D. each client selects a short-term craft activity from four available samples.

103. **The determination of an individual's Global Assessment of Functioning on the DSM-IV diagnosis is based on:**
    A. the degree of environmental and psychosocial problems the individual experienced.
    B. the medical conditions complicating the original diagnosis.
    C. the individual's level of psychosocial and occupational limitations.
    D. the person's maladaptive mechanisms.

104. **A picture of the self is drawn by a depressed adolescent and contains very lightly drawn facial features and very small ears. The most likely interpretation of this drawing is that the adolescent is uncomfortable with:**
    A. communication.
    B. his drawing ability.
    C. following directions.
    D. his immortality.

105. **Using an activity-based evaluation group in evaluation is consistent with the:**
    A. model of human occupation.
    B. analytic frames of reference.
    C. sensory integration frames of reference.
    D. developmental and acquisitional frames of reference.

106. **The occupational therapist is working with a 20-year-old man diagnosed with schizophrenia. He states that his main goal is to "have a girlfriend." The short-term goal statement that is the best to begin addressing is:**
    A. The client will find a job and move into his own apartment within 8 months.
    B. The client will identify the ways in which his disability has interfered with his thinking processes following each group session.
    C. The client will initiate appropriate, casual greetings when beginning casual conversations with female staff.
    D. During one to two conversations with female group members, the client will make eye contact for 8 to 10 second periods two times in each half hour socialization group.

107. **The environmental modification that the OTR should recommend to the COTA for clients who are at risk for acting out sexually in an activity-based group is to:**
    A. provide a relatively active and stimulating environment with opportunities for the at-risk individuals to engage in real life activities.
    B. stand to the side of at-risk individuals instead of face to face during interactions with the client.
    C. avoid having at-risk individuals in close proximity to others to reduce physical contact with others.
    D. advise at-risk individuals in a calm, nonjudgmental manner about the behavior you expect.

108. **The intervention that reflects the habilitation approach to cognitive skills is:**
    A. teach the problem-solving process to the client for generalization to future situations.
    B. identify the clients existing and inactive approaches to solving problems before facilitating improvement of deficit strategies.
    C. adapt the client's environment to decrease the risk of harm.

    D. determine the client's problem solving abilities with the Allen Cognitive Level (ACL) assessment and then teach problem solving strategies to the caregiver.

109. **The assessment instrument that is best for recording observations about a client's task and inter-personal behaviors and how these behaviors remained stable or changed for 15 sessions is the:**
    A. Routine Task Inventory (RTI).
    B. Comprehensive Occupational Therapy Evaluation Scale (COTE).
    C. NPI Interest Inventory.
    D. Weekly SOAP Progress notes.

110. **The therapist who decides to use pictures, music, and discussion questions with a group of elderly clients to encourage them to verbalize their thoughts and feelings about their first ride in a car is using:**
    A. remotivation.
    B. reality orientation.
    C. compensatory cognitive approach.
    D. environmental modification.

Development of the Treatment Plan

111. **The treatment goal that addresses the psychosocial skill of self-expression is that the:**
    A. client will identify and pursue activities that are pleasurable to the self.
    B. client will use facial expressions and gestures that are consistent with stated emotions during assertive, passive, and aggressive role play situations.
    C. client will recognize his or her own behavior and possible negative and positive consequences.
    D. client will identify his or her own assets and limitations following a movement group.

112. **The occupational therapist wrote: "the client will identify two strengths and one limitation about task performance at the close of each group." This goal addresses the component of occupational performance referred to as:**
    A. problem solving.
    B. values.
    C. self concept.
    D. self expression.

113. **The occupational therapist is the group leader of an activity-based parallel level group. The best goal for the members of this group is that:**
    A. each member should take a leadership role within the session.
    B. members will share materials with at least one other group member.
    C. each member will express two positive feelings about themselves within the group session.
    D. each member will remain in the group without disrupting the work of others for 30 minutes.

114. **The occupational therapist's goal is to select a type of game that allows group members equal opportunities to win and can be played by a variety of functional levels. The best game type to select is:**
    A. games of strategy.
    B. hobbies.
    C. games of chance.
    D. puzzles.

115. **The occupational therapist who selects a treatment activity from a "games of chance" category would use:**
    A. baseball card collecting.
    B. bingo.
    C. charades.
    D. balloon volleyball.

116. **The general technique to use when working with client's diagnosed with organic mental disorders is to:**
    A. improve social skills in relating to others.
    B. create new habits of time use.
    C. teach compensatory strategies and manage the environment.
    D. facilitate resuming previous life roles.

117. **The best method to use in encouraging problem solving in a craft media group is to:**
    A. begin with activities that have obvious solutions and high probability of success.
    B. begin with activities that require gross motor responses before fine motor responses.
    C. structure the number and kinds of choices available.
    D. gradually increase the time used in the activity by 15 minute increments.

118. **A therapist bases activity selection upon Allen's Cognitive Disabilities frame of reference and provides step by step samples that the client's use for matching their work. This therapist's activity selection is consistent with cognitive level:**
    A. 3: manual actions.
    B. 4: goal directed actions.
    C. 5: exploratory actions.
    D. 6: planned actions.

119. **Sensory-motor methods advocated by L.J. King for treating adult clients with schizophrenia are considered to be interventions that focus on:**
    A. habilitation.
    B. rehabilitation.
    C. maintenance of function.
    D. remediating the cause of dysfunction.

120. **The goal of using pleasurable activities to change the client's attention away from negative, anger producing thoughts is:**
    A. consistent with the object relations views of reducing a client's anger.
    B. consistent with the cognitive disabilities view of the role of activity in treating angry outbursts.
    C. consistent with the cognitive behavioral views of anger intervention.
    D. contraindicated in working with client's learning to deal with anger.

121. **The occupational therapist is selecting an activity for an activity-based group of young men diagnosed with schizophrenia. The therapist's thinking sequence begins with "what are the types of activities I have found to be helpful with individuals with schizophrenia?" What is this type of clinical reasoning?**
    A. Procedural
    B. Conditional
    C. Interactive
    D. Narrative

122. **The occupational therapist is working in a psychosocial setting. In order to establish a safe environment in the craft area by reducing the risk of unaccounted tools at the start and close of groups, the therapist would:**
    A. keep track of the keys to storage cabinets and unit doors.
    B. have all materials and supplies ready before the group begins.
    C. only allow clients who have no behavioral risk precautions to attend groups.
    D. utilize a tool storage area that can be locked and that uses tool shadows or outlines.

123. **The occupational therapist is leading a grooming group for female clients in a psychosocial treatment setting. In order to comply with universal precautions, the therapist should:**
    A. use disposable cotton swabs and have clients bring their own cosmetics.
    B. use disposable gloves when combing client's hair.
    C. wash and dry make-up brushes between uses.
    D. avoid bringing cosmetics with glass containers to the group.

124. **The occupational therapist is working in a psychosocial setting with a client who is classified as a potential suicide risk. In selecting craft media, the craft that would be safest is a:**
    A. leather checkbook cover with single cordovan lacing.
    B. macrame plant hanger.
    C. ceramic ash tray.
    D. decoupage wood key fob.

Implementation of the Treatment Plan

125. **The following craft material requires the therapist to follow precautions for ingesting toxic substances:**

A. mirrors.
B. white craft glue.
C. permanent magic markers.
D. leather dyes.

126. **The occupational therapist using anger interventions based on cognitive-behavioral model would begin with this step in the treatment phase:**
    A. document the client's physiological responses to anger situations.
    B. develop the client's awareness of the link between anger and stress.
    C. improve the client's stress management skills.
    D. encourage the use of pleasurable activities to shift the client's thoughts from those that are provoking anger.

127. **The occupational therapist explains the purpose of a prevocational evaluation program to a client who is in a psychosocial setting. The best explanation for this program is:**
    A. "The program will help you to learn about your interests, talents, and skills for assembly jobs."
    B. "The program will help you to learn about the skills you have that are needed on most jobs and about your potential for work."
    C. "This program will help you identify the responsibility you have to your employer while you are in treatment and to inform your employer of these responsibilities."
    D. "This program will help you to develop skills in getting a job."

128. **The aspects of psychosocial performance that are important to emphasize in developing a client's work potential in a prevocational program are:**
    A. punctuality, accepting responsibility for oneself, accepting directions from a supervisor, and appropriately interacting with peer coworkers.
    B. memory, sequencing of the work tasks, and making decisions.
    C. standing tolerance, eye-hand coordination, and endurance.
    D. exploring ways to seek out available jobs and preparing a resumé.

129. **The occupational therapist is documenting a client's psychosocial responses to an activity. The most objective statement is:**
    A. "On 11-1-95, the client did not want to finish her stenciling activity."
    B. "On 11-1-95, the client was hostile to another client in the activity group."
    C. "The client demonstrated the ability to make a decision when she selected one of six craft designs presented."
    D. "The client demonstrated an appropriate level of frustration tolerance during most of the activity."

Case Study: Central Psychiatric Hospital

James D. Smith
#54321
11-1-95

Section I. *Mr. Smith attended a total of 24 occupational therapy groups throughout his hospitalization for depression 10-15-95 to 11-1-95.*

Section II. *Patient achieved the following goals:*

1. *Pt. has demonstrated four alternative, effective coping strategies for restating negative, automatic thoughts.*

2. *Pt. identified three former interests and specified plan for gradually resuming involvement in these after discharge.*

3. *Pt. has demonstrated improved assertiveness skills in refusing unreasonable requests from boss in simulated experiences.*

Section III. *Pt. is capable of resuming role of parent and spouse and part time worker at discharge. Mr. Smith will gradually resume his work activities to full time (40 to 45 hours per week) over the course of 2 weeks. On final evaluation, Mr. Smith's leisure interest checklist showed a 15 percent increase in quantity of interests and included three interests that he upgraded from casual to strong. Mr. Smith has agreed to take his journal of automatic thoughts, restatements, and activities for his first week after discharge to the outpatient group at the community mental health center.*

Section IV. *Mr. Smith was scheduled to attend the outpatient support group next Tuesday at 7:00 P.M. Mr. Smith completed the authorization to transfer occupational therapy treatment records to the CMHC.*

130. **The sample documentation is a(n):**
    A. reassessment.
    B. initial note.
    C. discharge summary.
    D. treatment plan.

131. **In the sample documentation, the section that contains Mr. Smith's follow-up plans is:**
    A. Section I.
    B. Section II.
    C. Section III.
    D. Section IV.

132. **In the preceding documentation sample, the section that contains Mr. Smith's home program is:**
    A. Section I.
    B. Section II.
    C. Section III.
    D. Section IV.

133. **The step in Mr. Smith's plan described in the preceding question that would be most appropriate for an entry-level COTA to carry out is:**

A. reporting the number of treatments in Section I.
B. making the referral to the community mental health center.
C. deciding that Mr. Smith no longer needed OT services and discontinuing the provision of services in his last week of treatment.
D. independently formulating the occupational therapy follow-up plans.

134. **Panic attacks associated with fears of specific objects are known as:**
A. agoraphobia.
B. hypochondriasis.
C. phobias.
D. obsessions.

135. **The Axis of DSM-IV that is used to note the stressors contributing to psychiatric diagnoses is:**
A. Axis II.
B. Axis III.
C. Axis IV.
D. Axis V.

136. **An individual who washes their hands ritualistically and repeatedly is engaging in:**
A. delusions.
B. compulsions.
C. obsessions.
D. activities of daily living.

137. **The following individuals are most likely to commit suicide:**
A. individuals under 35 years old.
B. men over the age of 65.
C. women over the age of 65.
D. men over the age of 80.

138. **The disorder that is most likely to be related to stressors such as divorce or loss of one's job:**
A. adjustment disorders.
B. posttraumatic stress disorders.
C. cyclothymia.
D. dissociative identity disorder.

139. **A person whose mood and behaviors vacillate between grandiosity and hostility several times within an hour is exhibiting:**
A. mania.
B. emotional lability.
C. paranoia.
D. denial.

Evaluation of the Treatment Plan

140. **The client's initial short-term goal for improving social conversation with peers was: "client will initiate two requests to other group members for sharing or using group materials within a 1-week period." Because the client was unable to meet this goal, the therapist grades the goal to make it more achievable. The best revised goal to select is:**
A. "Client will initiate two requests to other group members for sharing or using group materials within a 2-week period."
B. "Client will initiate one request to one other group member for sharing or using group materials within a 1-week period."
C. "Client will initiate two requests to each of the five group members for sharing or using one group tool within 2 weeks."
D. "Client will say hello to group leader at start of each group session."

141. **The therapist changes a tile trivet activity by providing blue-colored craft glue instead of white glue to clients who confuse the glue and the grout. The therapist is using:**
A. activity analysis.
B. activity adaptation.
C. activity sequencing.
D. conditional reasoning.

142. **Mr. Brown is a client with the diagnosis of bipolar disorder manic episode. His behavior has changed as the week has progressed. On Monday, he walked into occupational therapy, stated that his name was John F. Kennedy, and then walked out of the clinic. On Wednesday, he was able to sit briefly at the table in the OT clinic but was noticeably hypermanic and unable to work on any one craft. On Friday, Mr. Brown was able to sit with the other clients in the clinic, was cheerful yet jumped from topic to topic while conversing. He worked quickly on a short-term craft project. The best description of this client's overall course of change is:**
A. regression.
B. progression.
C. decompensation.
D. recovery.

143. **The thematic group that would be most appropriate for Mr. Brown (see question 142) to attend on Saturday:**
A. assertiveness group.
B. no thematic groups are appropriate at this time.
C. discharge planning group.
D. exercise group.

144. **The cient whose goal is related to increasing attention span often watches the person next to him at the work table. The two clients are working on different tasks. The therapist discusses this difficulty with the treatment team and describes the client's problem as:**
A. memory deficits.
B. spatial operations.
C. generalization of learning.
D. distractability.

Discharge Planning

145. The legal principle that impacts the occupational therapists discharge planning process within all mental health practice areas is:
A. least restrictive environment.
B. the licensure laws of the state.
C. Public Law 94-142 (1975).
D. the Tarasoff decision.

146. The occupational therapist is planning a group that prepares clients for discharge from an acute care inpatient psychiatric hospital to a variety of community programs. Which of the following general approaches would be most important to include?
A. Develop social skills.
B. Address approaches to disciplining children.
C. Teach problem solving and goal setting.
D. Improve self-esteem.

147. The comment made in a discharge planning group on a psychiatric inpatient unit that indicates a client's concern about stigma would be:
A. "The smoke from your cigarette is really making me uncomfortable. Please put your cigarette out."
B. "My medications make my eyes blurry. I want to stop taking it so I can see better."
C. "My relatives are always trying to tell me what to do with my life. They think I should continue seeing a psychiatrist."
D. "When I apply for jobs, what should I put down when it asks if you have been hospitalized or treated for anything in the past 6 months?"

148. The treatment team discusses their concerns about an individual with schizophrenia who is scheduled to be discharged from inpatient treatment next week. The information that best reflects the occupational therapist's viewpoint is:
A. "John has been coming to community meeting regularly and telling the others about his scheduled discharge date. I'm not sure he's ready, however, as he laughs to himself when he's talking."
B. "John's tendency to discontinue his medications may be less of a problem if I can get his referral to the outpatient day program completed before he leaves the hospital."
C. "John's medication should be changed from oral administration to the long acting intramuscular injection before he's discharged."
D. "I'm concerned abut John's ability to live on his own unless he is better able to structure his leisure time. Before admission, he was rarely in contact with others. Then his voices got worse."

149. The husband of an individual who is being treated for bipolar disorder describes his frustation with the ups and downs of his wife's problems. The best support group referral to recommend to this husband is:
A. Al-Anon
B. Family therapy
C. National Alliance for the Mentally Ill
D. Recovery, Inc.

150. The most appropriate recommendation to make for an individual functioning at (Allen's) cognitive level 4 and needing to take two different psychotropic medications twice daily after discharge:
A. No special recommendation is needed as client can take correct dosage at correct times.
B. Have client take "one white and one blue pill" with the morning and evening meals.
C. Instruct caregiver to remind client to take a white pill and a blue pill twice a day.
D. Instruct caregiver to place pills into client's hands at the designated times.

ADMINISTRATION AND MANAGEMENT QUESTIONS

Organize and Manage Services

151. An occupational therapist seeks out the manager to ask if a set of cones, which was utilized in a patient's room, needs to be sterilized prior to being replaced in the equipment closet. Based on universal precautions, the manager is most likely to respond:
A. "It doesn't really matter, whatever you think is best."
B. "Yes, all items used in the patients' rooms need to be sterilized before return to the equipment closet."
C. "No, even if a patient's body fluids got onto the cones, they only need to be washed in the ADL apartment sink."
D. "It depends. If body fluids have not come in contact with the cones, no. However, if at any time the cones came in contact with body fluids, they should be sterilized."

152. The occupational therapist is working with an individual in the ADL bathroom practicing wheelchair-to-tub transfers. During the transfer, the individual's external catheter is dislodged and urine spills onto the floor. The therapist notes that the urine appears to have blood in it. Based on her knowledge of universal precautions:
A. an exposure has occurred and she should use universal precautions.
B. an exposure has NOT occurred so she does not need to use universal precautions.
C. an exposure has occurred but is not severe enough to require universal precautions.
D. an exposure has NOT occurred but she will use universal precautions anyway.

153. **Functional supervision is defined as:**
    A. provision of information and feedback to coworkers.
    B. a continuum of supervision, which may include close, general, and routine supervision.
    C. supervision provided on an as needed basis.
    D. supervision provided by monthly contact or on an as needed basis.

154. **The mechanism to review the results of service interventions for a population is referred to as:**
    A. a process.
    B. an outcome.
    C. program evaluation.
    D. utilization review.

155. **The format in which the delivery of services is monitored in relationship to how cost effectively the services were provided is:**
    A. a process.
    B. an outcome.
    C. program evaluation.
    D. utilization review.

156. **A written plan that identifies problems, provides objective assessment of the problems, determines whether an intervention worked, reassesses interventions, and develops information that describes a program's effectiveness is most likely contained within a:**
    A. quality-improvement plan.
    B. peer review.
    C. utilization review.
    D. program evaluation.

157. **In the quality-improvement plan, "measures" are:**
    A. the degree to which objectives are achieved.
    B. the results a program aims to achieve.
    C. characteristics according to severity.
    D. the standards with which outcomes are compared.

Questions 158–160 refer to the following quality assurance plan

Section I	Compliance with facility documentation standards
Section II	Occupational therapist's documentation in the patient's chart
Section III	Clinical findings are clearly documented according to the discipline's standards
Section IV	85 percent
Section V	25 patients
Section VI	Quarterly

158. **In the quality assurance plan, section I is representative of a(n):**
    A. indicator.
    B. monitor.
    C. threshold.
    D. data source.

159. **Section II in the quality assurance plan represents:**
    A. an indicator.
    B. a monitor.
    C. a threshold.
    D. the data source.

160. **Section VI of the quality assurance plan represents the:**
    A. time frame.
    B. sample size.
    C. threshold.
    D. data source.

161. **The manager of occupational therapy supervises an employee who demonstrates specialized skill in treatment and serves as an expert for her peers. This therapist has completed research, leadership training, and assisted in continuing education activities. The manager of the department is most likely to supervise this individual at what level?**
    A. close supervision
    B. intermediate supervision
    C. advanced supervision
    D. educator supervision

162. **The occupational therapist is establishing a department in a rural nursing home. As a part of developing the policies and procedures for documentation in the nursing home, the occupational therapist will MOST likely refer to:**
    A. the Uniform Terminology.
    B. the Occupational Therapy Code of Ethics.
    C. the Occupational Therapy Standards of Practice.
    D. The Occupational Therapy Roles.

163. **An occupational therapist is stopped in the hallway of an acute care hospital by the family of one of the patient's she is treating. The family asks if she will answer some of their questions while their mother is in the radiography room. The therapist indicates to the family that she has been seeing their mother twice a day for 30 minutes. The therapist reviews how their mother did that morning in her half-hour therapy session as well as her progress in therapy the past few days. The occupational therapist spends a total of 15 minutes with the family. Based on the Code of Ethics, the therapist will MOST likely:**
    A. charge the patient an additional 15 minutes of treatment for the time spent with the family.
    B. reduce the woman's time in therapy in the afternoon by 15 minutes and charge for one half-hour of treatment to cover the time spent with the family.

C. charge patient for 45 minutes of treatment.

D. treat the patient in the afternoon and charge for the 1 hour of direct time spent with the patient.

164. **The occupational therapist on an inpatient psychiatric unit calls in sick to work. The OT's schedule includes a task group and coping skills group. The treatment team includes nursing, an art therapist, and a therapeutic recreation specialist. What would be the best solution to provide activities in the absence of the OT?**

A. The art therapist will lead two task groups and bill for occupational therapy.

B. The TR will lead leisure awareness and skills groups and will bill for occupational therapy since it was during the regularly scheduled OT group time.

C. The TR will substitute recreational activities in the OT time, but will not bill for occupational therapy services.

D. The nurses will ask the patient to work on the assignments that they were given by the occupational therapist in this time and will be billed by the OT when she returns to work.

165. **The occupational therapist is working with an individual in redesigning the home environment to accommodate the individual's wheelchair. The therapist collaborates with the individual in identifying what aspects of the environment limit accessibility. This form of clinical reasoning would MOST likely be referred to as:**

A. procedural reasoning.

B. conditional reasoning.

C. interactive reasoning.

D. narrative reasoning.

166. **The occupational therapist is treating a 31-year-old man who experienced a T1-T2 spinal cord injury as a result of a motor vehicle accident. Prior to the injury, the young man worked as a computer programmer and played in basketball leagues in the evenings and on the weekends. The therapist shares this information with her colleagues and asks what they have done in similar situations. The form of clinical reasoning that the therapist is MOST likely to utilize in this scenario would be:**

A. procedural reasoning.

B. conditional reasoning.

C. interactive reasoning.

D. narrative reasoning.

167. **The occupational therapist has received a referral to treat a man who was diagnosed with lung cancer which has now metastacized to the brain. The therapist spends 15 minutes reviewing the patient's chart and talking to his nurse who indicates that he is preoccupied with finances. As the occupational therapist enters** the room, the man states that he does not want to be seen by any of the therapists because his insurance has run out and he cannot afford to pay for the treatment. Responding consistently with the Code of Ethics, the therapist will MOST likely:

A. treat the man per the physician's order and notify the nurse that the man's preoccupation with finances continues.

B. not treat the man based on his refusal and document the interaction in the chart.

C. treat the man but not charge or document the services.

D. not treat the man but charge for the time spent completing the chart review.

168. **The MOST effective action to identify health care benefits for a patient and ensure payment is to:**

A. copy the patient's insurance cards to submit to the health insurance provider when services are completed.

B. instruct the patient to sign documents which hold him or her responsible for the expenses incurred as a result of services.

C. gain prior authorization for services from the patient's health insurance provider.

D. request documentation of medical necessity from the physician.

169. **An occupational therapist works collaboratively with a COTA in an inpatient psychiatric program. Consistent with the Occupational Therapy Roles, the occupational therapist asks the COTA to complete which one of the following tasks:**

A. lead an unstructured evaluation group.

B. assess a client utilizing Allen Cognitive Level (ACL) Test.

C. develop goals for a client based on the occupational therapist's assessment.

D. supervise an aide leading an exercise group and bill for occupational therapy services.

170. **A basic request for occupational therapy services that may come from a nurse, social worker, or teacher is referred to as:**

A. a recommendation.

B. a plan of treatment.

C. an intervention strategy.

D. a referral.

171. **Upon completion of the level II fieldwork, the student:**

A. should be functioning slightly below entry level.

B. should be able to function at an intermediate skill level based on the Occupational Therapy Roles.

C. should be able to function at an advanced skill level based on the Occupational Therapy Roles.

D. should be able to function at an entry level or above the minimum entry level of competence.

172. **In order to provide direct supervision for a level II fieldwork student, the supervisor MUST:**
    A. be a registered occupational therapist with 6 months of experience.
    B. have at least 1 year of experience as a registered occupational therapist.
    C. be certified by the NBCOT.
    D. have supervised a level one student prior to the level II student.

173. **The term given to the practice of an organization acting as an intermediary between an insurance agency and a hospital is:**
    A. managed care.
    B. utilization review.
    C. peer review.
    D. prospective payment.

174. **The measure of the minimal level of performance that a student must meet in order to achieve the fieldwork expectations are:**
    A. goals.
    B. objectives.
    C. monitors.
    D. conditions.

175. **The setting in which referrals are most often received from physicians, employers, attorneys, rehabilitation counselors, case managers, and insurance companies is:**
    A. industrial rehabilitation settings.
    B. pediatric treatment programs.
    C. hospital inpatient rehabilitation programs.
    D. subacute rehabilitation programs.

176. **A therapist working in home health has received a referral from the agency she contracts with to provide occupational therapy services. Consistent with home health treatment guidelines, the therapist will respond to the referral within:**
    A. 24 hours.
    B. 48 hours.
    C. 72 hours.
    D. 96 hours.

177. **An occupational therapy department is working short staffed and the hospital administrator recommends that occupational therapists only do evaluations and COTAs provide all of the treatment and discharge planning independently. The occupational therapist in this department communicates to the administrator that:**
    A. this is an appropriate solution to the problem of being short staffed.
    B. they are concerned about this solution because it does not provide for adequate supervision. However, they will follow the administrators recommendation.
    C. this does not allow for adequate supervision of the assistant.

    D. this is not an appropriate solution. The occupational therapist must do the evaluation, progress, and discharge documentation on all patients.

Promote Professional Practice

178. **The supervisor of occupational therapy is off work and in a local establishment listening to a band with her friends. She observes one of the therapists she supervises at another table being intimate with a gentleman who is currently being treated on an outpatient basis by the therapist he is with. The supervisor's response that is consistent with the Occupational Therapy Code of Ethics will MOST likely be to:**
    A. indicate to the therapist that she may maintain the relationship as long as it does not impair the patient's treatment.
    B. notify the state licensure board and terminate the employee.
    C. notify the NBCOT of the situation and reassign the patient to a different therapist.
    D. discipline the employee and refer the patient to another outpatient center.

179. **An occupational therapist is preparing to discharge a patient home following 3 weeks of intensive rehabilitation. The patient hands the therapist a $50 bill as a gift of his appreciation. The therapist's response which is consistent with the occupational therapy Code of Ethics will MOST likely be to:**
    A. accept the gift and use it to purchase a new radio for her car.
    B. decline the gift but accept it if the patient is insistent.
    C. decline the gift and explain that she is unable to accept gifts.
    D. accept the gift and use it to purchase a textbook for the department.

180. **A writing that encompasses the underlying values and basic beliefs to be used by occupational therapists is the:**
    A. *Standards of Practice.*
    B. *Uniform Terminology System for Reporting Occupational Therapy Services, ed. 3.*
    C. licensure guidelines.
    D. *Occupational Therapy Code of Ethics.*

181. **An occupational therapist working in home care has received a referral to treat a Medicare patient. Within this setting, the one component of the referral that the therapist cannot treat without is:**
    A. identification of the deficits that impair functional abilities.
    B. expected duration and frequency of treatment.
    C. a physician's order identifying services to be provided.
    D. the individual's history of the current illness.

Questions 182–183 refer to this statement of purpose

This document is to outline the hiring procedure for Central City Hospital.

1. *Once contact has been made with a candidate, the Department Manager will contact the candidate within 1 week to set up an appointment for a tour and interview.*

2. *At the completion of the tour and interview, the manager will request, as appropriate, proof of licensure, certification, and three references. If mutual interest is evident, continue to step 3. If employment will not be pursued, contact Human Resources at ext. 111 and provide documentation.*

3. *The manager is responsible for sending feedback forms to individuals identified as personal and professional references. It is the manager's discretion to make hiring decisions based on information gained from the references. The manager is to contact Human Resources at ext. 111 with the employment decision. If an offer will be extended, the Human Resource Department will contact the candidate and schedule a preemployment physical.*

182. The above is an example of:
   A. a personnel policy.
   B. an institutional policy.
   C. a departmental policy.
   D. a credentialing policy.

183. The purpose of a plan such as the one outlined in the example is to:
   A. ensure equal opportunity for all individuals in the hiring process.
   B. provide criteria for the process of hiring individuals.
   C. define the manager's responsibilities.
   D. verify qualified candidates for occupational therapy positions.

184. Continued professional education after certification has been achieved MAY be required by:
   A. AOTA.
   B. NBCOT.
   C. Individual state occupational therapy associations.
   D. State licensure.

185. A federal and state program that covers the poor and indigent is:
   A. Medicare.
   B. Medicaid.
   C. Workers Compensation.
   D. Education for all Handicapped Children Act.

186. A federal program funded by the government and implemented by over 200 plans is:
   A. Medicare.
   B. Medicaid.
   C. workers' compensation.
   D. Education for all Handicapped Children Act.

187. An occupational therapist is confronted with an ethical decision when she takes a rehab patient out of the hospital to complete a home evaluation. While en route to the home, the hospital vehicle carrying the patient sustained a flat tire on the highway. (The therapist was traveling in her own vehicle behind the hospital vehicle.) The driver indicates that fixing the tire will take approximately half an hour. By hospital policy, the therapist is not allowed to transport the patient in her own car. However, the only other two alternatives were to have the patient remain with the hospital vehicle until it was repaired or to send for another vehicle, which will take at least another 20 minutes. The therapist decides to drive the patient in her personal vehicle to the home since it is only another 5 minutes, and to leave directions with the driver to meet them at the home after the tire of the vehicle is repaired. While in the above situation, the form of ethical tension involved was:
   A. ethical uncertainty.
   B. ethical distress.
   C. an ethical dilemma.
   D. unethical behavior.

188. Individuals who are over the age of 65 or have renal failure usually have the primary health care costs covered by:
   A. Medicaid.
   B. Medicare.
   C. third party payors.
   D. private pay.

189. A therapist is completing a home assessment and making recommendations for equipment to be used in the home. He recommends a hospital bed, lightweight wheelchair, bedside commode, reachers, a long handled sponge, and a shower chair with a hand-held shower. The item(s) that would be considered as durable medical equipment would be:
   A. lightweight wheelchair and reachers.
   B. shower chair with a hand-held shower and bedside commode.
   C. hospital bed and shower chair with a hand-held shower.
   D. lightweight wheelchair and hospital bed.

Case Study

In establishing an occupational therapy department, the therapist makes three separate lists of items. The first list contains a power board, one adjustable work table, two chairs with arm rests, two chairs without armrests, one mat table, one desk, and one filing cabinet. The sec-

ond list includes weights, a three-speed vibrator, a skate board, a bulb dynamometer, and a pinchmeter. The third list includes long handled sponges, reachers, long handled shoe horns, therapeutic band, and putty. Use the above information for the following questions:

190. **The items on the first list would be considered:**
    A. capital equipment.
    B. expendable equipment.
    C. adaptive equipment.
    D. supplies.

191. **The items listed on the second list would be considered:**
    A. capital equipment.
    B. expendable equipment.
    C. adaptive equipment.
    D. supplies.

192. **The following practice trend that is most descriptive of occupational therapy practice in mental health is that:**
    A. there is an increasing shortage of occupational therapy practitioners in the area of mental health.
    B. occupational therapy services are not required services in most mental health settings.
    C. inpatient programs, more than community programs, are an area of future growth for occupational therapists in mental health.
    D. the majority of occupational therapists practice in the area of mental health.

193. **Service competency is:**
    A. the concept that two therapists performing the same procedure will gain the same results.
    B. established when a therapist passes the NBCOT exam.
    C. achieved through an individual attaining a minimum number of continuing education credits.
    D. the theory that individual competency is gained each year that the therapist practices.

194. **The section of the Occupational Therapy Code of Ethics that addresses the patient-therapist relationship, including those served being involved in the goal planning, and confidentiality is:**
    A. beneficence and autonomy.
    B. competence.
    C. compliance with laws and regulations.
    D. public information.

195. **The age range most frequently treated by occupational therapists is:**
    A. 0 to 19 years of age.
    B. 20 to 64 years of age.
    C. 65 years of age and older.
    D. mixed ages.

196. **Occupational therapists most frequently see individuals with the diagnosis of:**
    A. cerebrovascular accident.
    B. cerebral palsy.
    C. developmental delay.
    D. neuromuscular disorders.

197. **Therapists employed in community settings are most likely employed in:**
    A. private practice.
    B. school systems.
    C. home health agencies.
    D. residential care facilities.

198. **Volunteers utilized in an occupational therapy setting will MOST likely:**
    A. independently transport patients to and from therapy.
    B. independently work with a patient once the therapist has set up the activity.
    C. assist with stock and inventory control.
    D. complete chart reviews.

199. **The principle of the Occupational Therapy Code of Ethics that addresses a therapist accurately representing his or her educational background and training is:**
    A. beneficence and autonomy.
    B. competence.
    C. compliance with laws and regulations.
    D. public information.

200. **The occupational therapist is describing to a group of occupational therapy students observing treatment the scientific basis for her treatment approach and the anticipated change in function. This therapist is MOST likely describing a:**
    A. philosophical base
    B. professional model
    C. theoretic base.
    D. function-dysfunction continuum.

ANSWERS FOR SIMULATION EXAMINATION 4

1. (B) Form constancy perception. Answer B is correct because form constancy refers to the ability to match similar shapes regardless of change in their orientation in space. Answer A is not correct because figure-ground perception refers to the ability to distinguish a form or shape against a distracting background. Answer C is not correct because visual sequencing requires the ability to copy the same sequence of shapes or objects presented to the child. Although the latter is required when stringing the geometric beads, the error described refers to a form constancy error. See reference: Kramer and Hinojosa (eds): Todd, VR: Visual perceptual frame of reference: An information processing approach.

2. (D) Accommodation. Answer D is correct because the child demonstrates a problem with visual accommodation, or the ability to focus from near to far distance, and vice versa, efficiently. Answer A, ocular motility, refers to the ability to pursue an object visually in an efficient and smooth manner. Answer B, binocular vision, is described as the ability to focus the eyes on an object at varying distances and on seeing a single object clearly. Answer C, convergence, is not correct because convergence is the ability to move the eyes inward or outward with continued focus on the object. See reference: Kramer and Hinojosa (eds): Todd, VR: Visual perceptual frame of reference: An information processing approach.

3. (C) Constructional. The correct answer is C because constructional play involves building and creating things and it is in this area of play that the child develops a sense of mastery and problem-solving skills. Answer A is not correct because sensorimotor play generally develops a child's body awareness and sensory experiences. Answer B, imaginary play, is not correct because this type of play involves manipulating people and objects in fantasy as a prelude to dealing with reality. Answer D is not correct because the child is primarily learning rules through game and play. See reference: Kramer and Hinojosa (eds): Olson, L: Psychosocial frame of reference.

4. (B) Help the child develop cognitive strategies for anxiety-producing activities. The correct answer is B because the child with innate temperament problems needs cognitive strategies that will help him or her to overcome anxiety and be more likely to approach and participate in the activities. Answer A is not correct because the parents need to understand the innate temperament problem and the discomfort the child feels during activities. Answer C is not correct because the child will find a predictable routine helpful when activities are disorganized. Answer D is not correct because the parent and child need to learn mutual play in an environment that will promote positive engagement. See reference: Kramer and Hinojosa (eds): Olson, L: Psychosocial frame of reference.

5. (A) Physical guidance. The correct answer is A because physical guidance requires the least cognitive ability and provides the child the opportunity to learn through a sensory-motor experience. Answer B is not correct because verbal cues require understanding of language. Answer C is not correct because visual cues, such as pictures, require understanding the meaning of pictures. Answer D is not correct because forward chaining requires that the first step of a sequence be completed by the child. See reference: Hopkins and Smith (eds): Humphrey, R, and Jewell, K: Mental retardation.

6. (C) Provides enjoyable activities in a safe and accepting environment. Answer C is correct because children who learn to enjoy activities alone will be more likely to cooperate with peers in a group activity. Answer A is not correct because the child will not initiate and develop social interaction in an environment that inhibits independence (such as an authoritarian environment). Answer B is not correct because children with peer interaction problems will need to be taught some basic social skills in order to increase peer interaction. Answer D is not correct because the children will more likely learn and accept rules and limits established by their group. See reference: Kramer and Hinojosa (eds): Olson, L: Psychosocial frame of reference.

7. (A) Attention-deficit hyperactivity. The correct answer is A because his behavior indicates the excessive fidgeting and restlessness, inattention, and impulsiveness characteristic of ADHD. Answer B is incorrect because although some of the symptoms of overactivity and impulsiveness are part of a mood disorder of the manic type, there usually are also symptoms of grandiosity and inflated self-esteem. Answer C is incorrect because there is no evidence of interference with the basic rights of other children or societal rules. Answer D is not correct because the child showed no signs of uneasiness, apprehension, or dread associated with anticipation of danger. See reference: Hopkins and Smith (eds): Florey, LL: Psychiatric disorders in childhood and adolescence.

8. (D) Joint contracture. The functional ADL problems of children with arthrogryposis multiplex congenita disorder are caused by the presence of joint contractures at birth. Independent feeding is often an initial concern. Answer A is not correct. Obstetric paralysis refers to brachial palsy occurring at birth. Answer B is incorrect as hip dislocation is not a usual part of this disorder; when the lower extremities are involved, the characteristic problem is also joint contracture. Answer C is not correct because joint inflammation is characteristic of juvenile rheumatoid arthritis, not arthrogryposis. See reference: Hopkins and Smith (eds): Atkins, J: Neural tube defect.

9. (C) Make a report to appropriate authorities. In many states, the therapist, as a health professional, is in the position of being a "mandated reporter" who must make a report if there is reason to believe a child has been abused. A report of the injury should be made to appropriate authorities (answer C is correct). Answers A, B, and D delay or prevent proper assistance to a family involved in the occurrence of child abuse and therefore are wrong answers. All agencies serving children have policies and procedures for reporting injury in these situations. See reference: Hopkins and Smith (eds): Simon, CJ: Child abuse and neglect.

10. (A) Teenage parents. Answer A is correct because "children of teenagers are more likely to suffer from inadequate health care, personal hygiene, and nutrition; injuries were more likely to be severe." Teenage parents frequently lack parenting skills, as well as having a poor concept of appropriate expectations for their children. Answer C, therefore is not correct because it is very young parents who may be most prone to these problems. Although socioeconomic problems may be part of abuse and neglect, child abuse and neglect occurs at all economic levels of a society. Therefore, answers B and D are not correct. See reference: Hopkins and Smith (eds): Simon, CJ: Child abuse and neglect.

11. (B) Developmental stimulation. Because these children are confined at a very young age and are restricted for repair of the hip dislocation, a primary concern of the therapist should be to evaluate and provide a developmental program (answer B is correct). These children are therefore at risk for developmental delay. Although answers A, C, and D could be worthy secondary goals as time proceeds. Initial goals should be focused on dealing with the child's risk for developmental delay and ability to deal with restriction. See reference: Hopkins and Smith (eds): Atkins, J: Neurologic and orthopedic conditions: Congenital deficiencies.

12. (C) Slow and predictable movement. Sensory integration treatment is a highly complex and individualized form of treatment. Within this consideration, Kinnealy and Miller describe the use of sensory input with the therapy ball for children with vestibular hypersensitivity as providing "slow predictable rhythmic movement tolerance, heavy bounce tactile input simultaneously all pressure." Answer A is not correct because movement in any position or direction is used with children who have vestibular hyposensitivity. Answer B is not correct because adaptation to movement will be an important goal for comfort in the child's life activities. Answer D is not correct because it describes the type of movement most likely to be used in therapy when children are hyposensitive to movement. See reference: Hopkins and Smith (eds): Kinnealey, M, and Miller, L: Sensory integration/ learning disabilities.

13. (A) Arrhythmic and unexpected. The characteristics of facilitatory sensory input are unexpected, arrhythmic, uneven, or rapid input. Therefore, answer A is correct because it contains two of these four features (arrhythmic and unexpected). Answer B is not correct because, although arrhythmic input is excitatory, slow sensory input is inhibitory. Answer C is not correct because sustained and slow sensory input is inhibitory. Answer D is incorrect because although facilitatory input is unexpected,

rhythmic input is inhibitory. Also, sensory integration treatment is complex and highly individualized and must be monitored carefully to observe the effects of sensory input of varying types on the individual child. See reference: Hopkins and Smith (eds): Kinnealey, M, and Miller, L: Sensory integration/learning disabilities.

14. (C) Design an individualized program that requires advanced training. Sensory integration is a complex treatment modality, and is a highly individualized form of treatment carried out by a therapist with advanced training. Answer A is incorrect because the child's program is not being "individualized" but is included in a group program. Answer B is not correct because sensory integration treatment is active and requires an adaptive response from the child. Answer D is not correct because sensory integration is directed at improving underlying neurologic functioning, rather than skill development. See reference: Hopkins and Smith (eds): Kinnealey, M, and Miller, L: Sensory integration/learning disabilities.

15. (D) Decrease abnormal muscle tone by positioning and moving shoulder, arm, and wrist in a reflex-inhibiting pattern. The first step in treatment of the upper extremities, according to a neurodevelopmental approach, is to "normalize muscle tone, either increasing or decreasing, in positions where inhibition works best . . ." Answer A is not correct because application of a quick stretch to spastic flexor muscles will increase the spastic pattern and interfere with the development of arm extension. Answer B is not correct because facilitation of cocontraction will increase spasticity and interfere with movement. Answer C is not correct because strengthening of the flexor muscles will also increase spasticity in the flexor muscles. See reference: Hopkins and Smith (eds): Erhardt, R: Cerebral palsy.

16. (B) Begin with passive movement (placing and holding). Placing or holding is the beginning point for therapy. Answer A is not correct because it will follow passive movement. Answer C is not correct because active movement will follow passive movement. Answer D is not correct because when abnormal patterns occur, the program should be adjusted to a lower level, postural support should be increased, or external control should be increased. See reference: Hopkins and Smith (eds): Erhardt, R: Cerebral palsy.

17. (C) Somatosensory system. Many children who use an excessively tight grip on the writing tool and press too hard with the pencil on their paper have poor proprioceptive awareness (somatosensory). Answer A, vestibular system, is not correct (although it is difficult to completely separate any sensory system from another) because it primarily affects balance and general motor coordination. Answer B, the auditory system, is not correct because this system interprets sound for use in language. Answer D is not correct because, although the visual system can monitor motor control such as pencil grip and pressure, use of the pencil requires unconscious awareness of body position and pressure at times when the task is not monitored visually. See reference: Case-Smith, Allen, and Pratt (eds): Amundson, SJ, and Weil, M: Prewriting and handwriting skills.

18. (D) Cut the paper in two following a straight line. Scissors skills develop from cutting snips to a single straight line next. Answer A is not correct because cutting a heavier material such as cardboard or cloth develops last in the above sequence. Answer B is not correct because the ability to cut along curved lines develops after cutting a straight line. And answer C is not correct because cutting along straight lines to cut a triangle develops after a single straight line, and before cutting a curved line. See reference: Case-Smith, Allen, and Pratt (eds): Exner, CE: Development of hand skills.

19. (A) 1-2-3. Since central-to-peripheral refers to development occurring from the center of the body outward to the extremities, answer A would be correct. Postural stability would be developed first, then shoulder stability, and lastly grasping patterns. Answers B, C, and D would not be correct as they do not follow this order. See reference: Case-Smith, Allen, and Pratt (eds): Exner, CE: Development of hand skills.

20. (C) Direct selection mode. The picture board is classified, along with typewriter keyboards, as a direct selection mode. Answer A is not correct because the scanning mode classification includes indicating "yes" and "no" to different options presented to the child. Answer B is not correct because encoding refers to an augmentative communication system that requires higher level cognitive ability in order to remember and use a code system. Answer D is not correct because the output mode is only the message presentation part of the augmentative communication system, such as visual display, speech output, and so on. See reference: Case-Smith, Allen, and Pratt (eds): Struck, M: Augmentative communication and computer access.

21. (C) Individual Family Service Plan (IFSP). Answer C is correct because the service plan developed under federal law (I.D.E.A. 99-457, Part H) and provided through early intervention programs is called an "Individual Family Service Plan." Answer A is not correct because the title refers to a service plan provided for children of school age. Answer B is not correct because there is no service plan called "Least Restricted Environment Plan." Answer D is not correct because there is no service plan entitled "Early Intervention Service Plan" under federal law. See reference: Case-Smith, Allen, and Pratt (eds): Stephens, LC, and Tauber, SK: Early intervention.

22. (D) Peabody Scale of Motor Development. Answer D is correct because it will test the developmental motor skills of a child who is Jason's approximate age. The test measures motor skills in children from birth to 7 years, and Jason is 2.5 years of age. Answer A is not correct because the Southern California Sensory Integration and Praxis Test is designed to be used with children from 4 to 8.11 years. Answer B is not correct because the

Bruininks-Oseretsky Test of Motor Proficiency is used with children from ages 4.5 to 14.5 years. Answer C is not correct because the Motor-Free Visual Perception Test is used with children from 4 to 8 years of age. See reference: Case-Smith, Allen, and Pratt (eds): Hunter, JG: The neonatal intensive care unit.

23. (A) Hips and legs flexed, shoulders protracted. The best feeding position for a child with extensor hypertonicity in the hips, shoulders, and legs is the opposite, reflex-inhibiting pattern of hips and legs flexed, shoulders protracted. The child could be positioned in a feeding chair that provides this support or positioned on the lap and facing the feeder with back and shoulders supported. Answers B, C, and D are incorrect because each answer includes a pattern that would not be inhibitory to extensor tone in hips, legs, and shoulders; namely, shoulder retraction, hip and legs extended. See reference: Finnie: Feeding.

24. (B) Corner chair with head support and padded abductor post. Answer B is correct because a corner chair provides hip, knee and ankle flexion of 90 degrees, and the abductor post will keep the legs separated when or if extensor tone increases. The corner shape of the chair facilitates shoulder protraction or prevents shoulder retraction, which can prevent Jason's hands from coming forward to assist with eating. Answer A, the prone stander, by placing the child in a standing or extended position, would not be correct. Answer C is not correct because the supine position could encourage or facilitate extension. Answer D is not correct because Jason, due to poor head control and extensor tone, would be unable to sit without support. See reference: Finnie: Baby carriages, strollers, and chairs.

25. (B) Head. Develop head control first because this will provide a stable base for oral-motor control. Answer C, trunk control, is not correct because head control precedes trunk control in developmental progression. Although answer A, shoulder control, and answer D, hand control, will both contribute to improving eating and feeding skills by increasing the possibility of independence in eating through improved use of the arm and hand, head control needs to be emphasized first. See reference: Case-Smith, Allen, and Pratt (eds): Case-Smith, J, and Humphry, R: Feeding and oral motor skills.

26. (D) Upper lip control. The use of a shallow spoon will assist the child's development of upper lip control because it will be easier for the lip to remove all of the food on the spoon. This will hopefully increase Jason's oral-motor control during feeding. Jaw opening and closing will not be affected by the depth of the spoon (answers A and B are not correct). Lower lip control is not used to draw food off the spoon and therefore is not influenced by the use of a shallow spoon. See reference: Case-Smith, Allen, and Pratt (eds): Case-Smith, J, and Humphry, R: Feeding and oral motor skills.

27. (A) Nose and throat irritation. The special problems of nose and throat irritation, as well as the tongue bumping against the tube at the back of the throat, may create an unpleasant association with eating. (A tube has been inserted through the child's nose down into the stomach with the gavage method of feeding.) Answers B, C, and D can be problems associated with a gastrostomy, which means that the gastrostomy may produce fewer negative reactions in the child because of less unpleasant intrusion into the oral area. See reference: Case-Smith, Allen, and Pratt (eds): Case-Smith, J, and Humphry, R: Feeding and oral motor skills.

28. (D) Hold him firmly when picking him up. Answer D is correct because holding him firmly when it is necessary to touch him will inhibit responses to light touch (which are usually most uncomfortable for children with this problem). In line with this thinking, answers A and C are not correct because light touch is being used to tickle the child or stroke him lightly during bath time. Answer B is not correct because a strong sensory stimulus such as loud music would cause further startle and discomfort during a time when he is most vulnerable to the light touch of clothing being removed. See reference: Case-Smith, Allen, and Pratt (eds): Parham, LD, and Mailloux, Z: Sensory integration.

29. (C) Prone over a wedge. Considering the information given on Jason, answer C is probably the best answer because head control is isolated, with the trunk supported. Answer A is not the best answer because the trunk is not supported in standing. Answer B is not correct because, although the chest is supported by a sling, shoulders, arms, and hips must be able to control the position. Sitting on the therapy ball would be an appropriate activity if the trunk were given more support initially. For this reason, answer D is not the best answer. See reference: Hopkins and Smith (eds): Clark, F, Mailloux, Z, and Parham, D: Sensory integration and children with learning disabilities.

30. (C) Orthotist or prosthetist. Because Jason is part of a family where there is a single mother who is having difficulty supporting the family, a referral to a social worker should be made as early as possible. The social worker will be able to provide counseling for the family in dealing with these problems, as well as assistance in the area of financial and community resources. Although Jason may benefit from services of a psychologist (answer A) for further assessment of cognitive programming, it appears that family support may still be more essential at this time. Jason's need for an orthotist to provide splints or orthotic devices is not clear at this time as possible joint tightness has not been determined. See reference: Case-Smith, Allen, and Pratt (eds): Allen, AS: Relationships with other service providers.

31. (A) Polyarticular. Because Janet's condition had a sudden onset, she has several joints involved and has a low grade fever, she demonstrates the signs and symptoms of the polyarticular form of JRA. Answer B is not correct because the systemic type of JRA is characterized by a high grade fever and involvement of the lymph nodes and spleen. Answer C is not correct because there are only

a few joints involved with pauciarticular JRA. Also, because Still's disease is another name for systemic JRA, this answer is also not correct. See reference: Case-Smith, Allen, and Pratt (eds): Gordon, CY, Schanzenbacher, KE, Case-Smith, J, and Carrasco, RC: Diagnostic problems in pediatrics.

32. (D) 15 percent. Only 15 percent of children diagnosed with JRA have a remaining permanent disability. See reference: Case-Smith, Allen, and Pratt (eds): Gordon, CY, Schanzenbacher, KE, Case-Smith, J, and Carrasco, RC: Diagnostic problems in pediatrics.

33. (B) Information on juvenile rheumatoid arthritis. The most essential information for parents and teachers to receive from the occupational therapist is information on juvenile rheumatoid arthritis. Information on the occupational therapy evaluation and treatment program are of lesser importance, and may in fact be unimportant in terms of the child's functional problems. (Answers A, C, and D are less important.) See reference: Case-Smith, Allen, and Pratt (eds): Gordon, CY, Schanzenbacher, KE, Case-Smith, J, and Carrasco, RC: Diagnostic problems in pediatrics.

34. (C) Prevent deformity. A child with juvenile rheumatoid arthritis (JRA) will need splinting to prevent deformity and maintain range of motion. Answer A is not correct because hypertonus is not a characteristic of this condition. Answer B is not correct because, due to the active nature of the child's condition, increasing range of motion may be contraindicated. The correction of deformity may also be contraindicated with this child due to the active nature of her disease, therefore, answer D is not correct. See reference: Case-Smith, Allen, and Pratt (eds): Gordon, CY, Schanzenbacher, KE, Case-Smith, J, and Carrasco, RC: Diagnostic problems in pediatrics.

35. (C) Pencil gripper. These are all adaptive devices that can be used with a child who has JRA for various reasons. However, the correct answer is C, because the pencil gripper will probably make grasping the pencil easier and reduce hand grasp fatigue. Because of weak hands and because printing and handwriting is a common task for this child's age, it is important that fatigue be reduced with these children. The reacher, answer A, is not correct because it frequently requires grasp strength and does adapt for children who have problems with extended reach. The jar opener, answer B, is not incorrect in terms of its adaptation for hand strength problems with extended reach, but it is not a frequent task performed by a school-aged child (such as handwriting). The plate guard, answer C, will provide adaptation for coordination, one-handedness, and lack of hand and arm movements, but is not particularly necessary when hand strength is decreased (adapting the utensil would be more reasonable). See reference: Case-Smith, Allen, and Pratt (eds): Gordon, CY, Schanzenbacher, KE, Case-Smith, J, and Carrasco, RC: Diagnostic problems in pediatrics.

36. (B) Club foot. Equinovarus, or talipes equinovarus, is also called "club foot." This is a deformity involving forefoot adduction and supination, heel varus, equinus through the ankle, and medial deviation of the foot in relationship to the knee. See reference: Case-Smith, Allen, and Pratt (eds): Gordon, CY, Schanzenbacher, KE, Case-Smith, J, and Carrasco, RC: Diagnostic problems in pediatrics.

37. (D) Intermittent headaches. The major signs of shunt malfunction in the older child are irritability, short attention span, increased paralysis, decreased upper extremity strength, decreased school performance, and intermittent headaches. Answers A and B, increased head size, and nausea and vomiting, respectively, are major signs of shunt malfunction in very young children, and therefore are not correct answers. Answer D, back pain, is not among the symptoms given for this problem, and therefore is incorrect. See reference: Hopkins and Smith (eds): Atkins, J: Neural tube defect.

38. (D) Development, ADL, and sensory integration. Occupational therapy testing for Megan should include tests of development, self-care, and sensory integration, based on the problems listed in her case study. Answer A is not correct because it does not consider the possibility of sensory integration problems, and children with myelomeningocele, often "exhibit sensory integrative problems, poor fine motor coordination, and immature sensory systems." Answer B is not correct because it does not consider the possibility of developmental problems, as according to Atkins, these children should be tested regularly in the area of development through childhood since new problems can occur due to complications such as shunt malfunction or meningitis. Answer C is not correct because it includes the option of vocational testing, which is not appropriate at Megan's age of 7 years. See reference: Hopkins and Smith (eds): Atkins, J: Neural tube defect.

39. (B) Renal failure. The major cause of death in children with myelomeningocele is urinary infection with renal failure. Answers A, C, and D can contribute to the vulnerability of these children; however, respiratory infection, spinal cord degeneration, and hydrocephalus are usually not the major cause of children with this condition. See reference: Hopkins and Smith (eds): Atkins, J: Neural tube defect.

40. (A) Practice regular skin inspection. Answer A is correct due to the level of her paralysis. Because of problems with sensation, there is the possibility of the development of decubitus ulcers or burns due to contact with hot water or objects. Answer B is not correct because generally, children with melingeomyocele do not have oral-motor or eating problems, unless Arnold Chiari deformity is present. Answer C is not correct because generally, apnea episodes are not present with children who have spina bifida unless Arnold-Chiari deformity is present. Tactile defensive behaviors and other sensory-integrative disorders can be present in children like Megan with spina bifida and myelomeningocele, but skin breakdown may

be an even more essential home instruction at this time. See reference: Hopkins and Smith (eds): Atkins, J: Neural tube defect.

41. (B) Joint hyperextensibility observation. By placing shoulder, elbow, and hand flexor muscles on stretch, it is possible to note the degree of hyperextension. Palpation of muscles can also show a soft quality, which indicates differences in muscle tone. Answer C is not correct because the arm extension test measures reflex integration and choreoathetosis. Answer B is not correct because the adiadokinesis test measures timing and sequencing of forearm rotation movements, and also demonstrates bilateral coordination. Answer D is also incorrect because the thumb-finger touching test provides observations of manual speed and coordination. See reference: Case-Smith, Allen, and Pratt (eds): Parham, LD, and Mailloux, Z: Sensory integration.

42. (D) Environmental. Mental retardation can be caused by toxins (such as lead exposure in children) in the environment. Because answers A, B, and C do not include toxins, none of these are the correct answer. Birth complications could include conditions such as anoxia. Congenital infection might include conditions such as maternal toxoplasmosis. An example of a genetic cause of mental retardation would be fragile X syndrome. See reference: Hopkins and Smith (eds): Humphrey, R, and Jewell, K: Mental retardation.

43. (C) Gravitational insecurity. Gravitational insecurity is described as "intense anxiety and distress in response to movement or to a change in head position." The child easily experiences a fear of falling and prefers to keep his or her feet firmly on the ground. Answer A, tactile defensiveness, is a term used to describe discomfort with various textures and with unexpected touch, and therefore is not correct. Answer C, developmental dyspraxia, is not correct because it is a term used to describe a problem with motor planning. Intolerance for motion, answer D, is incorrect because it refers to a very similar and often related problem of inhibition of vestibular impulses, but it is usually associated with sensory information received from the semicircular canals; whereas gravitational insecurity is associated with the utricle and saccule. See reference: Case-Smith, Allen, and Pratt (eds): Parham, LD, and Mailloux, Z: Sensory integration.

44. (D) Improve motor planning. Motor planning or praxis problems are often seen in young children when dealing with novel equipment. In Michael's case study, the rocking horse and scooterboard are probably new and different play equipment to him, and he must solve the motor problem of placing or positioning his body in accordance with the shape and the use of the equipment. This requires an adequate body percept and the ability to cognitively plan his movements. See reference: Ayres: Developmental dyspraxia: A motor planning problem.

45. (B) Improve vestibular processing. The vestibular system has "considerable influence on postural tone, ocular pursuits, the coordination of input from the two body sides, the establishment of laterality, language function, and visual perception." Answer A, C, and D are not correct because ocular pursuits, muscle tone, and postrotary nystagmus can all be affected by vestibular processing, and by emphasizing this sensory system, there may be a positive effect on these functions. In addition, it should be noted that answer D, "increasing postrotary nystagmus," is not an appropriate goal of sensory integration therapy, since it is regarded as an expression of only one aspect of intact vestibular functioning in response to rotary stimulation. See reference: Case-Smith, Allen, and Pratt (eds): Parham, LD, and Mailloux, Z: Sensory integration.

46. (C) Rolling in a carpeted barrel. Because tactile defensiveness is an area of sensory integration treatment that should be approached cautiously, the child-controlled rolling on a textured surface would be less intrusive to her nervous system than answer A, where the therapist is providing the sensory stimulation to the most sensitive areas of the body. In general, sensory integration therapy involves child-directed adaptive responses, and it is recommended that occupational therapists have consultation from a sensory integration therapist when applying direct sensory input. Answers B and D are not correct because balancing and swinging activities generally do not address a problem of tactile defensiveness. See reference: Ayres: Developmental dyspraxia: A motor planning problem.

47. (D) Flushing, blanching, or perspiration. These responses are autonomic nervous system signs of sensory overload. Answers A, B, and C are probably not correct because they do not describe autonomic responses to the activity. See reference: Case-Smith, Allen, and Pratt (eds): Parham, LD, and Mailloux, Z: Sensory integration.

48. (D) Test of Visual Perceptual Skills (Gardner). The Test of Visual Perceptual Skills by Gardner measures seven areas of visual perception for children of Martha's age (8 years). The Purdue, the Denver, and the Test of Visual Motor Integration do not define the areas of visual perception, although drawing of geometric forms is included in each of these tests. See reference: Case-Smith, Allen, and Pratt (eds): Schneck, CM: Visual perception.

49. (B) Crawl on top of a rope taped to the floor. Answer B is the most correct because the crawling activity provides either reciprocal or bilateral movements. Weight-bearing emphasized proprioceptive input, and having the rope between arms and legs develops awareness of body sidedness from a visual standpoint. The remaining choices each do not provide reciprocal or bilateral movements, which would develop coordination of the body sides in rhythmical patterns. See reference: Case-Smith, Allen, and Pratt (eds): Parham, LD, and Mailloux, Z: Sensory integration.

50. (A) Best responder. Research shows that a bilateral and sequencing sensory integration disorder responds best to this type of therapy. See reference: Case-Smith, Allen, and Pratt (eds): Parham, LD, and Mailloux, Z: Sensory integration.

51. (C) Manual Muscle Test. The manual muscle test is an example of a nonstandardized test. It has instructions for the administration and scoring of the test, however, it lacks validity and reliability. The results or interpretation of a nonstandardized test often depend on the skill, judgment, and bias of the evaluator. A standardized test has instructions for the administration and scoring, as well as information regarding the validity and reliability, which have established norms from a specific population. The Motor Free Visual Perception Test (answer A), the Minnesota Rate of Manipulation Test (answer B), and the Purdue Pegboard Evaluation (answer D) all have information available regarding the reliability and validity based on the established norms. See reference: Pedretti: Occupational therapy evaluation of physical dysfunction.

52. (B) Jebsen-Taylor Hand Function Test. This test uses seven subtests of functional activities such as writing, card turning, picking up small objects, simulated feeding activity, stacking objects, and picking up light objects and heavy objects that are large. This test may be constructed by the facility. The Purdue Pegboard Evaluation, answer A, uses a prefabricated kit. The Minnesota Rate of Manipulation, answer C, and the Crawford Small Parts Dexterity Test, answer D, are all prefabricated kits. The Purdue Pegboard Evaluation and the Crawford Small Parts Dexterity Test involve assembly tasks using pins and collars with other items. The Minnesota Rate of Manipulation uses colored plastic disks that nest in a board. See reference: O'Sullivan and Schmitz: Schmitz, T: Coordination assessment.

53. (B) Two. A person in stage two of Brunnstrom's level of recovery would have weak, associated movements seen usually in a flexor synergy. Also, there may be little or no finger flexion occurring. A person in stage one, answer A, would have no movement or spasticity on the affected side of the body. Stage three, answer C, has all movements occurring in synergy with definite spasticity noted and mass grasp in the affected hand. In stage four, answer D, a person would be able to have decreasing spasticity with some deviation from synergistic patterns with the person's hand demonstrating lateral prehension and partial finger extension. See reference: Rothstein, Serg, and Wolf: Neuroanatomy, neurology, and neurologic therapy.

54. (C) 6 weeks. During the acute stage of injury, healing will take place from 1 to 3 weeks (answers A and B, respectively). By 6 weeks, answer C, healing should have occurred enough to allow a resumption of most functional activities with pain noted as discomfort if it is present. If significant pain with impairment continues after 6 weeks, then this contributes to a diagnosis of chronic pain made by the physician. After trauma has occurred at 9 weeks, answer D, there would have been enough healing after the initial acute trauma so that only an occasional twinge of discomfort may be felt. See reference: Cailliet: Subluxations of the cervical spine.

55. (B) A dynamometer. A dynamometer is used to measure hand grasp. Usually three trials are averaged together and compared with a standardized norm. See reference: Hunter, Schneider, Mackin, and Callahan (eds): Swanson, A, Swanson, G, and Goran-Hagert, C: Evaluation of impairment of hand function.

56. (C) Jebsen-Taylor Hand Function Test. This test is easily constructed within the hospital and includes such subtests as writing, card turning, using a spoon, and grasping cans. Answers A, B, and D are all prefabricated tests. Answer A, the Minnesota Rate of Manipulation Test, measures manual dexterity with five different subtests that may be used individually; however the patient only manipulates one type of object. Answer B, The Purdue Pegboard Evaluation, is a test of fingertip dexterity using four different subtests. Answer D, the Valpar Work Sample, has 19 different work samples to assess the specific physical demands. The Valpar Upper Extremity Range of Motion Work Sample assesses the patient's ability to manipulate objects without use of vision. See reference: Hunter, Schneider, Mackin, and Callahan (eds): Swanson, A, Swanson, G, and Goran-Hagert, C: Evaluation of impairment of hand function.

57. (C) Volumeter. A volumeter is a container used to measure edema in the hand by measuring the amount of water displaced when the hand is placed into the container. A goniometer is used to measure movement at a joint by two arms. One arm is held stationary while the other arm moves around an axis of 360 degrees. An anesthesiometer measures two-point discrimination with a moveable point attached to a ruler that has a stationary point at one end. A dynamometer measures grip strength through gross hand grasp. See reference: Trombly (ed): Zemke, R: Remediating biomechanical and physiological impairments of motor performance.

58. (D) Developing a treatment plan. The treatment plan is developed after the person's problems have been identified, and at that time the specific approaches or methods are selected. The initial interview (answer A) assists the occupational therapist in deciding which evaluation procedures or specific assessments to use. The performance of assessments (answer B) gathers information to identify problem areas and plan treatment. After the assessments are complete, the occupational therapist uses clinical reasoning skills to analyze data (answer C) and to identify the person's strengths and weaknesses. See reference: Pedretti: Occupational therapy evaluation of physical dysfunction.

59. (B) Pain management techniques. A work hardening program is focused toward returning a person to work in a physically appropriate setting as quickly as is feasible by reconditioning the person. As part of that program, pain management techniques (answer B) are included to assist the person with managing and coping with pain during work-related activities. A work hardening program would not include recreational activities (answer A) since the focus is on work activities. A person who would

need driver re-education (answer C) would have physical impairments beyond the scope of treatment for work hardening and would be more appropriate for a physical rehabilitation program. A work hardening program would teach proper body mechanics to prevent further injury rather than focus on joint protection techniques, which is usually taught to someone who has joint pain caused by arthritis. See reference: Pedretti (ed): Burt, C, and Smith, P: Work hardening.

60. (A) Sequencing of picture symbols. A person would need to use picture symbols to indicate a two or more part thought or sequence of activities. For example, pointing to pictures of a shoe and a closet would indicate the place to find a shoe in response to a question from someone. Understanding letters or words (answers B and C) and then sequencing them (answer D) are significantly higher level skills than recognizing and sequencing pictures. See reference: Church and Glennen: Glennen, S: Augmentative and alternative communication

61. (D) A frame of reference. A frame of reference (answer D) is the concept on which a program of treatment is based and directs what methods or techniques are used in treatment by a therapist. A treatment technique (answer A) is based on the frame of reference or treatment approach and is a specialized activity or method used to improve a person's performance. An exercise (answer B) is an activity to improve the mind or body and is a generic term to describe an activity without referring to the treatment approach. A treatment plan (answer C) includes the specific techniques, methods, or approaches used to reach a goal for a person who is receiving treatment. See reference: Pedretti: Occupational performance: A model for practice in physical dysfunction.

62. (B) Sip and puff switch. A sip and puff switch (answer B) is operated by breath control and would be unaffected by random movements of the extremities. An infrared switch (answer A) sends an infrared beam from the switch to some surface that would reflect the light back to the switch. When the beam is broken, the switch would be activated. The switch may be activated by an eye blink or finger twitch. Random movements of the extremities may misalign the person's head or body causing false activation. A p-switch is a piezoelectric sensor that is activated by a muscle tensing and being relayed to the switch. A rocking lever switch activates a device when one side is pushed off the switch and turns the device off when the other side of the switch is pushed. An infrared switch, a p-switch, and a rocking lever switch could all be activated by random movements of the extremities moving or pushing the rest of the body out of alignment. See reference: Church and Glennen: Adaptive toys and environmental controls.

63. (D) The therapist has the man trace letters through a pan of rice with his fingers. This method involves a larger input of sensory information to the brain by performing a gross movement in a more stimulating environment. A verbal description of how to make a letter (answer

A), watch his grip (answer B), or perform strengthening exercises (answer C) would not give the man proprioceptive feedback on his letter formation through tactile input. See reference: Fisher, Murray, and Bundy: Cermak, S: Somatodyspraxia.

64. (A) Terminal behavior. The terminal behavior is the behavior or performance that is expected to be demonstrated by the patient. Answer B, the condition, is the circumstances under which performance of the patient will be evaluated. Answer C, the criteria, is the degree of competence of a patient's performance, which is stated in specific, measurable terms. Answer D, the plan, is the method or approach used to achieve a treatment objective as a proposal of treatment. See reference: Pedretti: Treatment planning.

65. (C) Moderate assistance of one person. The criteria is the degree of competence by which performance is specifically measured, which would be moderate (50%) assistance of one person. Answer A describes the conditions or circumstances under which the evaluation of the objective will occur by using a reacher, a long shoe horn, and a sock aid. Answer B, the individual, is the person who will demonstrate the change. Answer D, dress himself, is the terminal behavior or performance to be demonstrated, which will result in the treatment objective. See reference: Pedretti: Treatment planning.

66. (C) Inferior to the anterior superior iliac spine. A seat belt placed across the lap inferior to the anterior superior iliac spine prevents the hips from being extended into a posterior pelvic tilt. If the seat belt is placed at an angle inferior to the ischial tuberosity (answer A), it would go across the thighs and allow a posterior pelvic tilt. The belt placed superior to the iliac crest or the posterior superior iliac spine (answers B and D, respectively) would be too high, allowing hip extension with posterior pelvic tilt to occur below the seat belt. See reference: Rothstein, Serge, and Wolf: Harrymann, S, and Warren, L: Positioning and power mobility.

67. (D) An arm trough. An arm trough that slides onto the wheelchair armrest would provide a stable surface, which would keep the man's arm supported without the arm or trough sliding off from the pressure applied when he leans to the left. Also, the arm trough approximates the humeral head into the glenoid fossa at a more natural angle. If the man has edema in his hand, a foam wedge may be placed in the trough to elevate his hand and a foam strap used to keep the wedge and arm in place. A half lap tray (answer A) provides support, but the arm or lap tray could be pushed off by the weight bearing arm on the edges of the half lap tray when the man leans to the left side. The wheelchair armrest (answer B) would provide only a temporary means of support, because the man's arm would only remain in place until he shifted his weight causing the arm to fall off the armrest. Answer C, an arm sling, would provide support for the arm; however, this positioning immobilizes the arm in adduction and internal rotation. The sling provides support for the shoulder when walking; however, it should not be used when the man is sitting to allow a more functional position of the arm when possible. See reference: Trombly (ed): Linden, C, and Trombly, C: Orthoses.

68. (C) A lateral trunk support. A lateral trunk support, in the frontal plane, provides stabilization at the side of the man to maintain correct alignment of the pelvis and trunk in the chair, against asymmetric muscle tone. This also prevents improper loading onto the unstable shoulder joint through the upper extremity support. Answer A, a reclining wheelchair, will shift the man's weight to the posterior, but will not prevent the lateral shift of the trunk. An arm trough (answer B) may help maintain a more centered position of the trunk, but the weight to the affected extremity would be extremely unstable, causing improper alignment of the shoulder and could result in shoulder pain. A lateral pelvic support (answer D) provides stabilization of the pelvis to prevent it from shifting sideways, but this support is too low to prevent the trunk from moving laterally. See reference: Rothstein, Serge, and Wolf: Harrymann, S, and Warren, L: Positioning and power mobility.

69. (C) A toothpaste container with a flip-open cap. A person who frequently drops small items would be able to manage a toothpaste cap much more easily when it flips open, answer C, than a cap that must be removed completely from the tube. Also, flip-open toothpaste caps are available in a larger diameter, which would make them easy to manage. A shirt with contrasting buttons, answer A, would be easier to fasten for someone with visual or perceptual impairments, but not for someone who drops small things. A spray deodorant, answer B, would have a small button to push, which would be difficult for someone with incoordination to operate. Pants with a drawstring waist, answer D, would be difficult to tighten or tie with someone who has incoordination. See reference: Pedretti (ed): Foti, D, and Pedretti, L: Activities of daily living.

70. (B) Fold laundry and place in a basket. A prevocational activity is an activity when performed by a person that could lead to the evaluation or training of work related skills. A cashier would be standing for much of the job, removing clothing from hangers, folding the clothing to place in a bag, and then running the price tags through the scanner before finally totaling them on the cash register and making change. Activities performed while sitting, such as making a grocery list, answer A, or adding a column of numbers by hand, answer D, would not be activities related to her present employment. Washing dishes while standing, answer C, incorporates the standing aspect of her job; however, washing dishes would not be related to it. The activity that incorporates the most components of her job is folding laundry and placing in a basket while standing. See reference: Pedretti (ed): Foti, D, and Pedretti, L: Activities of daily living.

71. (C) Is performed in a comfortable position. An activity is performed for a greater length of time and more effectively when the person is able to perform the activity in a comfortable position. If the activity is adapted in a complicated manner, answer A, is monotonous, answer D, or needs frequent adjustment by the occupational therapist, answer B, then the activity will appeal to the person for a shorter length of time and cause frustration sooner to the person and the therapist. See reference: Pedretti (ed): Pedretti, L, and Wade, I: Therapeutic modalities.

72. (D) Batting a balloon. An activity such as batting a balloon may be graded for improving a strength by adding resistance to the arm in the form of weights, and endurance may be improved by adding more repetitions of the movement. Passive range of motion, answer A, and Codman's exercises, answer B, are both using passive movements of the upper extremities. A person who pops a balloon, answer C, would be able to increase the resistance needed for upper extremity performance by adding weight to the arms or using a balloon with thicker rubber. However, there would not be an appropriate method to increase the number of repetitions, since the repeated noise would be annoying. See reference: Pedretti (ed): Pedretti, L, and Wade, I: Therapeutic modalities.

73. (B) Physician's written consent and medical precautions. No part of the work hardening evaluation or treatment program may begin without a physician's written consent and medical precautions for the patient, because the patient's physical abilities and tolerances are analyzed through the program. Answers A and D are incorrect, since information regarding patient's work history and job site may be obtained after the program has been initiated. Answer C is incorrect, because insurance information is obtained by the business office when the referral is made and the evaluation is scheduled. This information is passed on to the therapist as necessary. See reference: Pedretti (ed): Burt, C, and Smith, P: Work hardening.

74. (B) 118 degrees F to 126 degrees F. At 118 degrees F to 126 degrees F (47.8 degrees C to 52.2 degrees C) the paraffin stays melted without forming a film on the surface, but it is not too hot to burn the skin. A temperature of 108 degrees F to 116 degrees F (answer A) would be comfortable to a person's skin, however, a film of cooling paraffin would form on the top and interfere with the proper coating of the hand. Temperatures of 128 degrees F to 136 degrees F (answer C) and 138 degrees F to 146 degrees F (answer D) would be too hot for the skin to tolerate comfortably and may cause a burn to sensitive skin. This modality is commonly used in the treatment of arthritis. See reference: Rothstein, Serge, and Wolf: Modalities.

75. (A) Isometric exercises. Isometric exercises involve contracting the muscles without joint movement or a change in muscle length (answer A). Isotonic exercises (answer B) shorten the muscle length with joint movement occurring. The progressive resistive exercises in answer C are a type of isotonic exercise that use an increase in weight during consecutive exercise repetitions. A person who has a cast obstructing movement would be unable to perform isotonic exercises. Passive exercises (answer D) are performed by an outside force to the arm with no muscle contraction, with joint motion occurring. Passive exercises could not be performed to a casted joint.

See reference: Pedretti (ed): Pedretti, L, and Wade, I: Therapeutic modalities.

76. (D) Independently without using equipment. A person with a spinal cord injury at the C8 level would have full upper extremity usage, and would be able to perform self feeding independently without using equipment. A person with an injury at C1, C2, or C3 levels would have no upper extremity movement and would not be able to perform self feeding at all (answer A). An injury at C4 or C5 levels would allow scapular elevation, and would allow the person to self feed using a mobile arm support independently (answer B). At the C6 and C7 levels, and injury would allow enough upper extremity function to use a universal cuff independently, (answer C). See reference: Trombly (ed): Hollar, L: Spinal cord injury.

77. (D) Passively by active motion of the body. Codeman exercises are completed with the body actively causing the dependent or passive arm to swing. Active movement, answers A and B, should not occur because this would elicit active cocontraction of the shoulder muscles. Irritation of the rotator cuff muscles would result in active movement, potentially causing an adhesion reaction at the joint. Answer C is incorrect in that passive movement of the shoulder would not exert enough force on the passive arm to counteract the adhesions. See reference: Cailliet: Tissue sites and mechanisms or shoulder girdle pain. In *Shoulder Pain.*

78. (D) In the upper cabinet to the left side. This pattern of movement promotes the greatest degree of weight shift to the affected side. Stretching in a diagonal to the upper left would also cause more shift in weight. Putting groceries on the counter directly in front of the person, answer A, or in the upper cabinet to the right side, answer C, would not cause enough weight to be shifted to the affected side and would even shift weight away from that side. When placing groceries on the counter to the left side, answer B, minimal weight shift occurs. See reference: Trombly (ed): Myers, B: Proprioceptive neuromuscular facilitation (PNF) approach.

79. (A) Bilateral reciprocal. A bilateral reciprocal pattern describes movement of the upper extremities in opposite directions at the same time. The movement of extension at the elbow and shoulder flexion would cause the other upper extremity to move in shoulder abduction and elbow extension, but in the opposite direction to balance the action, for example, placing an item on a high shelf or crawling. An ipsilateral pattern, answer B, describes movement of the upper and lower extremities on the same side moving in the same direction at the same time. A bilateral symmetric pattern, answer C, would be both of either the upper or lower extremities performing like movements at the same time, such as lifting a basket or hoping. A bilateral asymmetric pattern, answer D, would be both upper or lower extremities moving up or down, however both would be moving together right or left on the side of the body. An example is swinging a golf club or side sitting. See reference: Trombly (ed): Myers, B: Proprioceptive neuromuscular facilitation (PNF) approach.

80. (B) Medline. The computer access to a catalogue of information on dynamic splints is Medline, which is associated with The *Index Medicus*. The *Index Medicus*, answer A, is a book cataloguing articles found in many major medical health related journals in the world. The *American Journal of Occupational Therapy*, answer C, would provide only information about articles that have been published within the journal. Dissertation Abstracts, answer D, lists all currently published dissertations and is not part of a computer database. See reference: Bailey: Reviewing the literature.

81. (C) Biomechanic. The biomechanic approach is a treatment approach used when a person has a deficit in strength, endurance, or range of motion, but has voluntary muscle control during performance of activities. The biomechanic approach would focus on decreasing the deficit area to improve the person's performance of daily activities. The neurophysiologic approach, answer A, emphasizes an understanding of the nervous system in a person with brain damage and in how to elicit a desired response from that person. The neurodevelopmental approach, answer B, also uses an understanding of the nervous system, but uses this knowledge to elicit a response in a developmental sequence. The rehabilitative approach, answer D, teaches a person how to compensate for a deficit on either a temporary or permanent basis. See reference: Trombly (ed): Zemke: Remediating biomechanical and physiological impairments of motor performance.

82. (A) Administrative functions. The manager of the occupational therapy department uses the computer to compile information and reports as the primary administrative function. Most departments do not have the software available to use for treatment planning, answer B, patient evaluation functions, answer C, or patient and family education activities, answer D. The second most common area computers are used for would be cognitive rehabilitation because of their versatility in programming and ability to grade the activity. There are also few software programs available that offer treatment activities, patient evaluation formats, or patient and family education activities and the expense of software programs are a deciding factor when budgeting for a department. See reference: Cromwell (ed): Smith, R: Computers and the occupational therapy administrator.

83. (B) Second and third CMC joints. The second and third carpometacarpal joints act as a fixed axis based on the trapezoid and capitate bones, and are held together at the head by the transverse intermetacarpal ligament. The first CMC joint rotates to allow the thumb to form one side of the palmar arch by rotating against the second CMC joint, answer A. The fourth CMC joint rotates on the third, answer C, and the fifth CMC joint rotates from the fourth CMC joint, answer D. See reference: Norkin and Levangie: The wrist and hand complex.

84. (C) Lordosis and kyphosis. Lordosis is a result of excessive anterior pelvic tilt, which will also increase kyphosis of the thoracic spine to compensate for the increased lumbar curve. Scoliosis, in answers A and B, is a result of a lateral curve of the vertebral column and is unaffected by anterior pelvic tilt. Lordosis only, answer D, would result if an individual had increased muscle tone to the spinal extensors, which is not the result of normal muscle tone. See reference: Norkin and Levangie: The vertebral column.

85. (D) Cervical, thoracic, lumbar, sacral. The cervical and lumbar curves have developed from extending the head in prone and from standing. The curves in the thoracic and sacral areas developed to compensate for the curves developed in the cervical and lumbar vertebral areas. Answers A, B, and C do not list all of the curves in the spine of an adult. See reference: Cailliet: Functional anatomy. In *Shoulder Pain*.

86. (C) The placement of an object between the fingers and the thumb. A static grip of the hand, answer A, and the stabilization of an object between the fingers and the palm, answer B, are components of a power grip, answer D. Precision handling and a power grip are two types of prehension patterns. Precision handling involves the placement of an object between the fingers or the fingers and thumb for a dynamic manipulation of the object. See reference: Norkin and Levangie: The wrist and hand complex.

87. (C) Code of ethics. These are the moral guidelines that are used by a professional group to direct their behavior. Policies and procedures, answer A, are the guidelines set by the facility for how an activity or task is to be performed when working for the facility. Regulations, answer B, are determined by the federal or state government to define the rules for conduct of a professional group. Protocols, answer D, are the standard approaches to a problem that a professional may use in practice. See reference: O'Sullivan and Schmitz: Davis, C: Influence of values on patient care: Foundation for decision making.

88. (B) The man's written consent to take the photograph. A photograph of a person who is being treated at a health care facility would release privileged information and would violate his confidentiality just as much as releasing his name or diagnosis, answers A and D, respectively. No information about a person may be released without a written consent. Written consent is necessary to photograph a therapist, answer C, however it is not necessary to obtain permission of the department head to use a photograph to promote a positive image for the facility. See reference: Bailey: Writing and publishing.

89. (B) Reposition the person in the wheelchair to allow an optimal range of motion. When a person in a wheelchair who uses an augmentative communication device suddenly begins making errors, it is necessary to first check the positioning of the person. Improper positioning could result in the wheelchair interfering with access or with the range of motion when using the communication device. A person may be referred to a physician for a physical (answer A), however, it is best for the therapist to problem solve and seek a solution to the problem if the person's medical status remains unchanged. The person's communication abilities would not be reassessed (answer C) until the person has been optimally positioned in the wheelchair. A communication device would only need to be replaced (answer D) if there was a mechanical problem within the system causing the errors that could not be fixed. See reference: Church and Glennen: Harryman, S, and Warren, L: Positioning and power mobility.

90. (B) Increase the number of repetitions to 40. The woman's endurance is improved by increasing the number of repetitions, so the muscle has to work over a longer period of time. The angle of the board changing to 15 degrees, answer A, or pushing down the incline board, answer C, decreases the difficulty of the activity and does not lengthen the period of time needed to improve endurance by proving more repetitions. The arm could be strengthened by adding 1 pound of weight to each arm, answer D, but that will not increase the repetitions needed to improve endurance. See reference: Pedretti (ed): Pedretti, L, and Wade, I: Therapeutic modalities

91. (C) Interrater reliability. The student was checking interrater reliability. Interrater reliability is how similarly two people perceive a subject's performance or a characteristic. Split-half reliability, answer A, is how closely two parts of an instrument or other form of measurement will measure the same thing. Test-retest reliability, answer B, is how reliable a test is over a period of time. The test would be given, and after a period of time has passed, the test is repeated to compare the scores. Intrarater reliability, answer D, is the consistency of a person with administering the same test after an interval of time to the same subject or characteristic. See reference: Bailey: Collecting and analyzing qualitative data.

92. (D) A rotator cuff tear. The test for a rotator cuff tear is to place the arm in 90 degrees of shoulder abduction and ask the person to maintain this position against gravity. The arm will begin to drop slowly without pressure. With pressure, the arm will drop immediately. Carpal tunnel syndrome, answer A, would be evidenced by wrist pain and tingling with impaired hand function. If the woman had deltoid weakness, answer B, she would be able to maintain shoulder abduction without pain. Also a rotator cuff tear is differentiated by weak resistance to external rotation, which the deltoid muscle would be unable to perform. A dislocated clavicle, answer C, usually occurs at the acromioclavicular joint, with pain and subluxation in that area with pain during shoulder abduction and overhead elevation. See reference: Cailliet: Rotator cuff tear: Partial and complete. In *Shoulder Pain.*

93. (B) A key guard. A key guard is a hardware device that covers the keys and provides a guide for a finger or stick without punching extra keys. A moisture guard, answer A, is a flexible plastic cover that protects the keys from any drool, moisture, or dirt that could be spilled or settle onto the keyboard. An auto-repeat defeat mechanism, answer C, stops any repetition of letters or numbers when the keys are pressed too long or accidently. One-finger access software, answer D, allows an automatic lock of keys, such as shift or enter, to allow someone

using one finger or a stick to type capital letters or any other commands that would require multiple keys to be pressed. See reference: Church and Glennen: Church, G: Adaptive access for microcomputers.

94. (C) Swing away leg rests, removable arm rests. After swinging away the leg rests and removing the armrests, the individual can transfer without being blocked by the wheelchair. These allow removal from the patient's way when performing a sliding board transfer. Answers A and B are incorrect, because they would not facilitate a sliding board transfer. Answer D is incorrect because a removable armrest may make transfers easier, but elevating leg rest would not. A leg rest would need to be detachable or swing away in order for it to be moved out of the way. See reference: Pedretti (ed): Adler, C, and Tipton-Burton, M: Wheelchairs assessment and transfers.

95. (D) 82 cm. A minimum accessible width would be 82 cm or 32 inches to allow a wheelchair to pass through easily. All the other widths, answers A, B, and C, respectively, would be too narrow to allow a wheelchair to pass through a door into the next room. Answer A, 46 cm, would be too narrow to allow a standard walker entry easily even if the person side stepped. See reference: Rothstein, Serge, and Wolf: Wheelchairs and standards for access.

96. (C) The mother on the first floor and the grandmother in the basement. A master bedroom should be placed on the first floor to allow easy access for the woman with as few steps as possible. The grandmother would also want to use as few steps as possible, but there would not be room for a grandmother's suite on the first floor since the kitchen, dining area, living room, and master bedroom with bath would be located on that floor. The most available area with the least steps would be in the basement for the grandmother's suite. This would allow her access to the basement from the exterior basement door (no steps) or the interior door (one flight of steps). This would also place her living quarters close to the recreation area where her grandsons would be able to play after school. Placing the mother and grandmother on the second floor, answer A, would cause too many trips for them to reach the main living areas on the first floor. Placing the mother on the first floor and the grandmother on the second, answer B, eliminates steps for the mother, but not the grandmother. The mother and grandmother in the basement, answer D, would place them close to the boys play area, but would involve steps for the mother. See reference: O'Sullivan and Schmitz: Schmitz, T: Environmental assessment.

97. (D) 5 feet by 5 feet. An outward opening door needs a space of 5 feet by 5 feet to allow for the wheelchair to be maneuvered around the door. A standard wheelchair requires 5 feet of turning space for a 180 or 360 degree turn. An area that is 3 by 5 feet, answer A, 4 feet by 4 feet, answer B, or 4.5 feet by 3 feet, answer C, would not provide enough space to allow the wheelchair to be turned. See reference: Rothstein, Serge, and Wolf: Wheelchairs and standards for access.

98. (B) 33 to 36 inches. This is the proper height for grab bars to allow for the upper extremities to lift the body with enough clearance to transfer onto the toilet seat. A height of 28 to 31 inches, answer A, would be too low to allow the body to clear the toilet seat when the arms are straightened. A height of 38 to 41 inches or 43 inches to 46 inches, answers C and D, would be too high to effectively push down with the arms to lift the body onto the toilet seat. See reference: O'Sullivan and Schmitz: Schmitz, T: Environmental assessment.

99. (C) Changes necessary for furniture arrangement. It is necessary to document how furniture should be arranged in order to give the individual greatest accessibility. A report will supply the necessary information to the other team members, the family, or the therapists who will treat the woman as an outpatient or in the home. The outpatient therapy recommendations, answer A, and the status of the woman at the time of discharge, answer B, would be information needed in the discharge summary. The appropriate method of transportation, answer D, would be determined by the woman's physical abilities and by what is available to the family, not by the home visit. See reference: O'Sullivan and Schmitz: Schmitz, T: Environmental assessment.

100. (A) Toilet paper dispenser should not be used as a grab bar. Toilet paper dispensers are not installed to bear the weight of a person. Answer C is incorrect because carpeting should be short pile for pushing a wheelchair because the deeper the pile, the harder it is to push a wheelchair. Answer D is incorrect because the stove controls should be placed in front to allow easy accessibility. Answer B, placing the mirror with the bottom 48 inches from the floor, would be above eye level for a person in a wheelchair. In order to use the mirror, it would need to be tilted at the top downward for better visibility. See reference: Palmer and Toms: Wheelchairs, assistive devices, and home modifications.

101. (B) Add the two new admissions and then divide the members into two groups of four. Maintaining groups of four to six clients enables the therapist to adequately observe the interpersonal relations of the members. Utilizing interviews and groups with three or fewer members will provide dyadic interaction information but not their group relations. Asking those originally asked to wait is counter therapeutic to those individuals. Both answers C and D do not allow the therapist to assess group interpersonal skills. See reference: Mosey: Activity-based groups.

102. (B) All group members construct one tower that incorporates all the pieces provided in a set of constructional materials (e.g., Legos, Tinkertoys, or Erector set). Activities used in evaluation groups should require group collaboration that can be done in approximately 45 minutes and emphasize process rather than end product. The collage and crafts are individual and do not demand group interaction. Pizza for lunch is an end product that serves the group as a whole and usually takes longer than 45 minutes. The pizza activity and format is typically not an evaluation group but is better suited as a task-oriented group activity where self awareness and self understanding are primary goals. See reference: Mosey: Activity-based groups.

103. (C) The individual's level of psychosocial and occupational limitations. Global Assessment of Functioning, Axis V, is an overall rating of an individual's psychosocial and occupational functioning. Answer A describes the emphasis of the Axis V diagnosis, answer B describes the Axis III diagnosis, and answer D describes the Axis II diagnosis. See reference: Bonder: Psychiatric diagnosis and the classification system.

104. (A) Communication. When using projective approaches such as drawing the self, the therapist can make interpretations about an individual based on how the drawing is organized. Small, lightly drawn lines can indicate a lack of confidence or comfort with the body part or its function. Drawing ability or cognitive ability are not assessed with projective methods. Bruce and Borg: Appendix F: Person Drawings.

105. (D) Developmental or acquisitional frames of reference. The developmental and acquisitional frames of reference both address interactions within group and are consistent with activity-based evaluation groups. The Model of Human Occupation and sensory integration frames of reference do not describe the use of groups in the evaluation process but do use groups within treatment. See reference: Mosey: Developmental frames of reference; Acquisitional frames of reference.

106. (D) During one to two conversations with female group members, the client will make eye contact for 8 to 10 second periods two times in each half-hour socialization group. The short term goal that describes appropriate verbal and nonverbal interactions with female peers is the best answer. Attempting to develop skills with staff can pose some confusing boundary and ethical questions in a long-term goal related to developing future personal relations. The goals of finding employment and housing are long-term goals and are not directly linked to the area of personal relationships. Identifying disability-related interferences is not related to the client's long-term goal. See reference: Early: Understanding psychiatric diagnosis.

107. (C) Avoid having at-risk individuals in close proximity to others to reduce physical contact with others. Avoiding close proximity situations is the recommended environmental modification for sexually acting out behaviors. Advising the client of your expectations is an appropriate use of self in such situations. Standing to the side is a recommended environmental modification for highly aggressive and hostile behavior risks. Providing real life activities in a stimulating environment has been found to be helpful with reducing some delusions. See reference: Early: Safety techniques.

108. (A) Teach the problem-solving process to the client for generalization to future situations. Teaching skills would be appropriate for clients who previously had no problem-solving skills. This is known as habilitation approaches. Rehabilitation is the identification and restoration of previous abilities. Maintenance approaches generally focus on changing the environment versus changing existent abilities. Using the ACL is an evaluation and not an intervention approach. See reference: Hopkins and Smith (eds): Simon, CJ, and Daub, MM: Human development across the life span.

109. (B) Comprehensive Occupational Therapy Evaluation Scale (COTE). The recording of a series of task and interpersonal behaviors is best done with the COTE scale. The COTE scale can be used to translate observations into numbers that indicate ranges of task behaviors. Approximately 15 sessions can be recorded on one COTE scale report form. The RTI is an evaluation of ADL's and the NPI is an evaluation of leisure interests. They are used primarily as evaluation instruments. SOAP notes record progress but are not specifically designed to address only task and interpersonal behaviors. See reference: Hopkins and Smith (eds): Smith, HD: Assessment and evaluation—An overview.

110. (A) Remotivation. Remotivation approaches are used to encourage the expression of thoughts and feelings related to intact long-term memories. The topic should be linked to the group's past experiences and is easy to understand. Reality orientation is designed to maintain or improve awareness of time, situation and place. The compensatory cognitive approach is a category of several approaches that can be used when cognitive problems are not expected to improve. Environmental modification is one method to compensatory strategies. See reference: Early: Cognitive and sensorimotor activities.

111. (B) Client will use facial expressions and gestures that are consistent with stated emotions during assertive, passive, and aggressive role play situations. Self expression is the use of a variety of styles and skills to express thoughts, feelings, and needs. It is also the ability to vary one's expressions, thoughts, feelings, and needs. Being able to vary one's expression during three different styles of expressing feelings is an example of this. Identifying pleasurable activities is an example of interests. Recognition of one's behaviors and consequences is self-control. Identifying one's own assets and limitations is related to self-concept. See reference: Bonder: Appendix B—Uniform terminology for reporting occupational therapy services, Third edition.

112. (C) Self concept. Self concept is defined as the value of one's physical and emotional self. Stating one's strengths and limitations about one's own performance is a reflection of an individual's self concept. Values are more globally stated ideas or beliefs such as being a "perfectionist." Problem solving would involve identifying one's limitations and then identifying alternate approaches. Termination of the activity involves knowing when to stop working on the activity. See reference: Bonder: Appendix B—Uniform terminology for reporting occupational therapy services, Third edition.

113. (D) Each member will remain in the group without disrupting the work of others for 30 minutes. People who are in parallel groups do not have the ability to interact with the other group members other than some casual greetings. Therefore, appropriate expectations for parallel groups focus on remaining in the group and working alongside others. Taking leadership roles is a goal consistent with egocentric-cooperative groups. Sharing materials with some of the other group members is a project group goal. Expressing feelings within a group is consistent with a cooperative group. See reference: Mosey: Recapitulation of ontogenisis.

114. (C) Games of chance. Because winning a game of chance is based essentially on luck, many functional levels have "equal" opportunities at winning. Hobbies are not considered a category of games. Puzzles and strategy games both require specific skills to succeed. See reference: Early: Leisure skills.

115. (B) Bingo. Luck is the key element in games of chance, and bingo is a game that uses chance in calling out numbers randomly. Baseball card collecting is considered to be a hobby versus a game. Charades and balloon volleyball are strategy and skill-based games. See reference: Early: Leisure skills.

116. (C) Teach compensatory strategies and manage the environment. Interventions directed toward "improvement" are typically unrealistic in working with individuals diagnosed with organic mental disorders. These disorders are characterized by a deteriorating course. A social skills emphasis is more appropriate for individuals with schizophrenia. Habit restructuring is more appropriate for substance use disorders. Role resumption is more appropriate for mood disorders. See reference: Early: Understanding psychiatric diagnosis.

117. (A) Begin with activities that have obvious solutions and high probability of success. Beginning with activities that have obvious solutions and are successful and gradually increase in complexity is effective in developing problem solving. Sensorimotor activities in a group can facilitate self awareness. Time increases facilitate attention span improvement. Grading the number and kinds of choices is used for developing decision making. See reference: Early: Analyzing, adapting and grading activities.

118. (B) 4: Goal directed actions. Cognitive level 4 is referred to as "goal directed actions" where the stimulus for action is the desire to produce an exact match of sample. Cognitive level 3 individuals rely primarily on manual actions. Cognitive level 5 individuals can experiment or explore a variety of ways to use materials. Cognitive level 6 individuals can make their own plans for materials. See reference: Allen, Earhardt, and Blue: Allen, CK: Modes of performance within the cognitive levels.

119. (D) Remediating the cause of dysfunction. Sensory-motor methods address the underlying causes or processes of a disorder such as schizophrenia. Sensorimotor approaches are thought to impact the underactive vestibular processing in some schizophrenics. Habilitation approaches focus on building abilities that were never developed due to illness. Rehabilitation approaches emphasize the restoration of lost function. Maintenance is an approach that guards remaining abilities. See reference: Mosey: Developmental frames of reference.

120. (C) Consistent with the cognitive behavioral views of anger intervention.   A model of anger intervention for occupational therapy based on the cognitive behavioral approach was described in the OT literature in 1988. The use of activities to divert attention from thoughts that were escalating the expression of anger were recommended. This view of activities is quite different than object relations views about "expressing" anger (see answers A and D). The cognitive disabilities view does not directly address anger interventions and is not considered to be a cognitive-behavioral frame of reference. See reference: Taylor: Anger intervention.

121. (A) Procedural.   Procedural reasoning involves thinking about a disability and deciding about treatment activities or procedures to use. Interactive reasoning occurs in face to face collaborative problem solving. Conditional and narrative reasoning approaches are used by experienced therapists in seeing the whole person and seeing future outcomes from the client's perspective. See reference: Hopkins and Smith (eds): Fleming, MH: Aspects of clinical reasoning in occupational therapy.

122. (D) Utilize a tool storage area that can be locked and that uses tool shadows or outlines. Organizing the tool cabinet with shadows or outlines to indicate where tools are to be kept is a very effective method to easily and accurately identify missing items. This method also facilitates clients being responsible for returning tools at the end of groups. Keeping track of keys is an overall safety strategy that is not specific to tools. Advance preparation is a strategy to reduce the therapists distractions during groups. Many clients treated for psychosocial problems would be excluded from OT treatment if they had to wait until all of their behavioral risks are being managed. Clients with severe suicidal or impulsive behaviors should rarely be involved with activities requiring tools that have harm potential. See reference: Early: Safety techniques.

123. (A) Use disposable cotton swabs and have clients bring their own cosmetics.   Using disposable cotton swabs and having clients use their own cosmetics would be effective in reducing the risk of infection. Combing someone's hair does not usually involve risks related to blood or bodily fluids. Washing equipment that is used near eyes and mouths by several individuals is inadequate. Avoiding glass containers is a safety precaution that is related to self harm and not universal precautions. See reference: Hopkins and Smith (eds): Pizzi, M: HIV infection and AIDS.

124. (D) Decoupage wood key fob.   A wood key fob with a decoupage finish is the safest craft choice as this is

free of sharp, toxic, and cordlike materials. Finished craft projects that contain parts or pieces that can be used as sharp and harmful objects and pieces that can be used in hanging should be avoided. Examples of such objects are ceramic objects that can be shattered and rope or cordlike lacing materials. See reference: Early: Safety techniques.

125. (D) Leather dyes.   Leather dyes are toxic when swallowed or ingested. The precaution for mirrors is related to sharp edges when shattered. White glue is nontoxic. The precaution with permanent magic markers is inhaling fumes with extended use. See reference: Early: Safety techniques.

126. (B) Develop the client's awareness of the link between anger and stress.   Treatment begins with having the client become aware of the link between anger and stress. Documentation of the client's responses is part of the assessment and reassessment phase. Stress management skills and alternate use of activities would follow the client's increased awareness between stress and anger. See reference: Taylor: Anger intervention.

127. (B) "The program will help you to learn about the skills you have that are needed on most jobs and about your potential for work."   Prevocational evaluation programs are organized to assess work skills that the client has and to identify his or her potential for work. Vocational evaluation programs identify the actual interests and skills for specific types of work, such as assembly line work. Work role maintenance programs are for individuals who are employed but their involvement in treatment has temporarily disrupted their carrying out their work responsibilities. Developing job search skills is for clients who have job skills but who have difficulty finding employment. See reference: Early: Treatment settings.

128. (A) Punctuality, accepting responsibility for oneself, accepting directions from a supervisor, and appropriately interacting with peer coworkers. Psychosocial components include time management, social conduct, and self-control. Punctuality, accepting responsibility, and accepting feedback are examples of prevocational skills within these psychosocial performance components and are important prevocational skills. Memory, decision making, and sequencing are considered to be cognitive components. Standing tolerance, endurance, and eye-hand coordination are categorized as sensory motor components. Grooming and adhering to safety precautions are work performance areas and not psychosocial performance components. See reference: Bonder: Appendix B—Uniform terminology for reporting occupational therapy services.

129. (C) "The client demonstrated the ability to make a decision when she selected one of the six craft designs presented."   The notation of the client's response to treatment that contains the most objective information is C. The notations that address the client's "wanting" and "hostility" are interpretations of behavior versus directly observable responses. The use of the words "appropriate" and "most" are vague and general. See reference: Early: Medical records and documentation.

130. (C) Discharge summary. The discharge summary is documentation that includes a summary of the client's entire treatment and the goals achieved and compares the initial and discharge status. Initial notes record the therapist's receipt and responses to the referral for service. Reassessments contain recommendations for continued OT treatment and specific evaluation results. Treatment plans contain measurable goals, treatment pro- cedures, and expected attainment dates. See reference: Hopkins and Smith (eds): Appendix E—Guidelines for occupational therapy documentation.

131. (C) Section III. Follow-up plans state the scheduled and specific plans upon discontinuation of services. Although Section IV contains some of this information, it focuses on referral information. Sections I and II contain the summary of treatment sessions and the goals achieved. See reference: Hopkins and Smith (eds): Appendix E—Guidelines for occupational therapy documentation.

132. (C) Section III. Home programs are the written programs that the client will follow after discharge. Mental health approaches frequently incorporate journals as an effective way of following through with "exercises" or methods that were introduced in the hospital. See reference: Hopkins and Smith (eds): Appendix E—Guidelines for occupational therapy documentation.

133. (A) Reporting the number of treatments in Section I. According to the 1991 Role Delineations for OTRs and COTAs can record factual information at the time of discharge. Making referrals to outside agencies, independently discontinuing treatment services, and independently making follow up plans are not within the entry level COTAs responsibilities. See reference: Hopkins and Smith (eds): Appendix E—Guidelines for occupational therapy documentation.

134. (C) Phobias. Phobias are defined as panic attacks associated with fears of specific objects. Hypochondriasis is the preoccupation with having a serious disease. Agoraphobia is the fear of places. Obsessions are intrusive thoughts versus about actions. See reference: Bonder: Anxiety disorders.

135. (C) Axis IV. Axis IV describes psychosocial and environmental problems. Axis II contains personality or developmental disorder information. Axis III describes the coexisting medical conditions. Axis V describes the highest and current levels of functioning within the past year. See reference: Bonder: Psychiatric diagnosis and the classification system.

136. (C) Obsessions. Compulsions are the behavior routines that are engaged in to try and decrease the obsession. Obsessions are the intrusive thoughts that the individual experiences. Delusions are fixed systems of belief versus more narrowly focused obsessions. Although washing one's hands is an ADL task, the ritualistic performance implies a problematic aspect to this activity. See reference: Bonder: Anxiety disorders.

137. (D) Men over the age of 80. The highest rate of completed suicide is for men who are 80 years old or older. Women over the age of 65 have a lower incidence of suicide than when they are 40 to 60 years old. Individuals under age 35 are more likely to attempt than commit suicide. See reference: Bruce and Borg: The suicidal patient.

138. (A) Adjustment disorders. Adjustment disorders can be directly related to a stressful event in an individual's life. Posttraumatic disorders also follow stressful events; however, the events are usually traumas beyond most people's experiences (i.e., wars and violent crimes). The onset of cyclothymia is generally not linked to the stressor of severe childhood abuse. Dissociative identity disorders may be linked to severe, repeated abuse in childhood. See reference: Bonder: Other disorders.

139. (B) Emotional lability. Emotional lability is the rapid shift of moods. Emotional lability may be one of the symptoms observed with individuals experiencing mania. Paranoia describes enduring beliefs about being harmed. Denial is not acknowledging the presence of information. See reference: Bonder: Mood disorders.

140. (B) "Client will initiate one request to one other group member for sharing or using group materials within a 1-week period." Reducing the number of requests and the variety or number of individuals the client is expected to interact with is the best way to simplify the initial goal. Extending the amount of time to accomplish the goal does not make the goal easier to achieve. Increasing the number of individuals, and subsequently the number of requests, to five makes the goal more difficult to achieve. Changing interactions to the group leader moves the goal away from the original problem area of "peer" social conversation to authority conversations. See reference: Early: Treatment planning.

141. (B) Activity adaptation. Modifying the directions that are provided is one way to adapt activities. Activity adaptions enable the individual to become more functional in his or her task performance. Activity analysis is the process of identifying aspects, steps, and materials used in performing an activity. Activity sequencing is one method of grading activities. Conditional reasoning is the problem-solving process that therapists use in thinking about a client's treatment. See reference: Early: Analyzing, adapting, and grading activities.

142. (D) Recovery. Tangential (topic jumping) speech, elated mood, and some hyperactivity are known as prodromal of first stages of manic depressive illness. People in recovery are moving back through the stages to the first stages of the disease. Regression and decompensation are both processes of decline. Progression is a general term of improvement, but is not specific enough to describe this client's changes. See reference: Bonder: Mood disorders.

143. (C) Discharge planning group. Discharge planning group is recommended because this client's progress is toward recovery that has been fairly steady and quick. Addressing issues relative to recurrence prevention are particularly important with individuals with a bipolar disorder. Although assertiveness group could be generally helpful, there is no information that indicates Mr. Brown is having difficulty with passive or aggressive communication styles. Exercise group is not considered to be a thematic group. See reference: Bonder: Mood disorders.

144. (D) Distractibility. Distractibility involves losing one's focus because of other stimulus. Memory problems have to do with remembering what to do. Problems with spatial operations are generally observed when individuals attempt to fit objects into specific spaces. To observe generalization, the client would demonstrate using existing knowledge in a new situation. See reference: Bonder: Appendix B—Uniform terminology for reporting occupational therapy services.

145. (A) Least restrictive environment. Mental health services are organized along a continuum of care that generally varies according to degrees of restrictiveness involved in providing services. Since 1970 (Wyatt v. Stickney), all psychiatric patients in the United States have rights that protect clients from receiving care that is more restrictive than their condition warrants. Therapists should be aware of the restrictiveness of other treatment environments when planning discharge. Professional licensure laws protect consumers but do not define treatment settings. PL94–142 enabled handicapped children to receive educational services. The Tarasoff Decision (1966) describes rules for sharing confidential material during threats of harm. See reference: Hopkins and Smith (eds): Gibson, D: Trends affecting occupational therapy.

146. (C) Teach problem solving and goal setting. Because each group member's situation differs, problem solving and goal setting are suggested approaches for preparing clients in the transition from hospital to community. It is recommended that the client become actively involved in the goal setting processes to improve aftercare compliance. Social skills and self esteem approaches are linked to assertiveness groups. Discipline approaches are linked to parenting groups. See reference: Hughes and Mullins: Discharge preparation.

147. (D) "When I apply for jobs, what should I put down when it asks if you have been hospitalized or treated for anything in the past 6 months?" Stigma are indications that one has a history of a disorder. Generally, psychiatric treatment involves negative reactions to such a history, especially from employers. Identifying potential situations where stigma occurs and problem solving around such issues is an important part of discharge planning. The cigarette smoke and complaining relative comments are linked to assertiveness. The medication comments are linked to the client's misunderstanding of

the strategies used for dealing with side effects. See reference: Hughes and Mullins: Discharge preparation.

148. (D) "I'm concerned about John's ability to live on his own unless he is better able to structure his leisure time. Before admission, he was rarely in contact with others. Then his voices got worse." The occupational therapist emphasizes functional information. Answer D is an example of functional information of self management within the leisure performance area. Answer A is consistent with concerns of varied team members. Answer B is consistent with aftercare referral concerns of social work. Answer C reflects the medication concerns of the physician or nurse. See reference: Hopkins and Smith (eds): Gibson, K, and Richer, GZ: The therapeutic process.

149. (C) National Alliance for the Mentally Ill. This is a support group that is open to clients and families and focuses on education and support related to all mental illnesses. Al-Anon, answer A, is a support group for alcohol use among family members. Family therapy, answer B, is not a support group. Recovery, Inc., answer D, is a self-help support group for clients with mental disorders. See reference: Hopkins and Smith (eds): Richert, GZ: Program planning, development, and implementation.

150. (B) Have the client take "one white and one blue pill" with the morning and evening meals. Cognitive disabilities levels of function distinguish the types of assistance an individual needs to safely complete everyday tasks. Cognitive level 4 functioning involves having a routine goal in mind. Linking medications with meals helps the goal become routine. Answer C is consistent with cognitive 3. Answer D is consistent with cognitive level 2. See reference: Allen, Earhart, and Blue: Allen, CK, Kehrberg, K, and Burns, T: Evaluative instruments.

151. (D) "It depends. If body fluids have not come in contact with the cones, no. However, if at any time the cones came in contact with body fluids, they should be sterilized." OSHA has set out strategies to protect an individual from potential exposure to possible infection of HIV or HBV. In this example, sending the items to be sterilized would be considered a work practice control. Work practice controls are policies that require a procedure be done a certain way so that potential for exposure may be reduced. See reference: Elder: Transmission of HIV and prevention of AIDS.

152. (A) An exposure has occurred and she should use universal precautions. OSHA has identified materials that require universal precautions to be blood, semen, vaginal secretions, cerebrospinal fluid, synovial fluid, pleural fluid, any body fluid with visible blood, any unidentifiable body fluid, and saliva from dental procedures. Since the urine did have blood in it, it would be considered an exposure. Answers B and D are incorrect because they indicate that an exposure has not occurred. Answer C is incorrect because any time an exposure occurs, universal precautions must be followed. In addition, it should be noted that items OSHA has identified as not needing universal precautions are feces, nasal secretions, sputum, sweat, tears, urine, and vomitus. See reference: Elder: Transmission of HIV and prevention of AIDS.

153. (A) Provision of information and feedback to coworkers. Functional supervision occurs between peers. This type of supervision is frequently observed as fieldwork educators provide guidance and direction to therapists who are supervising students. This is also the type of feedback that may occur on self-directed work teams who coordinate services without a formal supervisor. Answer B describes formal supervision, answer C describes minimal supervision, and answer D describes general supervision. See reference: AOTA: The Occupational Therapy Roles Task Force: Occupational Therapy Roles.

154. (C) Program evaluation. Program evaluation is the compilation of the intervention results for a population of individuals. One of the most frequently used program evaluation systems is the FIM (functional independence measure). FIM scores may be compiled and compared with regional and national norms. Answer A, a process, is the manner in which services are rendered. Each process has an order in which activities occur. An example of the process of interaction between the consumer and therapist may progress from initial interview, to evaluation, to treatment, to family training, and to discharge intervention. Answer B, outcome, is the results of service intervention that an individual receives. These measures are taken at the completion of service intervention. Answer D, utilization review, reviews the care that is provided to assure that services were appropriate and not over or under utilized. Overall, utilization review analyzes the services to assure that the interventions were provided in an economical manner. See reference: Hopkins and Smith (eds): Perinchief, JM: Service management.

155. (D) Utilization review. Utilization reviews assess the care that is provided to assure that services were appropriate and not over or under utilized. Overall, utilization review analyzes the services to ensure that the interventions were provided in an economical manner. Answer A, a process, is manner in which services are rendered. Each process has an order in which activities occur. An example of the processes of interaction between the consumer and therapist may progress from initial interview, to evaluation, to treatment, to family training, and to discharge intervention. Answer B, outcome, is the results of service intervention that an individual receives. These measures are taken at the completion of service intervention. Answer C, program evaluation, is the compilation of the intervention results for a population of individuals. One of the most frequently used program evaluation systems is the FIM. FIM scores may be compiled and compared with regional and national norms. See reference: Hopkins and Smith (eds): Perinchief, JM: Service management.

156. (A) Quality improvement plan. Quality improvement programs have emerged from what was known as quality assurance programs. These programs look at the aspects of service, provision of care, identification of problems, and evaluation of the effectiveness of interventions. Quality improvement plans take this concept a step further to the con-

tinual evolution of identifying issues and working towards resolution. In these programs, once the issue is resolved, the team selects, monitors, and works toward resolution of another issue. Answer B, peer review, is the system of other service providers assessing the provision of care to assure appropriate interventions and documentation practices. Answer C, utilization review, is the process of analyzing the provision of services to promote the most economic delivery of service. Answer D, program evaluation, is a systematic collection and reporting of outcome data to document program effectiveness and cost efficiency. See reference: Hopkins and Smith (eds): Perinchief, JM: Service management.

157. (D) The standards with which outcomes are compared. Measures are the standards, which are established based on expertise and knowledge of the service intervention. Answer B, the results a program aims to achieve, are objectives. Answer C, characteristics according to severity or barriers to success, is referred to as descriptors. Answer D, the standards with which outcomes are compared, are thresholds. See reference: Hopkins and Smith (eds): Perinchief, JM: Service management.

158. (A) Indicator. An indicator is an overall aspect of care that has set criteria that are established. Answer B, a monitor, is a specific area or criteria that will be systematically checked and compliance to the established standard will be measured. Answer C, a threshold, is a numerical measure of the level at which quality services are provided. Answer D, the data source, is the area or way in which information will be gathered. See reference: Jacobs and Logigian: Quality assurance.

159. (D) The data source. The data source is the area or way in which information will be gathered. Answer A, an indicator, is an overall aspect of care that has set criteria that are established. Answer B, a monitor, is a specific area or criteria that will be systematically checked and compliance to the established standard will be measured. Answer C, a threshold, is a numerical measure of the level at which quality services are provided. See reference: Jacobs and Logigian: Quality assurance.

160. (A) Time frame. The time frame indicates the period in which the sample of subjects who will be studied are taken. Answer B, a sample size, is the number of subjects or items that will be included in a study. Answer C, the threshold, is the minimum acceptable level of performance. Answer D, the data source, is the area or way in which information will be gathered. See reference: Hopkins and Smith (eds): Service management.

161. (C) Minimal supervision. Minimal supervision occurs on an as-needed basis and is appropriate for those therapists who have attained the highest levels of clinical skills and clinical reasoning. Close supervision is daily on-site supervision and is provided to any therapist who has attained baseline competency but is developing skills in a treatment area. Routine supervision describes on-site supervision that occurs every 2 weeks and is appropriate for therapists with well developed clinical competency. General supervision involves monthly contact. This form of supervision is appropriate for those therapists who demonstrate high levels of clinical competency. All forms of supervision should also include interim forms of written or verbal communication (i.e.: phone, E-mail, written memos, etc). See reference: AOTA: Intercommission Council: Occupational therapy roles.

162. (C) The Occupational Therapy Standards of Practice. Guidelines for documentation that may be used for reimbursement, research, education, or to provide legal information may be obtained in the Occupational Therapy Standards of Practice. This document was originally written in 1978 and later revised in 1992. The Uniform Terminology, answer A, is a document that defines occupational therapy in relationship to performance areas and performance components. This document is used throughout the practice of occupational therapy so that there may be uniform use of the definitions provided. The Code of Ethics, answer B, is incorrect because it is a document that outlines the standard for the conduct expected of an occupational therapy professional. Answer D is incorrect in that the Occupational Therapy Roles define the various educational levels and skills of occupational therapy professionals. See reference: Hopkins and Smith (eds): Appendix B—Revision: Standards of practice for occupational therapy.

163. (D) Treat the patient in the afternoon and charge for the 1 hour of direct time spent with the patient. This answer is correct in that this meeting was not part of the planned intervention and had occurred spontaneously and without measurable goals. Based on the Standards of Practice, if collaboration with the individual or family was included as a part of the intervention plan, the patient could be billed for the time. See reference: Hopkins and Smith (eds): Hansen, RA: Ethics in occupational therapy.

164. (C) The TR will substitute recreational activities in the OT time but will not bill for occupational therapy services. Answers A, B, and D are incorrect because they all involve billing for occupational therapy services when actual services performed by an occupational therapist were not completed. Therefore, the only correct answer was not billing for occupational therapy. See reference: Hopkins and Smith (eds): Gibson, D, and Richert, G: Mental health: The therapeutic process.

165. (C) Interactive reasoning. This form of reasoning occurs when the patient and therapist work together in a manner that allows the therapist to better understand the patient and how he or she function within his or her environment. Answers A, B, and D are incorrect in that they do not allow for the collaboration that occurs in the discussion of the home environment. See reference: Mattingly and Fleming: Fleming, MH: The therapist with the three-track mind.

166. (D) Narrative reasoning. Narrative reasoning is a form of "story telling" in which therapists share similar experiences, which allows problem solving to occur. Procedural reasoning is the process of identifying a particular treatment or procedure that meets the need of a condition. Conditional reasoning is a form of clinical reasoning that takes into account various systems and dynamics involved

with the patient and their illness or injury. This approach is more "holistic" in that takes into account the "whole patient" as they function and interact within their environment. Interactive reasoning is a process by which the therapist and patient collaborate so that the therapist may better understand the patient's environment or situation. See reference: Mattingly and Fleming: Fleming, MH: The therapist with the three-track mind.

167. (B) Not treat the man based on his refusal and document the interaction in the chart. As stated in Principle 1 of the Code of Ethics, "the individual shall inform those people served of the nature and potential outcomes of treatment and shall respect the right of potential recipients of service to refuse treatment." Answers A and C are incorrect in that the therapist proceeded to treat the patient. Answer D is incorrect because it does not meet with Principle 3 of the Code of Ethics, "The individual shall accurately record and report information." See reference: AOTA: Commission on Standards and Ethics: Occupational Therapy Code of Ethics.

168. (C) Gain prior authorization for services from the patient's health insurance provider. The wide variety of reimbursement sources within the United States provides for high variability of what services and or equipment items are covered. The most beneficial way to ensure what the patient's financial responsibility for services will be is to contact the carrier and gain preauthorization for services. This information will provide the therapist with the frequency and duration of treatments that will be covered by the carrier. This information is then shared with the individual so that an informed decision to health care may be made. Answers A, B, and D assist in gaining reimbursement for services or equipment but are NOT fundamental actions that identify health care benefits. See reference: Hopkins and Smith (eds): Levy, LL: The health care delivery system today.

169. (B) Assess a client utilizing Allen Cognitive Level (ACL) Test. The COTA may complete structured, standardized testing as a part of the evaluation. The ACL is a standardized screening tool. Answer A is incorrect because the group is unstructured. Answer C is incorrect because goal writing requires analyzing and interpreting the assessment data, which is an activity to be completed by the occupational therapist. Answer D is incorrect because it is not appropriate for an aide to lead a group and bill for occupational therapy services. See reference: AOTA: Intercommission Council: Occupational therapy roles.

170. (D) A referral. A referral is a basic request for an individual to be assessed by an occupational therapist. A referral generally includes information such as the patient's name, age, date of birth, address, physician, and diagnosis. An individual may be referred to occupational therapy for deficits in occupational performance of work, play, and leisure skills. Answer A, a recommendation, is an advisement that an individual may benefit from a service. A plan of treatment or intervention strategy, answers B and C, respectively, are completed by the therapist following the assessment. See reference: Hopkins and Smith (eds): Spencer, EA: Preliminary concepts and planning.

171. (D) Should be able to function at any entry level or above the minimum entry level of competence. Following completion of the coursework and level II fieldwork for occupational therapy students, the individual should be functioning at entry level. The NBCOT exam is designed to test entry level knowledge. Therefore, answers A, B, and C are incorrect. See reference: AOTA: Intercommission Council: Occupational Therapy Roles.

172. (B) Have at least 1 year of experience as a registered occupational therapist. Based on the Essentials for level II fieldwork, an occupational therapist supervising a level II OTR student is required to have a minimum of 1 year of experience. OTRs with 6 months of experience may supervise level I or II COTA students. See reference: AOTA: Commission on Education: Guide to Fieldwork Education.

173. (A) Managed care. Managed care companies act as intermediaries between insurance companies and health care providers with the intent to reduce overall health care costs by requiring the individual to utilize providers who have prenegotiated rates. In addition, the managed care entities work to reduce hospital lengths of stay by limiting hospital days or therapeutic visits. Managed competition is the concept of utilizing outcome data and charge efficiencies of health care providers to award health business to the systems with the best ratings. It is anticipated that the concept of managed competition will drive the cost of health care down and potentially put some facilities out of business. Medicare and Medicaid are governmental systems that are not currently under managed care systems. However, within the next decade, it is anticipated that the enrollees of these systems will be in some form of managed care system. See reference: Hopkins and Smith (eds): Hansen, RA: Ethics in occupational therapy.

174. (B) Objectives. Objectives are established by the individual fieldwork sites to reflect the facility's philosophy and scope of care. Objectives define what learning experiences will be provided in the facility as well as the performance expectations for the objectives. See reference: AOTA: Commission on Education: Guide to Fieldwork Education.

175. (A) Industrial rehabilitation settings. These referrals are made by the physician, employer, attorney, rehabilitation counselor, or case manager in an effort to identify the physical and functional capacities of an employee. Referrals to pediatric, inpatient hospitalization, and subacute units are not generally made by all of the disciplines identified in the question. See reference: Hopkins and Smith (eds): Jacobs, K: Work assessments and programming.

176. (B) 48 hours. Acknowledgment of the referral in home health must occur within 48 hours. Answers A, C, and D are incorrect. See reference: Hopkins and Smith (eds): Levine, RE, Corcoran, MA, and Gitling, LN: Home care and private practice.

177. (C) This does not allow for adequate supervision of the assistant. However, if they were allowed the time to provide general or routine supervision to the COTA, the COTA would then be able to treat the patients, do the progress notes, and evaluate the discharge status. Occupational therapy departments frequently are understaffed and need to operate as efficiently as possible. The collaborative teamwork between an OTR and a COTA is vital in treatment planning and implementation. When a collaborative relationship is operational, the COTA may carry out the roles of providing treatment, completing the progress notes and the discharge summaries. Answer A is incorrect because the solution does not allow for appropriate supervision of the COTA, because the administrator indicated that they would be functioning independently. Answer B is incorrect because it violates the standards of practice and code of ethics for the therapist to agree to provision of inappropriate services. Answer D is incorrect because the occupational therapist does not have to provide all of the treatment as well as do all of the documentation. See reference: Hopkins and Smith (eds): Perinchief, JM: Service management.

178. (C) Notify the NBCOT of the situation and reassign the patient to a different therapist. According to the Code of Ethics, therapists are responsible for "maintaining a goal directed and objective relationship with all people served," as well as not engaging in behavior that may constitute a "conflict of interest that adversely reflects on the profession." The patient/therapist relationship is compromised when the therapist enters into a social or intimate relationship with a patient. Every therapist is responsible to report behavior that is in conflict with the Code of Ethics to the NBCOT (whether they are a supervisor or not). See reference: Hopkins and Smith (eds): Hansen, RA: Ethics in occupational therapy.

179. (C) Decline the gift and explain that she is unable to accept gifts. Accepting gifts from patients would be perceived as poor professional conduct. Fees are established based on a cost analysis of the overhead, supplies, and time required to provide a service. Therefore, answers A, B, and D are incorrect. See reference: Hopkins and Smith (eds): Hansen, RA: Ethics in occupational therapy.

180. (A) Standards of Practice. Membership in the American Occupational Therapy Association is voluntary and the AOTA does not have jurisdiction over therapists who are not members. The *Standards of Practice* outlines the values and basic beliefs that are to be exemplified by occupational therapists. The Standards and Ethics Commission (SEC) is responsible for the Code of Ethics and Standards of Practice. The SEC monitors compliance with the ethics and standards from which members practice. However, the SEC does not have any recourse against nonmembers who do not follow these standards. Even though employers may otherwise benefit from employees being members of AOTA, accountability to the professional standards is by far the most beneficial. See reference: Hopkins and Smith (eds): Hopkins, HL: Scope of occupational therapy.

181. (C) A physician's order identifying services to be provided. Within the home-care setting, the therapist must have a physician's order, which identifies the services that are to be provided. Following the occupational therapist's assessment, identification of deficits as well as frequency and duration of treatment (answers A and B) are completed. The individual's history of the current illness, answer D, is contained within the initial assessment. See reference: Hopkins and Smith (eds): Levine, RE, Corcoran, MA, and Gitling, LN: Home care and private practice.

182. (B) An institutional policy. Within the "Statement of Purpose," the document is defined as a procedure for Central City Hospital, thus making the policy an institutional policy. A personnel policy, answer A, is specific to the behavioral and performance expectations of an employee. A department policy, answer C, would be specific to the hiring of occupational therapy personnel. A credentialing policy, answer D, would specifically relate to the verification of personnel credentials. See reference: Hopkins and Smith (eds): Perinchief, JM: Service management.

183. (B) Provide criteria for the process of hiring individuals. Answers A, C, and D are technically correct. However, they are both a part of the criteria for hiring individuals. Thus, the MOST correct answer is B. A reference is not available for this question.

184. (D) State licensure. Many states are now requiring that a specified number of contact hours be achieved for renewal of licensure. Even though it is recommended, it is not currently required by AOTA, NBCOT, or state associations. See reference: Hopkins and Smith (eds): Perinchief, JM: Service management.

185. (B) Medicaid. Medicaid is a joint federal and state program. Because it is a joint program, benefits vary widely from state to state. These programs must include Aid to Families with Dependent Children (AFDC) and Supplementary Security Income (SSI). Medicare, answer B, is a federal program for health coverage for individuals 65 years or older, disabled individuals, or people in the end stages of renal disease. Workers' compensation, answer C, is a state-supported program into which employers pay. Beneficiaries will receive coverage for those services that are identified to be covered within their respective state. The Education for All Handicapped Children, answer D, is assisted through the provision of state and federal grants. See reference: Bair and Gray (eds): Scott, SJ, and Somers, PF: Payment for occupational therapy services.

186. (A) Medicare. Medicare is a federal program for health coverage for individuals 65 years or older, disabled individuals, or people in the end stages of renal disease. Medicaid, answer B, is a joint federal and state program. Because it is a joint program, benefits vary widely from state to state. These programs must include AFDC and SSI. Workers' compensation, answer C, is a state-sup-

ported program into which employers pay. Beneficiaries will receive coverage for those services that are identified to be covered within their respective state. The Education for All Handicapped Children, answer D, is assisted through the provision of state and federal grants. See reference: Bair and Gray (eds): Scott, SJ, and Somers, PF: Payment for occupational therapy services.

187. (C) An ethical dilemma. Ethical situations are clearly defined in the Occupational Therapy Manager. They define an ethical dilemma as "two or more equally unpleasant alternatives that are mutually exclusive." Ethical uncertainty is described as "uncertainty of what moral principles apply or if a problem is indeed a moral problem." Ethical distress is "knowing the right course of action but feeling constrained to act by institutional rules." Unethical behavior is behavior that is in conflict with the Occupational Therapy Code of Ethics. See reference: Bair and Gray (eds): Opacich, KJ, and Welles, C: Ethical dimensions in occupational therapy.

188. (B) Medicare. Medicare is a federal program for health coverage for individuals 65 years or older, disabled individuals, or people in the end stages of renal disease. Medicaid, answer B, is a joint federal and state program. Because it is a joint program, benefits vary widely from state to state. These programs must include AFDC and SSI. Workers' compensation, answer C, is a state-supported program into which employers pay. Beneficiaries will receive coverage for those services that are identified to be covered within their respective state. The Education for All Handicapped Children, answer D, is assisted through the provision of state and federal grants. See reference: Hopkins and Smith (eds): Levy, L: The health care delivery system today.

189. (D) Lightweight wheelchair and hospital bed. Durable medical equipment is defined by Medicare as "that which can withstand repeated use, is primarily and customarily used to serve a medical purpose, and generally is not useful to a person in the absence of illness or injury." Answers A, B, and C are incorrect because they included items that are not considered as "durable medical equipment" (e.g., reachers, a shower chair, or a hand held shower). Depending on the patient's medical condition, a bedside commode may be covered. See reference: Bair and Gray (eds): Scott, SJ, and Somers, PF: Payment for occupational therapy services.

190. (A) Capital equipment. Equipment pieces that cost in excess of $500, are considered capital equipment and will generally last for more than 2 years (i.e., filing cabinet). Items that cost less than $500 are considered expendable, answer B, may last up to approximately 2 years (i.e., pinch meter). Adaptive equipment, answer C, such as reachers may be utilized during therapy or sold to a patient. Supplies, answer D, are items such as forms and pens, which may be utilized by staff. See reference: Bair and Gray (eds): Scammahorn, G: Program planning.

191. (B) Expendable equipment. Items that cost less than $500 are considered expendable and may last up to approximately 2 years (i.e., pinch meter) Equipment pieces that cost in excess of $500 are considered capital equipment and will generally last for more than 2 years (i.e., filing cabinet). Adaptive equipment, answer C, such as reachers may be utilized during therapy or sold to a patient. Supplies, answer D, are items such as forms and pens, which may be utilized by staff. See reference: Bair and Gray (eds): Scammahorn, G: Program planning.

192. (A) There is an increasing shortage of occupational therapy practitioners in the area of mental health. Current trends in mental health to utilize recreational, music and art therapists has reduced the demand for occupational therapists in the mental health environment. In addition, an increasing number of therapists are pursuing positions in pediatrics and physical disabilities. These two issues combined are causing a current shortage of occupational therapy practitioners in the mental health setting. The inverse is true of answers B, C, and D, therefore making them incorrect. See reference: Hopkins and Smith (eds): Levy, L: The health care delivery system today.

193. (A) The concept of two therapists performing the same procedure will gain the same results. The term service competency indicates an interrater reliability between two occupational therapy professionals. Therefore answers C and D are incorrect. In addition, service competence is not gained through passing the certification examination. Service competency is necessary as an entry level therapist begins to function in an occupational therapy department to establish the same procedure for those tasks that may require more skill. This concept is also vital in the COTA and OTR relationship in that the OTR is ultimately responsible for the information gained and reported by the COTA. See reference: AOTA: Intercommission Council: Occupational therapy roles.

194. (A) Beneficence and autonomy. Principle 1 of the Occupational Therapy Code of Ethics speaks to the concern that is to be demonstrated by the therapist towards patients. This includes provision of services without discrimination, providing appropriate information to patients regarding education and research, and involvement of the patient in treatment planning. Answer B, principle 2, is competence. This refers specifically to credentialing and the therapist functioning within the parameters of their skill level. Therapists are guided to refer patients to other service areas when the skills required to not fall within their expertise. This includes provision of services without discrimination, providing appropriate information to patients regarding education and research, and involvement of the patient in treatment planning. Answer C, compliance with laws and regulations, is principle 3. This principle refers to therapists following state, local, and federal in addition to facility specific guidelines and requirements for accreditation. Answer D, public information, addresses the therapist accurately representing their expertise as well as not partici-

pating in any fraudulent statements or claims. See reference: Hopkins and Smith (eds): Hansen, RA: Ethics in occupational therapy.

195. (A) 0 to 19 years of age. The age range of patients most frequently seen in occupational therapy is 0 to 19 years of age. This represents 32.3 percent of all referrals. Answer B, 20 to 64 years of age, represents 30.5 percent. Answer C, 65 years of age and older, represents 14.9 percent. Mixed ages represents 22.3 percent. See reference: Punwar: Current trends in the field.

196. (A) Cerebrovascular accident. The diagnosis most frequently seen by occupational therapists is cerebrovascular accident at 28.2 percent. Answer B, cerebral palsy, is 11.2 percent. Answer C, developmental delay, is the second most frequent diagnosis seen by occupational therapists at 16.5 percent. Answer D, neuromuscular disorders, are seen by occupational therapists fairly infrequently at 0.6 percent. See reference: Punwar: Current trends in the field.

197. (B) School systems. 16.3 percent of occupational therapists in the community settings are employed in the school system. Answer A is incorrect because 6.0 percent are employed in private practice. Answer C is incorrect because 4.5 percent are employed in home health agencies. Answer D is incorrect because 3.5 percent are in residential care facilities. See reference: Punwar: Current trends in the field.

198. (C) Assist with stock and inventory control. Volunteers may actively participate in support functions of occupational therapy departments once training has been completed. However, answers A, C, and D conflict with components of the of the occupational therapy Code of Ethics and therefore would be incorrect. See reference: AOTA: Commission on Standards and Ethics: Occupational Therapy Code of Ethics.

199. (D) Public information. Public information addresses the therapist accurately representing their expertise as well as not participating in any fraudulent statements or claims. Answer A, beneficence and autonomy, speaks to the concern that is to be demonstrated by therapist towards patients. This includes provision of services without discrimination, providing appropriate information to patients regarding education and research, and involvement of the patient in treatment planning. Answer B, principle 2 of the Occupational Therapy Code of Ethics, is competence. This refers specifically to credentialing and the therapist functioning within the parameters of their skill level. Therapists are guided to refer patients to other service areas when the skills required do not fall within their expertise. Answer C, compliance with laws and regulations, is principle 3. This principle refers to therapists following state, local, and federal in addition to facility specific guidelines and requirements for accreditation. See reference: Hopkins and Smith (eds): Hansen, R: Ethics in occupational therapy.

200. (C) Theoretic base. The rational or theory base is to provide a foundation of knowledge from which a treatment approach may be selected (i.e., biomechanical, neurodevelopmental, behavioral, and so on). See reference: Bailey: Introduction.

SIMULATION EXAMINATION **5**

> **Directions:** Circle the correct answer to the following questions. When you have completed this examination, check your answers against the answer key that follows. As you will see, an explanation is given for each answer along with a reference for further study. The book author is listed as well as the chapter author. See the bibliography for complete references.

1. **The Milani-Comparetti Motor Development Screening Test measures the following in children:**
   A. primitive reflexes and postural reactions.
   B. developmental prehension skills.
   C. cognitive skills.
   D. language skills.

2. **The occupational therapist is assessing an individual with the diagnosis of a cerebrovascular accident. The most appropriate technique to be used in assessing sensory awareness is to:**
   A. test the individual's affected extremity before the unaffected extremity.
   B. demonstrate the procedure on the unaffected extremity, then occlude the individual's vision.
   C. demonstrate the procedure on the affected extremity then establish rapport with the individual.
   D. interview the individual and assess only the areas that they report are impaired.

3. **In the assessment of individuals diagnosed with early and middle stages of most dementias, the functional ability that will MOST likely remain intact for the longest duration is:**
   A. the ability to read written information.
   B. the ability to write down basic information.
   C. the ability to engage in superficial social conversation.
   D. the ability to dress and undress oneself.

4. **OSHA has defined four strategies to help prevent work place exposure to bloodborne pathogens. What is the strategy that teaches the concept of all blood and some body fluids being handled as if contaminated with HIV or HBV?**
   A. Engineering controls
   B. Work practice controls
   C. Personal protective controls
   D. Universal precautions

5. **At a team planning meeting for a 2-year-old child with multiple handicaps, it is decided that the occupational therapist will also fulfill the roles of other therapies needed. This includes a "role release" from the teacher, physical therapist, and speech therapist. Which of the following team approaches for young children does this method describe?**
   A. Unidisciplinary
   B. Multidisciplinary
   C. Interdisciplinary
   D. Transdisciplinary

6. **An individual who had a cerebrovascular accident and is dependent with self care and transfers with the assistance of two people, has expressed the goal of returning home with a transfer status of only needing the assistance of one person. A long-term goal would be that:**
   A. the individual will complete upper extremity sponge bathing with set up of equipment and verbal cues.
   B. the individual will perform lower extremity dressing with maximal assistance of one person.
   C. the individual will complete upper extremity self care with supervision of a family member and use appropriate adaptive equipment.
   D. the individual will complete a modified sit pivot transfer to the commode with moderate assistance of two people.

7. **The occupational therapist is planning treatment for individuals with a variety of personality disorders who have inaccurate perceptions of others and unrealistic perceptions of themselves. The treatment method that best addresses these problem areas is a:**
   A. small group that provides a wide range of craft activities from which the members are encouraged to select.
   B. session focused on understanding and changing the individual's way of relating with the therapist.

C. social skills training program completed in small groups.

D. cooperative group activity that both provides and elicits consistent and accurate feedback about interactions within the group.

8. **Upon completion of the level II fieldwork, the student:**

A. should be functioning slightly below entry level.

B. should be able to function at an intermediate skill level based on the Occupational Therapy Roles.

C. should be able to function at an advanced skill level based on the Occupational Therapy Roles.

D. should be able to function at an entry level or above the minimum entry level of competence.

9. **While in occupational therapy, a child has a seizure that barely interrupts activity performance. This would be reported as what type of a seizure?**

A. Grand mal

B. Psychomotor or tonic-clonic

C. Petit mal

D. Akinetic

10. **When planning a therapeutic program for a child who has visual discrimination problems, the first step would be to provide "matching" activities, which require discrimination in the areas of:**

A. object function.

B. object characteristics or details.

C. object color, shape, and position.

D. object recognition.

11. **An individual who had a stroke is copying a picture of a clock. The drawing appears as a lopsided circle with a flat side on the left. The numbers one through eight are written in numerical order around the right side of the clock. The hands are correctly drawn on the clock to represent three o'clock. The individual's performance demonstrates:**

A. right hemianopia.

B. left unilateral neglect.

C. cataracts in the left eye.

D. bitemporal hemianopia.

12. **A rating scale for head injured individuals that uses a numerical scale to rate three types of response by the head injured individual is the:**

A. Rancho Los Amigos Levels of Cognitive Functioning.

B. Claudia Allen Scale of Cognitive Functioning.

C. Braintree Hospital Cognitive Continuum.

D. Glasgow Coma Scale.

13. **Occupational therapists working in early intervention have frequent contact with a child's parent. Which of the following statements BEST describes how parents should be involved in the occupational therapy program?**

A. Parents should not be present during occupational therapy sessions.

B. Parents should be trained as substitute therapists.

C. Parents' needs and wishes should be included in program planning.

D. Only one parent needs to be present when the occupational therapy program is discussed.

14. **A power grip would MOST likely be used to hold:**

A. a sewing needle while it is being threaded.

B. a tall glass half filled with water.

C. a heavy handbag held by the strap.

D. a key while it is being placed in a lock.

15. **Inability to begin a task or activity may denote problems with:**

A. attention.

B. concentration.

C. initiation.

D. apraxia.

16. **The name of the standardized test that uses seven tasks of daily living to assess hand function is called the:**

A. Purdue Pegboard.

B. Jebson-Taylor Hand Function Test.

C. Minnesota Rate of Manipulation.

D. Crawford Small Parts Dexterity Test.

17. **Occupational therapists can contribute their assessment and planning information to an Individual Educational Plan (IEP). In which of the following settings is an IEP used as the central plan for a child?**

A. Rehabilitation center

B. Public school system

C. Outpatient care center

D. Home health agency

18. **According to Brunnstrom, a person who demonstrates developing spasticity on the hemiplegic side of the body with weak, associated movements in synergy and little active finger flexion, would be in which stage of recovery?**

A. One

B. Two

C. Three

D. Four

19. **The part of a treatment objective that describes the method by which the individual's performance will be measured is the:**

A. terminal behavior.

B. condition.

C. criteria.

D. plan.

20. **An example of a prevocational activity, involving a woman who had worked as a cashier in a clothing store, would be having the woman:**

A. Make a grocery list while sitting

B. Fold or put laundry on a hanger while standing

C. Wash dishes while standing

D. Add a column of numbers by hand while sitting

21. **An occupational therapist who uses splints with children may find the most controversy over use of hand splints for children who have:**

A. abnormal muscle tone.

B. muscle weakness.

C. traumatic injury.

D. joint inflammation.

22. **The therapist has determined that the main problem for an individual is increased neck and shoulder tension, which leads to headaches. This primarily occurs while the individual is at work as a word processor in a recently restructured corporation. The BEST stress management approach for this situation is:**

A. assertiveness training focusing on increasing the individual's assertiveness with their boss.

B. EMG biofeedback training combined with relaxation training.

C. training in cognitive reappraisal to decrease the frequency of the individual's tendency to generalize and exaggerate the negative side of work events.

D. teaching the individual more effective problem-solving strategies.

23. **The group format that is used most often by occupational therapists:**

A. cooking groups.

B. activity of daily living groups.

C. arts and crafts groups.

D. exercise groups.

24. **Why does the occupational therapist decide to respond to an individual by paraphrasing?**

A. To refocus or redirect an individual's comments.

B. To show acceptance and understanding to the individual.

C. To repeat what an individual has said.

D. To encourage additional information from an individual.

25. **An 11-month-old child who was born 3 months prematurely is being reevaluated through the occupational therapy outpatient clinic. The child's abilities in all areas should be compared with a normal child of:**

A. 11 months.

B. 14 months.

C. 8 months.

D. 10 months.

26. **Occupational therapists working in mental health are most likely to address these patient problems:**

A. Adjustment disorders

B. Affective disorders

C. Alcohol use disorders

D. Anxiety disorders

27. **The therapist is working with an individual on a goal of enhancing the individual's self esteem. The individual is diagnosed with depression. This person refuses to participate in the treatment activities today. Which refusal is MOST LIKELY to be linked to their depression?**

A. "I can't."

B. "I don't know how."

C. "I'm just too tired."

D. "I'm waiting for my visitors to come."

28. **Which of the following community vocational services are adults with mental retardation most likely to be referred?**

A. Adult activity centers

B. Supported employment

C. Job coaching

D. Sheltered workshops

29. **A 7-year-old child with a learning disability is unable to focus on a blackboard 20 feet away from him and refocus on his paper in order to copy a mathematics problem. The therapist also observes the same problem during clinical observations requiring the child to focus on a pencil at 12 inches and refocus on the wall clock at 20 feet. The therapist should conclude that the child has a visual problem with:**

A. ocular motility.

B. binocular vision.

C. convergence.

D. accommodation.

30. **Directive group treatment is the MOST appropriate approach in acute care mental health for individuals with:**

A. substance abuse.

B. eating disorders.

C. adjustment disorders.

D. disorganized psychosis.

31. **The advantage of asking a closed question is that the question:**

A. allows the therapist to obtain facts.

B. avoids emphasizing feelings being expressed by the patient.

C. can help the therapist who is in a hurry.

D. forces the person to give the answer that the therapist needs.

32. **The occupational therapist is treating a 31-year-old man who experienced a T1-T2 spinal cord injury as a result of a motor vehicle accident. Prior to the injury, the young man worked as a computer programmer and played in basketball leagues in the evenings and on the weekends. The therapist shares this information with her colleagues and asks what they have done in similar situations. The form of clinical reasoning**

that the therapist is MOST likely to use in this scenario would be:

A. procedural reasoning.
B. conditional reasoning.
C. interactive reasoning.
D. narrative reasoning.

33. **The therapist is carrying out a sensory integration program using activities to improve sensory processing. If she is working with a child who has underreactive sensory processing, the activities should have the following facilitory characteristics:**

A. arrhythmic and unexpected.
B. arrhythmic and slow.
C. sustained and slow.
D. unexpected and rhythmic.

34. **A child with a severe physical disability and no cognitive delays does not have a form of functional mobility. At what age could a powered wheelchair first be considered for this child?**

A. 2 years
B. 4 years
C. 6 years
D. 8 years

35. **The determination of an individual's Global Assessment of Functioning (GAF) on the DSM-IV diagnosis is based on:**

A. the degree of environmental and psychosocial problems the individual experienced.
B. the medical conditions complicating the original diagnosis.
C. the individual's level of psychosocial and occupational limitations.
D. the individual's maladaptive mechanisms.

36. **The treatment goal that addresses the psychosocial skill of self expression is that the:**

A. client will identify and pursue activities that are pleasurable to the self.
B. client will use facial expressions and gestures that are consistent with stated emotions during assertive, passive, and aggressive role play situations.
C. client will recognize own behavior and possible negative and positive consequences.
D. client will identify own assets and limitations following a movement group.

37. **The thematic group that would be most appropriate for mental health settings that treats a wide variety of diagnoses:**

A. Self expression through poetry
B. Evaluation group
C. Discharge planning group
D. Exercise group

38. **The comment made in a discharge planning group on a psychiatric inpatient unit that indicates a client's concern about stigma would be:**

A. "The smoke from your cigarette is really making me uncomfortable. Please put your cigarette out."
B. "My medications make my eyes blurry. I want to stop taking it so I can see better."
C. "One of my relatives is always trying to tell me what to do with my life. They think I should continue seeing a psychiatrist."
D. "When I apply for jobs, what should I put down when it asks if you have been hospitalized or treated for anything in the past 6 months?"

39. **An individual who is 70 years old is hospitalized after a cerebrovascular accident. The acute care stay for this individual will most likely be paid under:**

A. a diagnostic related group (DRG).
B. a functional rehabilitation group (FRG).
C. Medicaid.
D. third-party reimbursement.

40. **The concept of the federal government making a standard payment for health care services for individuals in diagnostic categories is known as:**

A. DRGs.
B. PROs.
C. UB-82s.
D. cost shifting.

41. **Benefits paid under Medicare Part A would include:**

A. inpatient hospitalization.
B. in-home occupational therapy services (psychiatric).
C. outpatient occupational therapy.
D. comprehensive outpatient rehabilitation facility.

42. **The therapist is treating an adult whose medical coverage is provided by a state payment system. The system most likely to be involved would be:**

A. Medicaid or Medicare.
B. Medicaid, the Education for All Handicapped Children, or workers' compensation.
C. workers' compensation or Medicaid.
D. Education for all Handicapped Children or workers' compensation.

43. **In the majority of states, acute care orders for occupational therapy services must come from:**

A. a patient's self referral.
B. a physician's referral.
C. a referral from a significant other.
D. a referral from physical therapy.

44. **Quality improvement plans include a model for identifying quality indicators or areas that should be monitored. An area that should be monitored regardless of reaching 100 percent compliance would be one with:**

A. high volume.
B. high risk.
C. high incidence.
D. problems.

45. **Volunteers used in an occupational therapy setting will MOST likely:**
    A. independently transport patients to and from therapy.
    B. independently work with a patient once the therapist has set up the activity.
    C. assist with stock and inventory control.
    D. complete chart reviews.

46. **The profession of occupational therapy is continually evolving and developing. As health care changes through the next century, the focus will move more toward health status and away from health care. The occupational therapists' role in this trend to enhance wellness through education, behavioral change and cultural support is called:**
    A. occupational behavior.
    B. synchrony.
    C. self efficacy.
    D. health promotion.

47. **The following practice trend that is most descriptive of occupational therapy practice in mental health is:**
    A. there is an increasing shortage of occupational therapy practitioners in the area of mental health.
    B. occupational therapy services are not required services in most mental health settings.
    C. inpatient programs, more than community programs, are an area of future growth for occupational therapists in mental health.
    D. the majority of occupational therapists practice in the area of mental health.

48. **Service competency is:**
    A. the concept that two therapists performing the same procedure will gain the same results.
    B. established when a therapist passes the NBCOT exam.
    C. achieved through an individual attaining a minimum number of continuing education credits.
    D. the theory that individual competency is gained each year that a therapist practices.

49. **The manager of occupational therapy is writing to report to justify additional staff. The information that would provide the STRONGEST support for additional staff would be:**
    A. a cost accounting report.
    B. definition of Relative Value Units (RVUs) report.
    C. a productivity report.
    D. a market analysis

50. **The occupational therapist is preparing to discharge a 6-year-old child who was initially referred for treatment for developmental dyspraxia. The child's new teacher asks: "What does dyspraxia mean?" The best description would be:**

    A. a problem with learning new motor skills.
    B. a neuromuscular problem.
    C. a lack of development of higher order reflex reactions.
    D. a problem of poor balance.

51. **Assessment of a child indicates a normally developing infant. The occupational therapist documents presence of a postural reaction associated with development of the extensor tone needed for sitting and standing. This reaction would be:**
    A. tonic labyrinthine in prone.
    B. asymmetrical tonic neck.
    C. neck righting.
    D. Landau reaction.

52. **The occupational therapist is preparing to complete an evaluation for an individual with the diagnosis of cerebrovascular accident. The sensory portion of the test would be invalid for an individual with which one of the following impairments?**
    A. Expressive aphasia
    B. Receptive aphasia
    C. Agnosia
    D. Ataxia

53. **The assessment instrument designed for use as a screening of self-care, physical, and social behaviors through the observations of caregivers familiar with the individual's daily care is the:**
    A. Bay Area Functional Performance Evaluation (BAFPE).
    B. Comprehensive Occupational Therapy Evaluation (COTE).
    C. Role Checklist.
    D. Parachek Geriatric Rating Scale.

54. **The occupational therapist is working in a collaborative relationship with the certified occupational therapy assistant. The teamwork between the two professionals would be exemplified by:**
    A. the occupational therapist completing the assessment and then telling the COTA what treatment to provide.
    B. the COTA updating the occupational therapist on the improvements that the patient has made in the past week and both therapists providing information to update the goals.
    C. the COTA giving her progress note to the occupational therapist and the occupational therapist writing the discharge summary from the progress note.
    D. the occupational therapist telling the COTA what type of equipment to order for the patient and the COTA arranging for the equipment from a durable medical equipment company.

55. **When planning treatment for a child with high tone or spasticity, the occupational therapist**

would MOST likely use the neurodevelopmental treatment (NDT) principle of:
A. weight-bearing and compression with movement.
B. small movements with stability.
C. stability, reduction of movements, and development of midline orientation.
D. passive movement followed by slow, rhythmical movement.

56. **After evaluation, the goal for an individual who had a total hip replacement was minimal assistance with verbal cues for memory. After 2 weeks of treatment, the individual is able to dress with standby assistance. What skills does the this person need to demonstrate prior to changing the goal?**
A. Less time needed to perform dressing.
B. Improved concentration.
C. Ability to remember two of three hip precautions.
D. Consistent and appropriate use of adaptive equipment.

57. **Comprehensive psychiatric rehabilitation services often include recreational therapy. The primary role that is expected of recreational therapy is to:**
A. provide a variety of therapeutic sports, arts, crafts, music, and recreation activities to develop and reinforce healthy interest patterns.
B. provide specially designed learning experiences that stimulate awareness of social skills and behaviors.
C. provide acting-doing experiences that enable the individual to acquire leisure, work, and self-care skills at a maximum level of independence and a sense of self satisfaction and personal worth.
D. support the work-related behaviors and habits of time management, organization, and dependability through a variety of activities.

58. **The term that mandates the confidentiality of patient information and holds the therapist to remain faithful to the patient's best interest is:**
A. informed consent.
B. fidelity.
C. beneficence.
D. nonmaleficence.

59. **During treatment, the occupational therapist is providing activities that assist the child in integrating rotary motion. Sensory receptors for this type of vestibular processing are located in the:**
A. semicircular canals.
B. utricle.
C. saccule.
D. cochlea.

60. **Using a visual perceptual frame of reference, the first step in planning a program for a child with visual perceptual problems would be to consider:**

A. visual memory skills.
B. visual attention skills.
C. general visual discrimination skills.
D. specific visual discrimination skills.

61. **Scapulohumeral rhythm is defined as:**
A. a ratio of 2:1 as the humerus moves on the scapula.
B. a ratio of 2:1 as the scapula moves on the humerus.
C. a ratio of 5:1 as the scapula moves on the humerus.
D. a ratio of 1:5 as the humerus moves on the scapula.

62. **An individual with a left hemisphere cerebro-vascular accident is given a paper typed with letters of the alphabet randomly dispersed. The individual is instructed to cross out all of the Ms. After completing the task, the missed letters are in a random pattern throughout the page. This person demonstrates:**
A. a left visual field cut.
B. a right visual field out.
C. functional illiteracy.
D. decreased attention.

63. **During assessment of a 13-month-old child with congenital blindness, the child demonstrates a Moro reflex to loud noise and loss of position. This evaluation tells the occupational therapist that:**
A. reflex maturation is occurring at a normal rate.
B. reflex maturation is slightly delayed.
C. reflex maturation is significantly delayed.
D. reflex maturation is advanced for the child's age.

64. **Hypersensitivity training is graded from:**
A. soft to hard to rough.
B. tap to rub to touch.
C. light to medium to heavy.
D. rough to hard to soft.

65. **Rood facilitation techniques include which of the following:**
A. fast brushing, slow icing, and slow stroking.
B. light stroking, fast brushing, and quick stretch.
C. slow brushing and slow rolling.
D. slow brushing, fast icing, and slow rolling.

66. **An individual with a head injury is impulsive during self feeding. This is exemplified by placing too much food in her mouth at one time. What method may be used to control the rate of intake during self feeding?**
A. Cut the food into smaller pieces.
B. Have the individual count to 10 between bites of food.
C. Have the individual set the utensil down until the mouth is cleared.
D. Serve food in separate containers on the meal tray.

67. An occupational therapist is developing a treatment plan for a child with mild cerebral palsy who has difficulty with in-hand manipulation. The skill that needs remediation is linear movement of an object from the palm to the fingers or fingers to the palm. Of the three types of in-hand manipulation this type is called:
    A. translation.
    B. shift.
    C. rotation.
    D. stabilization.

68. An individual stops after performing only one part of a self-care task and requires prompting to continue, although the individual is correctly able to list the next steps in the activity. This individual demonstrates difficulty with:
    A. impulsivity.
    B. initiation.
    C. memory.
    D. attention.

69. A person may be diagnosed with chronic pain from cervical disk disease when the symptoms of acute pain with impairment and disability have lasted longer than the acute stage of pain had disappeared by how many weeks?
    A. 1 week
    B. 3 weeks
    C. 6 weeks
    D. 9 weeks

70. The second level of use in an augmentative communication hierarchy after understanding picture symbols and their use would be:
    A. sequencing of picture symbols.
    B. recognizing letters of the alphabet.
    C. recognizing whole words.
    D. spelling letter by letter.

71. The adaptation on a chair that will usually inhibit extensor tone or pattern and make sitting in a chair possible is a:
    A. lateral trunk support.
    B. seat belt at the hips.
    C. wedge-shaped seat which is higher in front.
    D. lapboard.

72. An activity may be effectively used when the adaptation:
    A. is complicated.
    B. needs to be adjusted frequently.
    C. is performed in a comfortable position.
    D. is monotonous.

73. An activity that may be graded to improve a person's arm strength and endurance would be:
    A. passive range of motion.
    B. Codman's exercises.
    C. popping a balloon.
    D. batting a balloon.

74. Asking a middle-aged individual about the grade school he or she attended is one way of obtaining data about this individual's:
    A. retention.
    B. remote memory.
    C. orientation.
    D. recent memory.

75. The occupational therapist selects a pie-of-life activity to use with a group of individuals in a stress management group. The therapist states: "I see that at least half of you have drawn your pie of life with too little time for rest and relaxation. Why don't we spend some group time exploring some ways to add more relaxation and rest into our days? Why don't we each give one suggestion?" The phase of group development this therapists' interaction describes is called:
    A. opening the group.
    B. processing the group.
    C. developing the group.
    D. group closure.

76. Which of the following side effects of neuroleptic medications would the therapist want to take precautions for when planning a community outing in the summer that involves walking outdoors between the bus stop, the bank, a utility company, and a grocery store.
    A. Hypotension
    B. Photosensitivity
    C. Excessive perspiration
    D. Weight gain

77. In psychosocial areas of occupational therapy, the therapist's relationship with an individual is best described as:
    A. the central focus of occupational therapy treatment.
    B. a therapeutic device in helping.
    C. a friendship.
    D. sympathy for the individual's problems.

78. In the review of an adolescent individual's chart, the DSM IV, Axis V diagnosis shows a score of 35. The BEST interpretation of functioning with this score is:
    A. slight impairment in social and school functioning (e.g., falls behind in schoolwork).
    B. moderate difficulty in social or school functioning (e.g., few friends).
    C. major impairment in several areas (e.g., defiant at home and failing at school).
    D. serious impairment in communication or judgment (e.g., suicidal preoccupations).

79. A 10-year-old child with a behavior disorder is being evaluated by the occupational therapist for the development of play skills. The child has considerable difficulty with problem solving during any play activity. She becomes

frustrated and gives up easily. In terms of development of play skills, the therapist can conclude that this child's major play problem is in the area of:
A. sensorimotor.
B. imaginary.
C. constructional.
D. game.

80. The medication listed in an individual's chart considered to be an antipsychotic agent:
A. Lithium carbonate
B. Elavil
C. Xanax
D. Thorazine

81. The occupational therapist is planning to demonstrate and then involve a group of individuals in practicing "broken record" behaviors. "Broken record" is part of:
A. music therapy activities.
B. self-awareness activities.
C. assertiveness training.
D. psychodrama approaches.

82. An example of a group norm is when:
A. one member contributes superficial comments.
B. members role play.
C. there is improved self esteem among members.
D. smoking during the group is prohibited.

Case Study

Janet is a 12-year-old girl with a diagnosis of juvenile rheumatoid arthritis (JRA). She has normal intelligence and although she misses school occasionally, she is able to maintain her age group grade level. Onset was sudden and she has periodic episodes of acute inflammation, which primarily affect her knees, hips, elbows, and hands, and there is a slight loss of range of motion in these joints. Besides a low-grade fever, she is frequently listless and irritable. There is no lymph node or spleen involvement. Hand strength has become weaker in the past year, and her right dominant hand now shows 1 to 2 pounds of grasp strength. Answer the following five questions regarding this child:

83. What type of JRA is described by Janet's symptoms?
A. Polyarticular
B. Systemic
C. Pauciarticular
D. Still's disease

84. Janet's therapist is planning for discharge and needs to consider the possibility of permanent disability. What percentage of children with JRA will not recover completely from this condition?
A. 100 percent
B. 75 percent

C. 50 percent
D. 15 percent

85. When planning for discharge, Janet's therapist would like to focus on the most important information to share with Janet's classroom teacher. This would be the:
A. child's level of visual perceptual skills.
B. information on JRA.
C. degrees of range of motion in involved joints.
D. occupational therapy treatment plan in general.

86. Janet's therapist is designing a splint for Janet's right wrist. Considering her problems, what would be the most appropriate goal for her splint?
A. Inhibition of hypertonus
B. Increase range of motion
C. Prevent deformity
D. Correct deformity

87. Janet is being discharged from occupational therapy in an outpatient clinic. Although the active nature of her condition is gone, there is remaining hand strength weakness. Which of the following pieces of adaptive equipment would be most important to prevent hand fatigue in Janet's situation?
A. Reacher
B. Jar opener
C. Pencil gripper
D. Plate guard

88. The occupational therapist wrote: "The client will identify two strengths and one limitation about task performance at the close of each group." This goal addresses the component of occupational performance referred to as:
A. termination of activity.
B. values.
C. self concept.
D. self expression.

89. The occupational therapist is the group leader of an activity-based parallel level group. The best goal for the members of this group is:
A. each member should take a leadership role within the session.
B. members will share materials with at least one other group member.
C. each member will express two positive feelings about themselves within the group session.
D. each member will remain in the group without disrupting the work of others for 30 minutes.

90. The occupational therapist is working in an acute care, inpatient psychiatric program with children between 6 and 12 years old. The following play activities would be recommended by the OT to the parents of an 8-year-old who is being discharged at the end of the week:

A. board games where the parents focus on "playing only by the rules."
B. board games where the parents don't interfere with the variety of rules modifications made by the children playing the game.
C. participation in organized competitive sports.
D. encouragement to begin involvement in girl or boy scouts.

91. **When an individual's discharge from a psychiatric inpatient service is delayed, he or she may risk:**
    A. disruptions in the clients continuity of care.
    B. counter-transference.
    C. posttraumatic stress disorder.
    D. regression.

92. **The manager of an occupational therapy department is approached with an ethical dilemma by an occupational therapist. In utilizing The Savage Model of Ethical Contemplation, her first response will be to:**
    A. identify problems to be solved.
    B. sort decisions to be made.
    C. ascertain facts and impressions.
    D. verify information with key players.

93. **Health care coverage for disabled individuals, people with end stage renal disease, or those over 65 is most likely paid for by:**
    A. Medicare.
    B. Medicaid.
    C. third-party payors.
    D. private pay.

94. **The therapist is treating a middle-aged woman who is being seen for carpal tunnel syndrome. The employer's industrial nurse indicated that the condition was a result of repetitious fine motor movement required as an essential job function. The payment program MOST likely to provide payment of occupational therapy services is:**
    A. Medicare.
    B. Medicaid.
    C. workers' compensation.
    D. Education for all Handicapped Children Act.

95. **A writing that encompasses the underlying values and basic moral beliefs to be used by occupational therapists is the:**
    A. Standards of Practice.
    B. Uniform Terminology System for Reporting Occupational Therapy Services, ed 3.
    C. licensure guidelines.
    D. Occupational Therapy Code of Ethics.

96. **Materials that require universal precautions are listed by OSHA to be:**
    A. nasal secretions and blood.
    B. sputum, nasal secretions, and blood.
    C. blood, semen, and saliva from dental procedures.
    D. urine, vomitus, and nasal secretions.

97. **General supervision is defined by the AOTA as:**
    A. contact with supervisor once a day.
    B. contact with supervisor once a week.
    C. contact with supervisor once a month.
    D. contact with supervisor on an as needed basis.

98. **Studies that support the benefit of occupational therapy based on a comparison of the outcomes with the costs incurred are referred to as:**
    A. efficacy studies.
    B. quality improvement studies.
    C. market survey studies.
    D. expenditure studies.

99. **The occupational therapist is working with an individual in the ADL bathroom practicing wheelchair to tub transfers. During the transfer, the individual's external catheter is dislodged and urine spills onto the floor. The therapist notes that the urine appears to have blood in it. Based on her knowledge of universal precautions:**
    A. an exposure has occurred and she should use universal precautions.
    B. an exposure has NOT occurred so she does not need to the universal precautions.
    C. an exposure has occurred but is not severe enough to require universal precautions.
    D. an exposure has NOT occurred but she will use universal precautions anyway.

100. **A 5-year-old child diagnosed with autism is being discharged to a school program for children with severe emotional impairments. The occupational therapist is recommending a preparatory vestibular activity to be used in the classroom. This activity will decrease arousal so that this child will be able to concentrate on simple activities. A therapeutic activity that would meet this criterion would be:**
    A. bouncing while sitting on a large therapy ball.
    B. manual rocking while in prone on a therapy ball.
    C. spinning in supine while on a hammock swing.
    D. rolling down a large wedge.

101. **In assessing a child diagnosed with cerebral palsy resulting in spastic diplagia, the occupational therapist would anticipate involvement in the following extremities:**
    A. both upper limbs.
    B. both legs.
    C. lower extremity, trunk, and mild upper extremity.
    D. all extremities.

102. **A woman with a head injury has been referred for occupational therapy services. Assessment of her affected extremity indicates that she is capable of performing gross movement combinations with minimal evidence of synergy. However, flexion synergy is evident when she attempts activities that are strenuous for her. This patient is in what stage of return?**

A. Stage 3
B. Stage 4
C. Stage 5
D. Stage 6

103. **The occupational therapy frame of reference that is consistent with psychoanalytic perspectives used by other members of the health care team is:**
    A. occupational behavior.
    B. human occupation.
    C. object relations.
    D. role acquisition.

104. **The most common example of utilizing the problem-oriented medical record would be:**
    A. completed patient checklists included in the medical record.
    B. SOAP notes.
    C. facility-specific documentation forms to be completed and placed into the patient chart.
    D. narrative notes that do not follow a structured format.

105. **In discussions with a child's caregiver, the occupational therapist explains that the normal development pattern of infants is to sit without support:**
    A. before they lift their heads in prone.
    B. after back extension in prone develops.
    C. before primitive reflexes disappear.
    D. after they are able to walk alone.

106. **According to Brunnstrom, a head-injured individual in stage two of muscle return would be most likely to demonstrate the following movement in treatment:**
    A. isolated joint movement.
    B. voluntary gross motor movements 25 percent of range.
    C. flexor synergy and voluntary or associated reactions.
    D. gross motor movements such as reaching arm forward to 90 degrees and pronating and supinating the forearm.

107. **When planning a meal preparation activity with an individual who is receiving a MAO inhibitor for depression, the safest food item to include would be:**
    A. aged cheddar cheese.
    B. smoked turkey.
    C. chocolate chips.
    D. rice.

108. **The ADA set out regulations that include providing "reasonable accommodations." This term that BEST describes this is:**
    A. making physical modifications to the environment to allow for wheelchair accessibility.
    B. any modification to a job that will allow a disabled worker to perform the essential functions.

C. standard job task that is fundamental to the position.
D. providing support personnel so that an employee may complete the essential functions with assistance.

109. **The occupational therapist has set up an unstructured play setting to reassess a child. This method of evaluation is MOST effective for a(n):**
    A. observation.
    B. interview.
    C. performance-based screening test.
    D. standardized test.

110. **A child with a learning disability has difficulty attending to visual stimuli (i.e., textbook and chalkboard reading). The appropriate therapeutic approach would be to:**
    A. provide visual tasks of low interest to the child.
    B. increase stimulation surrounding the visual task.
    C. provide visual tasks that lack novelty.
    D. prepare the child mentally and physically for visual tasks.

111. **In assessment of an individual with rheumatoid arthritis, the occupational therapist has her raise her left arm. Range is limited to 85 degrees of shoulder flexion. While in this position, the patient is able to tolerate moderate resistance. The therapist evaluates passive range of motion to be the same as active range of motion. Her manual muscle test score would be:**
    A. normal (5).
    B. good (4).
    C. fair (3).
    D. fair minus (3–).

112. **What approximate Celsius temperature range is recommended for hot and cold sensation testing?**
    A. Hot is 40 to 45 degrees; cold is 5 to 10 degrees
    B. Hot is 45 to 50 degrees; cold is 10 to 15 degrees
    C. Hot is 30 to 35 degrees; cold is 0 to 5 degrees
    D. Hot is 25 to 30 degrees; cold is –5 to 0 degrees

113. **During assessment of a 10-month-old child with Down syndrome, the occupational therapist notes hyperextensibility of all joints. This means that the child probably has:**
    A. increased muscle tone.
    B. decreased muscle tone.
    C. anterior horn cell disease.
    D. muscle and joint disease.

114. **Teaching a task one step at a time and gradually adding more steps is called:**
    A. repetition.
    B. cueing.
    C. rehearsal.
    D. chaining.

115. **Which two tactile senses are the earliest to recover after a peripheral nerve injury?**
   A. Vibration and pain
   B. Temperature and pain
   C. Light touch and proprioception
   D. Tactile localization and proprioception

116. **The occupational therapist is training an individual in the principles of joint protection prior to discharge. These principles would include:**
   A. using the strongest joint, avoiding positions of deformity, and ensuring correct patterns of movement.
   B. massaging a joint before exercise.
   C. practicing vivid imagery and relaxation exercises during difficult functional activities.
   D. application of heat before treatment and application of cold after range of motion treatment.

117. **A therapist planning treatment for a child with athetoid cerebral palsy is concerned about the child's inability to control flexion and extension of the arm when reaching for a toy. The child flexes too much or extends too much, which makes placement of the hand very difficult. The most appropriate goal for this type of hand function problem would be to:**
   A. improve ability to isolate movement.
   B. improve ability to grade movement.
   C. improve timing of movement.
   D. improve bilateral integration of arm movements.

118. **An individual with a high level spinal cord injury is returning home. What type of adaptive technology would the individual need to ensure safety?**
   A. An environmental control unit
   B. A call system for emergency and nonemergency use
   C. A remote control power door opener
   D. An electric page turner

119. **When an occupational therapist decides to use a neurophysiologic approach to treatment of a person with a cerebrovascular accident, the therapist has selected:**
   A. a treatment technique.
   B. an exercise
   C. a treatment plan.
   D. a frame of reference.

120. **A woman who had a CVA has random movements in all four extremities. What is the most appropriate switch to use on the controls for her wheelchair?**
   A. Infrared switch
   B. Sip and puff switch
   C. P-switch
   D. Rocking lever switch

121. **A treatment goal for a child with athetoid cerebral palsy is self-feeding. Which piece of** equipment would best solve the problem of food sliding off the plate when the child attempts to pick it up with a spoon?
   A. Swivel spoon
   B. Nonslip mat
   C. Mobile arm support
   D. Scoop dish

122. **Information the therapist will need before a work hardening program may begin is the:**
   A. evaluation of the individual's job site.
   B. physician's written consent and medical precautions.
   C. insurance information.
   D. individual's work history.

123. **The temperature range in which paraffin may be used comfortably without developing a film on top is:**
   A. 108 degrees F to 116 degrees F.
   B. 118 degrees F to 126 degrees F.
   C. 128 degrees F to 136 degrees F.
   D. 138 degrees F to 146 degrees F.

124. **The occupational therapist has completed the facility's assessment protocol, which includes a chart review, an interview, and a performance measure with an individual referred for psychiatric services. In writing the summary of the assessment results, the therapist will rely on the interview information to address:**
   A. the individual's diagnosis.
   B. the individual's current medications.
   C. the individual's ability to concentrate and problem solve.
   D. the individual's view of the problem and overall goal.

125. **The best performance measure for the occupational therapist observing an adult's performance. and determining that individual's sensory motor functions in a psychosocial setting is the:**
   A. Bay Area Functional Performance Evaluation (BaFPE).
   B. Schroeder Block Campbell (SBC).
   C. Southern California Sensory Integrative Test (SCSIT).
   D. Comprehensive OT Evaluation Scale (COTE).

126. **The food preparation activity that is the simplest is to:**
   A. prepare a can of soup.
   B. prepare a casserole.
   C. prepare brownies from a box mix.
   D. prepare a meal with two side dishes and an entree.

127. **An individual who is HIV positive cuts his or her finger while doing copper tooling. To follow universal precautions, the therapist should take this action:**

A. Throw the piece of copper tooling into the trash can and get the individual a new piece of copper to use.

B. Obtain the clinic's first aid kit and put a bandage on the individual's cut finger.

C. Locate a puncture resistant container that the copper piece could be placed into before disposing of it.

D. Wipe up any blood that is on the counter top with a paper towel.

128. **An adolescent individual diagnosed with this disorder is most likely to engage in aggressive and violent behavior:**

A. Asperger's disorder.

B. attention deficit disorder.

C. conduct disorder.

D. oppositional defiant disorder.

129. **The therapist working in an acute care hospital receives an occupational therapy referral for a 1-year-old child with congenital hip dislocation. The child has recently been hospitalized for skin traction prior to body casting. The initial concern of the therapist when developing a treatment plan should be:**

A. upper extremity strengthening.

B. developmental stimulation.

C. preacademic skill development.

D. activities of daily living.

130. **The approach that describes an occupational therapist's role when providing forensic psychiatry services is:**

A. helping individuals with criminal histories before they receive psychiatric medications and counseling.

B. planning and implementing recreational and leisure activities in a prison setting.

C. assessing and submitting reports determining an individual's ability to manage his or her own funds for a competency hearing.

D. providing treatment to individuals who are admitted to a locked psychiatric inpatient unit for individuals whose treatment is required by the court.

131. **Which individual's complaints and behaviors are characteristic of geriatric individuals with major depression?**

A. The individual has problems sleeping, difficulty with "thinking" or concentrating, describes oneself as "dumb" or "stupid," and feels very hopeless that things will improve.

B. The individual complains of feeling "blue" or sad, has lost interest in activities previously enjoyed, and reports decreased libido.

C. The individual's complaints focus on physical concerns, denies feeling depressed but feels less energy, has lost weight, and complains of some concentration and memory problems

D. The individual cannot correctly identify the date or their present location, does not recall where they were earlier in the day, and has difficulty sleeping during the night

132. **The occupational therapist wants to change the seating arrangement to facilitate the communication among members of a group. The best arrangement is to:**

A. provide enough chairs around a rectangle table.

B. provide enough chairs around a round table.

C. provide enough pillows to sit on the floor.

D. use the couches and chairs that are already in the room.

Case Study

Martha is an 8-year-old child who has recently been identified as having a learning disability. She had been referred to occupational therapy by an educational psychologist in the school system. Besides academic difficulties in reading and writing, she was distractible, frustrated, and easily discouraged in many of her school and home activities. Martha was given the Southern California Sensory Integration and Praxis Tests (SIPT) and the SIPT Clinical Observations of postural control and other neuromuscular responses. The results of the evaluation indicate the presence of bilateral sequencing disorder, with vestibular processing dysfunction (underreactivity). Martha showed depressed postrotary nystagmus, low muscle tone, inadequate equilibrium reactions, poor balance, difficulty with assumption of the prone extension posture, and irregular eye pursuits. There was also evidence of tactile defensiveness, and depressed visual perception scores. The school system provided sensory integration therapy through a private clinic, since her sensory integration dysfunction appeared to have a direct influence on her academic performance. Answer the following questions regarding this case study:

133. **Considering Martha's presenting sensory integration problems, which of the following goals should be considered first when developing her treatment plan?**

A. Improve eye pursuit skills

B. Improve vestibular processing

C. Improve muscle tone

D. Increase postrotary nystagmus

134. **Which of the following activities would be the most appropriate initial activity for Martha in the treatment of her tactile defensiveness?**

A. Therapist brushes her neck and face

B. Balancing on a therapy ball

C. Rolling in a carpeted barrel

D. Swinging in a hammock swing

135. **When planning treatment for Martha, the therapist should consider precautions when using a hammock swing as an activity. Which of the following observations would indicate autonomic responses indicating sensory overload during this activity?**

A. Suddenly scratching oneself
B. Spinning oneself very fast
C. Hitting one's head on the floor
D. Flushing, blanching, or perspiration

136. **The occupational therapist's goal is to select a type of game that allows group members equal opportunities to win and can be played by a variety of functional levels. The best game types to select are:**
   A. games of strategy.
   B. hobbies.
   C. games of chance.
   D. puzzles.

137. **The aspects of psychosocial performance that are important to emphasize in developing a client's work potential in a prevocational program are:**
   A. punctuality, accepting responsibility for oneself, accepting directions from a supervisor, and appropriately interacting with peer coworkers.
   B. memory, sequencing of the work tasks, and making decisions.
   C. standing tolerance, eye-hand coordination, and endurance.
   D. exploring ways to seek out available jobs and preparing a resumé.

138. **Outcome measures demonstrate the effectiveness and efficiency of a therapeutic program. What is the format generally used to collect, analyze, and report results of therapy in a rehabilitative program in relationship to costs?**
   A. Quality improvement
   B. Peer review
   C. Cost accounting
   D. Program evaluation

139. **A treatment plan or "plan of care":**
   A. specifies directions for the therapist.
   B. measures the progress towards an individual's goal.
   C. organizes the individual's priorities.
   D. summarizes the approach of management of an individual.

140. **Informed consent is:**
   A. the process of giving an individual sufficient information so that they may make an informed decision about their own health care.
   B. a clinical judgment by the therapist to implement a particular treatment on an individual.
   C. a verbal agreement made by the prospective employee to accept a job offer.
   D. written acknowledgment of ability to complete a job with or without accommodation.

141. **A program that ensures that disabled children receive educational services in the least restrictive environment is:**
   A. Americans with Disabilities Act.
   B. Education for all Handicapped Children Act.

C. Children's Protective Services.
D. Medicare.

142. **The term that best describes the relationship between an occupational therapist and a certified occupational therapy assistant is:**
   A. dependent.
   B. independent.
   C. collaborative.
   D. intuitive.

143. **An occupational therapist and a certified occupational therapy assistant share and coordinate therapy for a caseload. One of the roles that the COTA may assume would be to:**
   A. complete the chart reviews.
   B. complete the nonstandardized portions of the evaluation.
   C. interpret the results gained from the nonstandardized portion of the evaluation.
   D. independently design a treatment plan for the individual.

144. **The primary purpose of licensure is to:**
   A. delineate roles between occupational therapists and certified occupational therapy assistants.
   B. protect consumers of occupational therapy.
   C. ensure continued levels of competency of therapists.
   D. justify occupational therapy services for Medicare and Medicaid reimbursement.
   D. an exposure has NOT occurred but she will use universal precautions anyway.

145. **Functional supervision is defined as:**
   A. provision of information and feedback to coworkers.
   B. a continuum of supervision that may include close, general, and routine supervision.
   C. supervision provided on an as needed basis.
   D. supervision provided by monthly contact or on an as needed basis.

146. **The mechanism to review the results of service interventions for a population is referred to as:**
   A. a process.
   B. an outcome.
   C. program evaluation.
   D. utilization review.

147. **The format in which the delivery of services are monitored in relationship to how cost effectively the services were provided is:**
   A. a process.
   B. an outcome.
   C. program evaluation.
   D. utilization review.

148. **A therapist is completing a home assessment and making recommendations for equipment to be used in the home. He recommends a hospital bed, lightweight wheelchair, bedside commode,**

reachers, a long handled sponge, and a shower chair with a hand held shower. The item(s) that would be considered as durable medical equipment would be:
A. lightweight wheelchair and reachers.
B. shower chair with a hand held shower and bedside commode.
C. hospital bed and shower chair with a hand held shower.
D. lightweight wheelchair and hospital bed.

Case Study

In establishing an occupational therapy department, the therapist makes three separate lists of items. The first list contains a power board, one adjustable work table, two chairs with arm rests, two chairs without armrests, one mat table, one desk, and one filing cabinet. The second list includes weights, a three-speed vibrator, a skateboard, a bulb dynamometer, and a pinch meter. The third list includes long handled sponges, reachers, long handled shoe horns, therapeutic band and putty. Use the above information for the following two questions:

149. **The items on the first list would be considered:**
A. capital equipment.
B. expendable equipment.
C. adaptive equipment.
D. supplies.

150. **The items listed on the second list would be considered:**
A. capital equipment.
B. expendable equipment.
C. adaptive equipment.
D. supplies.

151. **If a 9-year-old child with sensory integration problems has not developed a preferred hand for printing or writing, the best option for the occupational therapist would be to:**
A. develop right hand skills as most children are right handed.
B. wait a few more years until the child decides for herself or himself on the preferred hand.
C. let the teacher decide on a preferred hand.
D. consider and treat underlying sensory integration problems as a possible cause.

152. **The SOAP note method of documentation is used in an acute care hospital setting to record information regarding an individual with dementia. Which statement is an example of subjective information?**
A. The therapist will establish a daily self-feeding routine using verbal and physical cues to encourage the individual to open containers on the lunch tray.
B. The individual has been able to identify closed liquid beverage containers on the meal tray for four of six presentations.

C. The individual is able to identify and drink liquids presented in cups without lids, but leaves beverages in closed containers untouched.
D. The individual asks for more beverages during meals, but appears surprised when beverages in closed containers are indicated on the meal tray.

153. **The occupational therapist selects activities appropriate for young adults on tricyclic antidepressant medications. The activity that is contraindicated is:**
A. counted cross stitch needlework projects.
B. cooking foods that include aged cheese or coffee.
C. a gross motor activity that can be graded between moderate to heavy metabolic equivalents (METS).
D. outdoor activities that include being in the direct sun.

154. **Occupational therapy services should be discontinued when:**
A. the goals have been met and the individual can no longer benefit from occupational therapy services.
B. the goals have not been met and the individual could benefit from continued occupational therapy services.
C. the goals have been met but the individual could benefit from continued occupational therapy services.
D. the individual feels that he or she has not made gains despite objective measures to the contrary.

155. **A child's caregiver asks the occupational therapist when a normal child begins to "cruise, walk sideways while holding onto a rail." The therapist reports that this is usually between the ages of:**
A. 3 and 5 months.
B. 6 and 8 months.
C. 9 and 12 months.
D. 13 and 15 months.

156. **Sensory retraining is:**
A. successful for hypersensitivity.
B. successful for hyposensitivity.
C. successful for both hyper and hyposensitivity.
D. unsuccessful for both hyper and hyposensitivity.

157. **The best description of stressors is:**
A. the process by which individuals adjust to daily stressful events within their environments.
B. the body's reactions to threat, often described as "fight or flight."
C. the precipitating conditions and events that elicit stress reactions.
D. the process of "fit" between the individual and his or her environment.

158. **When writing the results of a research project, the researcher should include:**

A. writing conclusions in the results section.
B. writing qualitative and quantitative facts in the results section.
C. writing subjective information in the results section.
D. interpretive and analytical information in the results section.

159. **Through treatment, the occupational therapist observes that the child is now developing a reflex or reaction that enables rotation of the trunk. This reflex or reaction is:**
A. neonatal neck righting.
B. asymmetrical tonic neck.
C. body righting.
D. tonic labyrinthine.

160. **A child with a learning disability has significant problems with visual memory. The therapist may use the following approach to enhance visual memory:**
A. provide memory tasks that are of low interest to the child.
B. decrease visual attention prior to memory tasks.
C. combine task with additional sensory input (i.e., tactile, proprioceptive, auditory).
D. repeat the visual memory task one time.

161. **An individual is placed on a blood thinning medication after surgery for an endarterectomy. What grooming tool will be recommended by his therapist to use in the hospital as well as after discharge?**
A. An electric razor
B. A single-blade safety razor
C. A straight razor
D. A double-blade safety razor

162. **When the therapist is assessing the sense of proprioception at an individual's joint, movement within the range should be performed:**
A. until pain is elicited.
B. until the stretch reflex is elicited.
C. at the end ranges of the joint.
D. at the midrange of the joint.

163. **A child diagnosed with autism is being evaluated by an occupational therapist. He demonstrates a decided craving for tactile stimulation by rubbing objects on his arms and legs. He also avoids being touched by others. What sensory integration problem is he demonstrating?**
A. Poor modulation of tactile input.
B. Hypersensitivity to tactile input.
C. Hyposensitivity to tactile input.
D. Poor modulation of proprioceptive input.

164. **What piece of equipment would continue to be used at home by a individual with a total hip arthroplasty?**
A. A wire basket attached to a walker
B. A padded foam toilet seat 1 inch in height
C. A short handled bath sponge
D. A long handled bath sponge

165. **An example of a nonstandardized test used by occupational therapists in a physical disabilities setting would be the:**
A. Motor Free Visual Perceptual Test.
B. Minnesota Rate of Manipulation
C. Manual Muscle Test
D. Purdue Pegboard Evaluation

166. **After a TIA, a man has demonstrated some impairments with proprioception, which has caused uneven letter formation during writing activities. Which activity would best improve his letter formation?**
A. The therapist verbally describes to him how to make a letter as he writes.
B. The man is encouraged to watch his grip during writing with a pen.
C. The man works with putty to strengthen his hand.
D. The therapist has the man trace letters through a pan of rice with his fingers.

167. **The treatment goal for a 4-year-old child with hypotonia is to improve grasp. Which of the following activities would be most appropriate to prepare the child's hand for grasp activities?**
A. Dropping blocks into a pail.
B. Placing pegs into a pegboard.
C. Weight bearing on hands.
D. Holding and eating a cookie.

168. **The part of a treatment objective that describes the performance of an individual to be changed is the:**
A. terminal behavior.
B. condition.
C. criterion.
D. plan.

169. **A man who has a fractured radial head has his elbow immobilized by a cast. He wants to maintain his strength in the affected arm, and has asked his therapist for some exercises. The therapist instructs him in performing:**
A. isometric exercises.
B. isotonic exercises.
C. progressive resistive exercises.
D. passive exercises.

Case Study

A 38-year-old woman who has been newly diagnosed with multiple sclerosis will be returning home in approximately 1 month. The woman's goal is to be performing activities from a wheelchair level within the home independently to conserve her energy. The woman plans to perform some walking in the home for short distances (10 to 15 feet) and is only able to do two to three steps with assistance.

The woman and her husband are in the process of having a house built. The husband has filled out a home assessment form for the occupational therapist to review and make suggestions for adaptations prior to the home visit. The form reveals a two-story home with a walk-in basement. The front door opens inward with an outward-opening storm door and has two steps in with a platform that is flanked by two bushes. The basement is unfinished at present with plans to finish part into a recreation room with a half bath. The unfinished area will contain a storage area, laundry room, and a place for the family's dog, an Irish setter. The first floor contains areas for the kitchen, formal dining room, breakfast nook, entry way, informal and formal living areas, office/library, and a half bath. There is also a door to the back yard with an area planned for a spa, and a changing area that is part of the garage. The second floor has four bedrooms and two full baths, with a sitting area at the top of the stairs.

The woman's 62-year-old mother, who is widowed, will be living with the family to assist her daughter as needed and to supervise the 8-year-old twin boys after school when the father and 18-year-old daughter are at work. The grandmother has arthritis in her knees, and had her right knee replaced 2 months previously, however she still uses a cane when walking. The grandmother would like to have her own separate living area to entertain her own friends.

170. The husband would like to know what the minimum width the doorways should be for adequate accessibility from either a wheelchair or a walker. The distance would be:
A. 46 cm.
B. 58 cm.
C. 70 cm.
D. 82 cm.

171. The family would like to know where to place the bedrooms for the mother and the grandmother:
A. The mother and the grandmother on the second floor
B. The mother on the first floor, the grandmother on the second floor
C. The mother on the first floor, the grandmother in the basement
D. The mother and the grandmother in the basement

172. How much space is needed around the front door to allow easy access by a wheelchair?
A. 3 feet by 5 feet
B. 4 feet by 4 feet
C. 4.5 feet by 3 feet
D. 5 feet by 5 feet

173. The family would like to place grab bars around the toilets in the house for easy access during transfers by the mother. At what height should they be placed?
A. 28 to 32 inches
B. 33 to 36 inches

C. 38 to 41 inches
D. 43 to 46 inches

174. After the occupational therapist has completed the home visit, the therapist should include in the report of the visit the:
A. outpatient therapy recommendations.
B. status of the woman at the time of discharge.
C. changes necessary for furniture arrangement.
D. appropriate method of transportation.

175. The therapist is working with an individual being treated for anxiety. The medication that the therapist would expect to see in the individual's home during an outreach home visit is:
A. Tegretol.
B. Tranxene.
C. Trilafon.
D. Tofranil.

176. What treatment program format emphasizes discharge planning in addressing mental health problems?
A. Club house
B. Community mental health center
C. Acute care hospitalization
D. Quarterway house

177. The group that is the MOST appropriate self-help group to recommend to an individual who has difficulty with alcohol:
A. Mothers Against Drunk Drivers (MADD).
B. Al-Anon.
C. Alcoholics Anonymous (AA).
D. group therapy.

178. The therapist is working in an acute care inpatient psychiatric facility. The FIRST step in planning for the discharge of a socially isolated individual is:
A. to provide community reentry activities to introduce the individual to community resources to use after discharge.
B. to evaluate the individual's occupational performance
C. to education the family about the individual's ability to return home.
D. to make a referral to an outpatient socialization program.

179. A child with sensory integration problems demonstrates hypersensitivity to movement activities by becoming nauseated and dizzy. Which of the following activities would be the most appropriate use of the large therapy ball for this child?
A. Movement in any position or direction.
B. No movement.
C. Slow and predictable movement.
D. Quick and unpredictable movement.

180. The therapist changes a tile trivet activity by providing blue-colored craft glue instead of white glue to clients who confuse the glue and grout. The therapist is using:
    A. activity analysis.
    B. activity adaptation.
    C. activity sequencing.
    D. conditional reasoning.

181. Mr. Brown is a client with the diagnosis of bipolar disorder manic episode. His behavior has changed as the week progressed. On Monday, he walked into occupational therapy and stated that his name was John F. Kennedy, and then walked out of the clinic. On Wednesday, he was able to sit briefly at the table in the OT clinic but was noticeably hypermanic and unable to work on any one craft. On Friday, Mr. Brown was able to sit with the other clients in the clinic and was cheerful, yet he jumped from topic to topic while conversing. He worked quickly on a short term craft project. The best description of this client's overall course of change is:
    A. regression.
    B. progression.
    C. decompensation.
    D. recovery.

182. Eisenmenger's complex is a life-threatening situation that must be monitored in children who have the following medical condition:
    A. rheumatic fever.
    B. ventricular septal defect.
    C. sickle-cell anemia.
    D. asthma.

183. A 6-month-old infant has begun to sit and is leaning forward onto his arms. The therapist assessing the child notes that this child is able to coactivate muscle groups around the shoulder and arm in order to bear weight on arms in sitting, or the child has developed:
    A. protective reactions.
    B. equilibrium reactions.
    C. rotational righting reactions.
    D. support reactions.

184. When adapting a tricycle for a child with cerebral palsy, the child's tendency to flex forward increases when the hip and lower extremities were positioned correctly. What further adaptation should solve this problem?
    A. Raise the seat height.
    B. Raise the handle bars.
    C. Lower the seat height.
    D. Lower the handle bars.

185. A 5-year-old child with spina bifida has developed daytime control of bowel and bladder, but not nighttime control. At what age for a typical child should the therapist consider lack of nighttime control as a delay and consider development of a therapeutic program?
    A. 2 years
    B. 3 years
    C. 4 years
    D. 5 to 6 years

186. While completing the assessment and treatment planning process, the occupational therapist confers with the individual to establish program goals. As the therapist writes these goals, they should be:
    A. specific measurable statements with time frames.
    B. time frames for what will be accomplished.
    C. specific measurements of the individual's skill and performance.
    D. activities to be completed that correspond with the goals and objectives.

187. Objectives are:
    A. specific measurable statements with time frames.
    B. time frames of what will be accomplished.
    C. specific measurements of the individual's skill and performance.
    D. statements of how the goals will be achieved.

188. After identifying a potential research question, the next step in the process is:
    A. stating the purpose.
    B. designing the research.
    C. completing a literature review.
    D. establishing boundaries for the study.

189. State organizations that were established to assure appropriate cost effective care and protect the consumer are:
    A. JCAHOs.
    B. CARFs.
    C. PROs.
    D. ARAs.

190. Changing trends in the provision of health care in society will cause:
    A. a reduction in home health services.
    B. an increase in the amount of hospitalizations.
    C. a reduction in the need of nursing homes.
    D. an increase in the amount of services available on an outpatient basis.

191. After a question or problem has been identified and a literature review completed, the researcher should:
    A. refine the question and develop the background.
    B. decide on methodology.
    C. establish boundaries for the study.
    D. collect and analyze qualitative data.

192. What type of feeding equipment would be MOST appropriate for an individual with a C5 spinal cord injury?

A. A wrist-driven flexor hinge splint
B. A mobile arm support
C. An electric self-feeder
D. Built up handled silverware

193. The therapist is working with a confused individual who has difficulty placing his feet into his pants legs. A prefunctional treatment activity would be:
A. pulling up pants during toileting activities.
B. teaching the individual to use a reacher to pull his pants up to knee level.
C. doffing socks using a dressing stick.
D. have him place his feet through loops of a therapeutic band.

194. The best assessment instrument to obtain data about an individual's stressors is:
A. to use biofeedback equipment to determine changes in muscle tension.
B. the Holmes-Rahe Life Change Index.
C. Axis V of DSM-IV.
D. the Type A Behavior Scale.

195. The occupational therapist works with an entry level COTA on an inpatient psychiatric unit. They each work 4 days a week, overlapping schedules only on Mondays. The task that would be inappropriate for the OTR to ask the COTA to do is to:
A. carry out leading the daily craft group.
B. begin the assessment process when individuals are admitted on the weekends. The OTR will finish the assessment on Monday.
C. assist individual's in carrying out their ADLs on Saturday and Sunday mornings.
D. carry out a leisure planning group on Saturday afternoon.

196. A school-aged child with residual visual perceptual problems is being discharged from occupational therapy. What compensatory technique would the therapist share with this child's teacher to assist with visual figure-ground problems?

A. Place a red line on the left side of the paper.
B. Use a timer for certain activities.
C. Teach the child to use lists and color coding of books and folders.
D. Blocks out all areas of the page except important words.

197. The primary objective of fieldwork education is to:
A. provide the student with the opportunity to apply theory to practice.
B. keep facilities abreast of state-of-the-art techniques.
C. provide financial support to the university in exchange for a student completing 3 months of affiliation.
D. support research activities.

198. A 7-year-old child with a visual perceptual problem is lacing a series of geometric beads from a stimulus card. She is unable to identify a triangle shape when the lacing bead is turned sideways on the table. This is called a problem with:
A. figure-ground perception.
B. form constancy perception.
C. visual memory.
D. visual sequencing.

199. In order to provide direct supervision for a level II fieldwork student, the supervisor MUST:
A. be a registered occupational therapist with 6 months of experience.
B. have at least 1 year of experience as a registered occupational therapist.
C. be certified by the NBCOT.
D. supervised a level one student prior to the level II student.

200. The term given to the practice of an organization acting as an intermediary between an insurance agency and a hospital is:
A. managed care.
B. utilization review
C. peer review
D. prospective payment

ANSWERS FOR SIMULATION EXAMINATION 5

1. (A) Primitive reflexes and postural reactions. The Milani-Comparetti test measures the disappearance of primitive reflexes and emergence of postural reactions. These reactions are linked to locomotor patterns. Neither cognitive nor language skills are included on this test. See reference: Case-Smith, Allen, and Pratt (eds): Nichols, DS: The development of postural control.

2. (B) Demonstrate the procedure on the unaffected extremity, then occlude the individual's vision. The presentation of stimuli in sensory evaluation is extremely important. Because of the compensation that may occur

with vision, it is necessary to occlude the individual's vision. Also, the unaffected extremity should be assessed before the affected extremity, which is the opposite of answer A, in order to reduce anxiety in the individual. Stimuli should be presented in a random proximal to distal pattern. A rapport, answer C, should be established before beginning any of the evaluation procedures to also reduce anxiety. An individual may not be aware of any deficit areas, answer D, so the whole extremity should be assessed to ensure accuracy. Picture cards are helpful in assessing individuals with expressive aphasia. See reference: Trombly (ed): Bentsel, K: Evaluation of sensation.

3. (C) The ability to engage in superficial social conversation. The onset of most dementias is slow and progressive. Cognitive abilities such as reading and writing are most often initially affected. Sensorimotor abilities such as dressing tend to follow. Superficial social abilities are often preserved until the last stages of dementia and often cover the earlier cognitive and sensorimotor changes. See reference: Bonder: Delerium and dementia.

4. (D) Universal precautions. Treating blood and some body substances as though they are contaminated is the concept of universal precautions. There are four strategies to protect an employee from potential exposure. Engineering controls modify the work environment to reduce risk of exposure. An example would be utilizing sharps containers, eye wash stations, and biohazard waste containers. Work practice controls are policies that require a procedure be done a certain way so that potential for exposure may be reduced. An example of such would be the technique for disposal of sharps using only one hand or frequent handwashing during and after patient contact. The primary prevention for exposure is handwashing. Personal protective equipment would include wearing the appropriate gear to prevent contact with blood or identified body substances. Equipment may include goggles, masks, and gowns. See reference: Hopp and Rogers: Elder, HA: Transmission of HIV and prevention of AIDS.

5. (D) Transdisciplinary. The concept of "role release" or one team member fulfilling the roles of others to ease communication with the family is called the transdisciplinary method of teamwork. Answer A is incorrect because a unidisciplinary team is not really a team since the term implies that there is only one member. Answer B is not correct because the multidisciplinary team uses several disciplines, but they may not work in a collaborative manner. Answer C is also incorrect because in the interdisciplinary team because, although it has group consensus regarding program planning, the members carry out their programs in their own environments. See reference: Case-Smith, Allen, and Pratt (eds): Humphry, R, and Case-Smith, J: Working with families.

6. (C) The individual will complete upper extremity self care with supervision of a family member and use appropriate adaptive equipment. A long-term goal is written in conjunction with the individual and family to specify the end result of a longer period of treatment. A short-term goal breaks the long-term goal into manageable steps to be accomplished by the individual within a certain time frame or number of treatment sessions. Performing upper extremity bathing, lower extremity dressing, or a commode transfer with clothing adjustment were all short increments toward the stated goal of the individual returning home with assistance of one person. See reference: Trombly: Planning, guiding, and documenting therapy.

7. (D) Cooperative group activity that both provides and elicits consistent and accurate feedback about interactions within the group. Because the underlying issues for most personality disorders are related to inaccurate perceptions of the self and others, the selected treatment approach should directly address these problems. A group format offers a wider variety of feedback about the specific interactions that occur. The group activity should be based on a central goal of reducing misperceptions. Social skills groups, answer C, are often used to address the interaction difficulties experienced with cluster C personality disorders. The question does not identify that cluster C personality disorders are included in the group. Answer B is best used for problems with individuals, not groups. Answer A addresses decision making and not inaccurate perceptions. See reference: Bonder: Personality disorders.

8. (D) Should be able to function at an entry level or above the minimum entry level of competence. It is recommended that entry level therapists practice in settings where they may be supervised by an experienced occupational therapist. Entry-level therapists are more likely to be able to receive coaching and mentoring in development of clinical skills while in settings that provide the opportunity to be supervised by an experienced OTR. See reference: AOTA: Commission on Education: Guide to Fieldwork Education.

9. (C) Petit mal. Petit mal is the correct name for a seizure that barely interrupts a child's performance. Answer A, grand mal, usually involves loss of consciousness. Answer B, psychomotor or tonic-clonic, affects automatic movements and is incorrect. Answer D, akinetic, involves loss of muscle tone and is also incorrect. See reference: Case-Smith, Allen, and Pratt (eds): Gordon, CY, Schanzenbacher, KE, Case-Smith, J, and Carrasco, RC: Diagnostic problems in pediatrics.

10. (D) Object recognition. A child must first be able to recognize an object before dealing with its specific visual attributes. Answer A is incorrect because, in developmental order, matching object characteristics or details will be the last of the visual discrimination abilities to develop. Answer C is not correct because color, shape, and position are details of visual objects that also develop last in terms of visual discrimination or ability to match objects. See reference: Kramer and Hinojosa: Todd, VR: Visual perceptual frame of reference: An information processing aproach.

11. (B) Left unilateral neglect. This is the inability to respond or orient to perceptions from the left side of the body. Evidenced as left unilateral neglect, this deficit will also be apparent in the draw-a-man test, copy a flower, house test, and completing a human figure or face puzzle. Unilateral neglect is contralateral to the side of a brain lesion, therefore, left unilateral neglect would result from right-side brain damage. Left neglect occurs most commonly in right hemisphere lesions. A cataract would cause a visual impairment with detail on both sides of a page. Bitemporal hemianopia (hemianopia is also referred to as "hemianopsia") is also known as "tunnel vision," with the individual's peripheral vision lost. The individual would still be able to cross midline with cataracts or bitemporal hemianopsia. A right neglect would not see the right side, and would draw all the figures on the left side of the page.

Visuospatial deficits are an important factor influencing functional independence outcomes. Visuospatial ability should be taken into account when establishing treatment goals as well as during discharge planning. See reference: Trombly (ed): Quintana, L: Evaluation of perception and cognition.

12. (D) Glasgow Coma Scale. The Glasgow Coma Scale rates the responses of the eye opening best motor response from 1 to 6 and verbal response from 1 to 5. The score for each area is totaled and the scale developers consider any person with a score of 8 or below to be in a coma and a score of 9 or above to be out of the comatose state. The Claudia Allen Scale of Cognitive Function is a measurement that uses task performance to evaluate a person's cognitive level of functioning. The Rancho Los Amigos Cognitive Scale uses a scale of eight levels to describe a person's behavior as he or she emerges from a coma and progresses beyond the confused state to a more purposeful and appropriate behavior. The Braintree hospital Cognitive Continuum rates a person in the five areas of arousal, attention, discrimination, organization, and higher level cognitive function. This scale demonstrates the recovery neurologically from a diffuse head injury and the person may be at a different place on the continuum according to the environment. See reference: O'Sullivan and Schmitz (eds): Mills, V: Traumatic head injury.

13. (C) Parents' needs and wishes should be included in program planning. Individual parents' needs and wishes should be considered when decisions about parental involvement in the occupational therapy program are discussed. Parents should be encouraged to observe their child in therapy so that they may better understand the program and their child's problems, therefore, answer A is incorrect. Although some parents may carry out therapy programs at home, many therapists and parents feel too much responsibility for the program may detract from normal family life and socialization. It is also recommended that both parents be present when an occupational therapy program is discussed, answer D, so that one parent does not become dependent on the other for information and communication. See reference: Case-Smith, Allen, and Pratt (eds): Humphry, R, and Case-Smith, J: Working with families.

14. (C) A heavy handbag held by the strap. The power grip is strongly based on the ulnar nerve and flexion of the ulnar fingers. The wrist is in a slightly extended position, which allows the object to be pressed firmly into the palm of the hand with the thumb in opposition. A needle would be held with two-point pinch while being threaded. A glass would be held with a cylindrical grasp. Finally, a key being placed in a lock would be held by a lateral pinch. See reference: Fess, Ewing, and Phillips: Strickland, JW: Anatomy and kinesiology of the hand.

15. (C) Initiation. Initiation or the ability to begin a task affects a person's spontaneity in performing activities and how much he or she is able to perform. An individual with initiation problems may be able to plan or carry out activities, but may be unable to begin until prompted by an-

other person. Problems with attention, concentration, or apraxia evidence as the incomplete or incorrect completion of an activity but no difficulty is noted with beginning the activity. See reference: Zoltan, Siev, and Freishtat: Cognitive deficits.

16. (B) Jebsen-Taylor Hand Function Test. This test uses seven subtests of functional activities such as writing, card turning, picking up small objects, simulated feeding activity, stacking objects, and picking up light objects and heavy objects that are large. This test may be constructed by the facility. The Purdue Pegboard Evaluation (answer A) uses a prefabricated kit. The Minnesota Rate of Manipulation (answer C) and the Crawford Small Parts Dexterity Test (answer D) are all prefabricated kits. The Purdue Pegboard Evaluation and the Crawford Small Parts Dexterity Test involve assembly tasks using pins and collars with other items. The Minnesota Rate of Manipulation uses colored plastic disks that nest in a board. See reference: O'Sullivan and Schmitz: Schmitz, T: Coordination assessment.

17. (B) Public school system. The IEP is the required plan for children receiving special education in public school systems. It is a document that incorporates the child's needs and the occupational therapist contributes his or her evaluation of the child as well as educational objectives. Answers A, C, and D are incorrect because they each have different methods of coordinating a plan for a child, none of which are called an IEP. See reference: Hopkins and Smith (eds): Kauffman, NA: Occupational therapy in school systems.

18. (B) Two. A person in stage two of Brunnstrom's level of recovery would have weak, associated movements usually seen in a flexor synergy. Also there may be little or no finger flexion occurring. A person in stage one, answer A, would have no movement or spasticity on the affected side of the body. Stage three, answer C, has all movements occurring in synergy with definite spasticity noted and mass grasp in the affected hand. In stage four, answer D, a person would be able to have decreasing spasticity with some deviation from synergistic patterns with the person's hand demonstrating lateral prehension and partial finger extension. See reference: Rothstein, Serg, and Wolf: Neuroanatomy, neurology, and neurologic therapy.

19. (C) Criteria. The criteria is the method by which the level of an individual's performance will be measured in the treatment objective. The terminal behavior is the change an individual must demonstrate through performance or behavior. The condition is the circumstances under which the individual will perform. The plan is the approach used to reach a treatment objective. See reference: Pedretti (ed): Foti, D, and Pedretti, L: Activities of daily living.

20. (B) Fold or put laundry on a hanger while standing. A prevocational activity is an activity when performed by a person that could lead to the evaluation or training of work related skills. A cashier would be standing for much of the job, removing clothing from hangers, folding the clothing to place in a bag, and then running the price tags through the scanner before finally totaling them on the cash register and making change. Activities performed while sitting, such as making a grocery list, answer A, or adding a column of numbers by hand, answer D, would not be activities related to her present employment. Washing dishes while standing, answer C, incorporates the standing aspect of her job; however, washing dishes would not be related to it. See reference: Pedretti (ed): Foti, D, and Pedretti, L: Activities of daily living.

21. (A) Abnormal muscle tone. The literature addresses splinting for adults with abnormal tone, but only a few articles have been written about children. More articles have been written about splinting of children's hands where muscle weakness, answer B, traumatic injury, answer C, and joint inflammation, answer D, exist. See reference: Case-Smith, Allen, and Pratt (eds): Exner, CE: Development of hand skills.

22. (B) EMG biofeedback training combined with relaxation training. All of the answers describe stress management techniques. EMG biofeedback provides the individual with information about his or her muscle tension levels, whereas relaxation techniques are strategies to reduce muscle tension. Answer A is for individuals who are unable to distinguish between assertive and aggressive behaviors, and therefore do not respond assertively when necessary. Answer C is for individuals whose irrational beliefs and thought processes lead to maladaptive behaviors. Answer D is for individuals who have difficulty selecting effective solutions or identifying the source of their problems. See reference: Christiansen and Baum (eds): Christiansen, C: Performance deficits as sources of stress—Coping theory and occupational therapy.

23. (B) Activity of daily living groups. Activity of daily living groups are used by 17% of therapists using a group format. This group format is most often used in psychosocial settings and rehabilitation centers. Concerns often addressed in these groups were self-care skill development and predischarge living skills. See reference: Howe and Schwartzberg: Current practice in occupational therapy.

24. (B) To show acceptance and understanding to the individual. Paraphrasing is used to clarify and relay acceptance of what an individual has communicated. Paraphrasing is in the therapist's own words versus repeating what the individual stated. Answer A is the purpose of clarifying whereas answer D is the purpose of probing. Answer C describes the paraphrasing technique but is not a purpose. See reference: Denton: Effective communication.

25. (C) 8 months. This is correct because 3 months (number of months premature) are usually subtracted from the child's chronologic age to adjust for prematurity. This child is then given the benefit of time lost because of a shorter gestation period. See reference: Dunn (ed): Cook, DG: The assessment process.

26. (B) Affective disorders. Affective disorders are problem areas addressed by 22 percent of mental health occupational therapists. Adjustment disorders and alcohol use make up approximately 5 percent of the problems treated. Anxiety disorders are problem areas with less than 1 percent of the patients. See reference: Hopkins and Smith (eds): Richert, GZ, and Gibson, D: Practice settings.

27. (C) "I'm just too tired." One of the main symptoms of depression is decreased energy, therefore, the response of "I'm too tired" indicates fatigue. Answers A and B are responses reflecting the individuals perceptions of their ability or competence. Answer D is a response reflecting interests or values that conflict with the proposed activity. See reference: Bonder: Mood disorders.

28. (D) Sheltered workshops. Sheltered workshops are the most available vocational service for adults with mental retardation. Although supported employment and job coaching may be preferred, they are not commonly available. Adult activity centers do not emphasize vocational goals. See reference: Hopkins and Smith (eds): Humphrey, R, and Jacobs, K: Mental retardation.

29. (D) Accommodation. The child demonstrates a problem with visual accommodation, or the ability to focus from near to far distance and vice versa efficiently. Answer A, ocular motility, refers to the ability to pursue an object visually in an efficient and smooth manner. Answer B, binocular vision, is described as the ability to focus the eyes on an object at varying distances and seeing a single object clearly. Answer C, convergence, is the ability to move the eyes inward or outward with continued focus on the object. See reference: Kramer and Hinojosa: Todd, VR: Visual perceptual frame of reference: An information processing approach.

30. (D) Disorganized psychosis. Directive group treatment is a highly structured approach that is used in acute care psychiatry for minimally functioning individuals. This approach is useful for disorganized and disturbed functioning with psychoses and other neurologic disorders. Task groups are more appropriate for substance abuse. Psychoeducation groups are appropriate for eating disorders and adjustment disorders. See reference: Hopkins and Smith (eds): Beck, NL: Substance abuse: Drug addiction and alcoholism.

31. (A) Allows the therapist to obtain facts. Fact gathering is the primary advantage to closed questions. The occupational therapist should be aware that posing mostly closed questions can lead to biased information gathering, as with answers B and D. Although you can generally ask more closed questions in a short amount of time, this is generally not a patient-focused goal. See reference: Denton: Effective communication.

32. (D) Narrative reasoning. Narrative reasoning is a form of story telling in which therapists share similar experiences, allowing for problem solving to occur. Procedural reasoning is the process of identifying a particular treatment or procedure which meets the need of a condition. Conditional reasoning is a form of clinical reasoning which takes into account various systems and dynamics involved with the patient and their illness or injury. This approach is more "holistic" in that takes into account the "whole patient" as they function and interact within their environment. Interactive reasoning is a process by which the therapist and patient collaborate so that the therapist may better understand the patient's environment or situation. See reference: Mattingly and Fleming: Fleming, MH: The therapist with the three-track mind.

33. (A) Arrhythmic and unexpected. The characteristics of facilitory sensory input are unexpected, arrhythmic, uneven, or rapid input. Therefore answer A is correct because it contains two of these four features. Answer B is not correct because, although arrhythmic input is excitatory, slow sensory input is inhibitory. Answer C is not correct because sustained and slow sensory input is inhibitory. Answer D is incorrect because although facilitory input is unexpected, rhythmic input is inhibitory. Also, according to these authors, sensory integration treatment is complex and highly individualized, and must be monitored carefully to observe the effects of sensory input of varying types on the individual child. See reference: Hopkins and Smith (eds): Kinnealey, M, and Miller, L: Sensory integration/Learning disabilities.

34. (A) 2 years. A powered wheelchair that provides rapid mobility to the nonambulatory child can be considered as early as 18 months. Because an 18-month-old child can direct his body through space safely, a nonambulatory child of the same age should also be able to direct a wheelchair. Answers B, C, and D are incorrect because the power wheelchair can first be considered at a much earlier age. See reference: Kramer and Hinojosa (eds): Colangelo, CA: Biomechanical frame of reference.

35. (C) The individual's level of psychosocial and occupational limitations. GAF is an overall rating of an individual's psychosocial and occupational functioning. Answer A describes the emphasis of Axis IV. Answer B describes the Axis III diagnosis. Answer D describes the Axis II diagnosis. See reference: Psychiatric diagnosis and the classification system.

36. (B) Client will use facial expressions and gestures that are consistent with stated emotions during assertive, passive, and aggressive role play situations. According to the Uniform Terminology, self expression is the use of a variety of styles and skills to express and vary thoughts, feelings, and needs. Being able to vary one's expression during three different styles of expressing feelings is an example of this. Identifying pleasurable activities is an example of interests. Recognition of one's behaviors and consequences is self control. Identifying one's own assets and limitations is related to self concept. See reference: Bonder: Appendix B—Uniform terminology for reporting occupational therapy services.

37. (C) Discharge planning group. Discharge planning group is a thematic group that helps patients gain knowl-

edge, skills, and attitudes needed for posthospital situations. Exercise group is considered to be an instrument group. Evaluation groups are not considered to be thematic groups. A self expression group with poetry is the cooperative level of a developmental group. See reference: Mosey: Activity-based groups.

38. (D) "When I apply for jobs what should I put down when it asks if you have been hospitalized or treated for anything in the past 6 months?" Stigma are indications that one has a history of a disorder. Generally, psychiatric treatment involves negative reactions to such a history, especially from employers. Identifying potential situations where stigma occurs and problem solving around such issues is an important part of discharge planning. The cigarette smoke and complaining relative comments are linked to assertiveness. The medication comment is linked to the client's (mis)understanding of what strategies for dealing with side effects. See reference: Hughes and Mullins: Discharge preparation.

39. (A) A diagnostic related group (DRG). DRGs are a part of the prospective payment system established by Medicare. Because this patient is over 65, she would qualify under Medicare. An FRG is not in effect as of the printing of this guide. However, this term relates to groups of patients categorized by diagnosis that are admitted to rehabilitation facilities. Medicaid, answer C, is incorrect because this population is poor and indigent. Answer D is partially correct because if the woman involved did have insurance, it would be used; however, it would be considered the secondary insurance and Medicare would be the primary provider. See reference: Bair and Gray (eds): Scott, SJ, and Somers, FP: Payment for occupational therapy services.

40. (A) DRGs. Diagnostic categories were defined in order to establish the level of payment per diagnosis. The intent of government was to impose constraints on health care spending for the beneficiaries of Medicare. PROs were established to numerically assess unnecessary procedures, client and patient deaths, and substandard care. UB-82s are forms that must be completed on each patient listing their diagnosis and comorbidity information for the purpose of reimbursement. Cost shifting is what occurs when a hospital increases its prices to all customers in order to make up for the shortfall of reimbursement by a few providers. See reference: Bair and Gray (eds): Scott, SJ, and Somers, FP: Payment for occupational therapy services.

41. (A) Inpatient hospitalization. Medicare was established in 1965 by an act of congress as Title VIII of the Social Security Act. The program consists of two parts. Part A pays for inpatient hospitalization, skilled care, and hospice services. Medicare part B covers answers B, C, and D. These are in home occupational therapy (psychiatric), outpatient occupational therapy, and comprehensive outpatient therapy. All of these services are physician and other professional medical services. See reference: Bair and Gray (eds): Scott, SJ, and Somers, FP: Payment for occupational therapy services.

42. (C) Workers' compensation or Medicaid. Workers' compensation is a state-supported program into which employers pay. Medicaid is a joint state and federal program that provides coverage for the poor and medically indigent. Medicare, answer A, is a federal program for health care coverage for individuals 65 years or older, disabled individuals, or people in end stage renal failure. The Education for All Handicapped Children is assisted through the provision of state and federal grants. Therefore, answers B and D are incorrect. See reference: Bair and Gray (eds): Scott, SJ, and Somers, FP: Payment for occupational therapy services.

43. (B) A physician's referral. Within acute care hospital settings, it is necessary to gain a physician referral to meet accrediting agency regulations and for third party reimbursement. Therefore, answers A, C, and D are incorrect. However, when in other settings, the occupational therapist may respond to a request for service and initiate services based on his or her own judgment. See reference: Reed and Sanderson: Referral or prescription.

44. (B) High risk. Because of the seriousness of high-risk areas, it is vital to continue monitoring secondary to the serious consequences. A consequence is a result of an occurrence within a specified monitor. An example would be a patient falling in the ADL shower. One incident could have serious consequences. Therefore, even if this area did not have any incidents, it may continue to be monitored on an ongoing basis. However, when high volume or incidence or problem prone areas achieve 100 percent, the quality issue is resolved. When this occurs, new monitors of quality care may be established. See reference: Hopkins and Smith (eds): Perinchief, JM: Service management.

45. (C) Assist with stock and inventory control. Volunteer interaction within an occupational therapy department should be limited so that it is in the direct line of vision of an occupational therapist. In addition, it is not appropriate for volunteers to treat a patient in that they lack the skill and expertise of an occupational therapist. Answer D is incorrect because it violates the confidentiality of the patient. See reference: Reed and Sanderson: Direct service functions.

46. (D) Health promotion. Health promotion is the advancement of healthy lifestyles, which may include education, behavioral change, and cultural support. Answer A, occupational behavior, is the developmental continuum of play to work. Answer B, synchrony, is actually the provision of treatment. Answer C, self efficacy, would be promoting the positive effects of occupational therapy services. See reference: Hopkins and Smith (eds): Levy, LL: The health care delivery system today.

47. (A) There is an increasing shortage of occupational therapy practitioners in the area of mental health. Current trends in mental health to use recreational, music, and art therapists has reduced the demand for occupational therapists in the mental health environment. In addition, an increasing number of therapists are pursuing positions in pediatrics and physical disabilities. These two issues combined are causing a current shortage of occupational therapy practitioners in the mental health setting. The inverse is true of answers B, C, and D, therefore making them incorrect. See reference: Hopkins and Smith (eds): Gibson, D, and Richert, G: Mental health: The therapeutic process.

48. (A) The concept of two therapists performing the same procedure will gain the same results. The term service competency indicates an interrater reliability between two occupational therapy professionals. Therefore answers C and D are incorrect. In addition, service competence is not gained through passing the certification examination. Service competency is necessary as an entry level therapist begins to function in an occupational therapy department to establish the same procedure for those tasks that may require more skill. This concept is also vital in the COTA/OTR relationship in that the OTR is ultimately responsible for the information gained and reported by the COTA. See reference: AOTA: The Occupational Therapy Roles Task Force: Occupational Therapy Roles.

49. (C) A productivity report. Productivity information is the primary indicator for need of additional staff. These data take into account the use of staff resources (productive hours versus nonproductive hours) compared with the services generated within a department. A cost accounting report, answer A, is a compilation of all of the services provided to an individual. This would include occupational therapy as well as any additional services provided. Because a cost accounting report includes other departments, it is not a good source of data for justifying additional occupational therapy support. A definition of Relative Value Units (RVUs) report, answer B, is often used as part of a cost accounting system. It includes data of the services provided, the cost per unit for time and materials, and the variable cost per unit. A market analysis, answer D, is an assessment of the ability of a facility to provide a service to a given population or region. See reference: Jacobs and Logigian: Logigian, M: Cost accounting.

50. (A) A problem with learning new motor skills. Answer A describes the central problem of dyspraxia—difficulty in performing skills not previously mastered, where motor planning is required. Answers C and D are incorrect because, although neuromuscular, reflex integration and balance problems may be present with developmental dyspraxia, they are not problems of praxis or motor planning. Answers C and D are also automatic motor activities and dyspraxia is a problem of mastering activities that must be learned. See reference: Case-Smith, Allen, and Pratt (eds): Parham, LD, and Mailloux, Z: Sensory integration.

51. (D) Landau reaction. The Landau reaction is stimulated by the lifting of the head when the child is suspended horizontally. Extensor tone is created throughout the body and is needed for sitting and standing. The tonic labyrinthine reflex in prone involves body flexion. The asymmetrical tonic neck reflex is characterized by flexion on the face side and extension on the skull side with head turning. The neck righting reaction is characterized by head and body alignment on the rotational axis. None of the latter answers develop normal extensor tone. See reference: Hopkins and Smith (eds): Simon, CJ, and Daub, MM: Human development across the lifespan.

52. (B) Receptive aphasia. Individuals with receptive aphasia are unable to comprehend spoken or written words and symbols. Therefore, they cannot accurately understand verbal directions or consistently respond to stimuli. Individuals with receptive aphasia may be able to imitate and follow demonstration. However, these techniques may not be used with a sensory evaluation. Expressive aphasia interferes with an individual's verbal or written expression but not comprehension of verbal or written information. An individual with expressive aphasia would be able to indicate the response by pointing to the stimulus used or a card that has been marked with the correct response. An individual who has agnosia or ataxia would be able to understand directions, but would be unable to accurately indicate an area due to impaired recognition of the body part or impaired coordination. The method of response may be adapted by using verbal description of an area or cue cards. See reference: Trombly (ed): Woodson, AM: Stroke.

53. (D) Parachek Geriatric Rating Scale. The Parachek Geriatric Rating Scale is a 10-item screening instrument that can be completed in approximately 5 minutes by those familiar with the individual's daily behaviors. The protocol for this assessment also contains suggested interventions appropriate for the score levels derived from this assessment. The BafPE and COTE are direct observations of an individual's performance. The Role Checklist involves a self-assessment format. See reference: Christiansen and Baum (eds): Christiansen, C: Occupational performance assessment.

54. (B) The COTA updating the occupational therapist on the improvements that the patient has made in the past week and both therapists providing information to update the goals. A collaborative relationship between an occupational therapist and the assistant supports sharing of information and utilization of each professional's skills. In this type of relationship, communication is two-way and both individuals work as a team to the benefit of the patient. Answers A and D demonstrate one-way communication with the therapist telling the assistant what to do. Answer C is incorrect in that the therapist only taking information off of the progress note does not allow for feedback or input of the COTA into the patient's discharge status or discharge disposition and recommendations. See reference: AOTA: The Occupational Therapy Roles Task Force: Occupational Therapy Roles.

55. (D) Passive movement followed by slow, rhythmical movement. Therapy for the child with spasticity should include the neurodevelopmental treatment principle of passive movement to reduce tone. This is important because this type of movement will initially elongate the muscles and prepare the child for gentle movement such as rocking on a therapy ball in prone to further reduce tone. Answer A is wrong because it is the treatment principle for children with low muscle tone, who need the additional tactile and proprioceptive input of weight bearing and compression with movement. Answer B is wrong because it is the principle underlying treatment of low to normal muscle tone or ataxia, where the child needs to move to develop righting and balance reactions, without losing stability. Answer C is wrong because it applies to the treatment of children with athetosis who move too much in very asymmetrical patterns. See reference: Hopkins and Smith (eds): Erhardt, RP: Cerebral palsy.

56. (D) Consistent and appropriate use of adaptive equipment. Many factors are considered when a long-term goal is reset. These factors may include items such as consistency, cognitive or perceptual impairments, the amount of time required, or any change in attention or concentration. For the long-term goal to be changed, the individual would need to be able to demonstrate consistency of performance, since improved memory and increased performance have already been demonstrated. The amount of time needed or concentration have not been problems or they would have been part of the goal originally. The ability to remember two of three hip precautions does not demonstrate improved memory, so the long-term goal would not change. See reference: Kovich and Bermann (eds): Head Injury: A Guide to Functional Outcomes in Occupational Therapy.

57. (A) Provide a variety of therapeutic sports, arts, crafts, music, and recreation activities to develop and reinforce healthy interest patterns. Differences among psychiatric service providers should be based on roles versus the media and modalities used. Answer B is the role of educational disciplines, answer C is the role of occupational therapy, and answer D is the role of vocational rehabilitation. Effective program planning is based on a clear understanding of the contributions of all the service providers within a team. See reference: Fidler: Program services.

58. (B) Fidelity. Fidelity is defined as "remaining faithful to the patient's best interest." This includes statements regarding the confidentiality of patient information. Answer A, informed consent, is in reference to the rights of individuals to be provided information regarding their health care as well as to make choices about their own health care. Answer C, beneficence, is the concept of striving to bring about the best possible outcome for patients served through treatment modalities. Answer D, nonmaleficence, is defined as the obligation of the therapist to deliberately create a situation or cause harm or injury to a patient. See reference: Jacobs and Logigian: Bloom, G: Ethics.

59. (A) Semicircular canals. Although the vestibular system functions are not completely understood, it is generally believed that the semicircular canals receive sensory information about motion. The utricle and saccule receive sensory information about gravity. The cochlea receives auditory sensory information. See reference: Ayres: The nervous system within.

60. (B) Visual attention skills. Development of visual attention skills should be worked on first as they prepare and provide foundation skills for other aspects of visual perception. Answer A is incorrect because visual memory skills can only be developed after visual attention skills are established. Answers C and D are incorrect because general and specific visual perceptual skills develop after visual memory. See reference: Kramer and Hinojosa: Todd, VR: Visual perceptual frame of reference: An information processing aproach.

61. (A) A ratio of 2:1 as the humerus moves on the scapula. This is accomplished as the arm is abducted. For every 20 degrees of movement in the humerus, 10 degrees of movement will occur in the scapula. See reference: Cailliet: Functional anatomy. In *Shoulder Pain.*

62. (D) Decreased attention. An attention deficit would be discovered if the person recognizes the letter, marks it accurately throughout the page on the right and left sides, but misses letters in a random pattern. Visual field cuts (answers A and B) would be evidenced by the missed letters appearing close together in one area. Functional illiteracy (answer C) would either be determined prior to the test, during the interview prior to evaluation, or from the chart review, and a more appropriate test would be administered. The person with functional illiteracy may also be able to complete the task accurately or mark additional letters depending on the level of illiteracy. See reference: Trombly (ed): Quintana, LA: Remediating cognitive impairments.

63. (C) Reflex maturation is significantly delayed. The Moro reflex should be integrated before 5 to 6 months of age. Because this child is 13 months old, this represents a significant delay. Answer A is incorrect because the child has not integrated a reflex at 13 months that should have been absent by 6 months. Answer B is incorrect because an 8-month delay in reflex maturation is a significant delay. Answer D is also incorrect because all primitive reflexes (including the Moro reflex) should have been integrated by 6 months. Therefore reflex integration could not be "advanced" when primitive patterns are still present at 13 months. See reference: Hopkins and Smith (eds): Simon, CJ, and Daub, MM: Human development across the lifespan.

64. (A) Soft to hard to rough. Hypersensitivity stimuli is graded by texture and force. Texture begins with soft, progresses to hard, and finally to rough. The force begins with touch, progresses to rub, and then to tapping. The texture and force of the stimuli are graded together. Light, medium, and heavy do not specify what the texture and force of the stimuli would be during training. A person with hypersensitivity would be unable to tolerate training beginning with a rough texture. See reference: Trombly (ed): Bentzel, K: Remediating sensory impairment.

65. (B) Light stroking, fast brushing, quick stretch. Facilitation techniques are used to stimulate the muscle to provide a specific response, such as to improve postural control or to evoke a movement. Some of the facilitory techniques are light stroking, fast brushing, and quick stretch. Any techniques that use slower movement or warmth act as inhibitory techniques in the Rood approach, such as slow stroking or rolling and neutral warmth. In addition, prolonged icing may act as an inhibitor. See reference: Trombly: Rood approach.

66. (C) Have the individual set the utensil down until the mouth is cleared. The individual needs to the establish a routine to pace him or herself during feeding. This skill may then be used after discharge from therapy. An individual with problems relating to the rate of intake will put too much food in the mouth in spite of the size of the pieces. An impulsive person who eats too fast will also have difficulty counting slowly enough to have the mouth cleared by the time the count of 10 is reached. Food in separate containers would slow the meal down if they were presented one at a time, but not slow the rate of food intake. See reference: Kovich and Bermann (eds): Van Dam-Burke, A, and Kovich, K: Self-care and homemaking.

67. (A) Translation. Translation is the linear movement of the object from the palm to fingers. Answer B, shift, is incorrect because this type of in-hand manipulation is the movement of an object between or among the fingers. Answer C, rotation, is incorrect because this type of in-hand manipulation rolls the object horizontally or end-over-end between the finger pads. Answer D, stabilization, is incorrect because it is not one of the three types of in-hand manipulations. See reference: Case-Smith, Allen, and Pratt (eds): Exner, CE: Development of hand skills.

68. (B) Initiation. Initiation problems are often seen when an individual is unable to perform the first step of an activity without requiring prompting. A problem with impulsiveness during self-care would be seen by attempting to complete many steps of an activity rapidly, requiring slowing the rate for safety reasons. Memory or attention problems are seen by skipping the steps of an activity either because he or she does not remember the steps or is distracted by internal or external stimuli. Memory deficits are also evidenced as steps of a task not performed in sequence. The lack of initiation (the ability to begin a task) will affect a person's spontaneity in performing activities. The individual with initiation problems may be able to plan or carry out activities, but may be unable to begin until prompted by someone else. An individual who has difficulty with impulsivity, memory, or attention would have no difficulty with beginning the activity, but would have difficulty listing the steps. See reference: Kovich and Bermann (eds): Bermann, D: Treatment of sensory-perceptual and cognitive deficits.

69. (C) 6 weeks. During the acute stage of injury, healing will take place from 1 to 3 weeks (answers A and B, respectively). By 6 weeks, answer C, healing should have occurred enough to allow a resumption of most functional activities with pain noted as discomfort if it is present. If significant pain with impairment continues after 6 weeks, then this contributes to a diagnosis of chronic pain made by the physician. After trauma has occurred, at 9 weeks, answer D, there would have been enough healing after the initial acute trauma so that only an occasional twinge of discomfort may be felt. See reference: Cailliet: Subluxations of the cervical spine: The whiplash syndromes. In *Shoulder Pain.*

70. (A) Sequencing of picture symbols. A person would need to use picture symbols to indicate a two or more part thought or sequence of activities. For example, pointing to pictures of a shoe and a closet would indicate the place to find a shoe in response to a question from someone. Understanding letters or words (answers B and C, respectively) and then sequencing them (answer D) are significantly higher level skills than recognizing and sequencing pictures. See reference: Church and Glennen: Glennen, S: Augmentative and alternative communication.

71. (C) Wedge-shaped seat that is higher in front. A wedge-shaped seat insertion will increase hip flexion more than 90 degrees, which is inhibitory to an extensor pattern. Answer A is incorrect because lateral trunk supports will support the trunk from sideward movement only. Answer B is incorrect because a seat belt at the hips will hold a child in a chair, but cannot inhibit an extension pattern. Answer D is incorrect because although it may contribute to holding a child in a chair, it does not affect the angle of the hip joint, which is necessary to decreasing extensor tone in sitting. See reference: Case-Smith, Allen, and Pratt (eds): Shepherd, J, Procter, SA, and Coley IL: Self-care and adaptations for independent living.

72. (C) Is performed in a comfortable position. An activity is performed for a greater length of time and more effectively when the person is able to perform the activity in a comfortable position, answer C. If the activity is adapted in a complicated manner, answer A, is monotonous, answer D, or needs frequent adjustment by the occupational therapist, answer B, then the activity will appeal to the person for a shorter length of time and cause frustration sooner to the person and the therapist. See reference: Pedretti (ed): Pedretti, L, and Wade, I: Therapeutic modalities.

73. (D) Batting a balloon. An activity such as batting a balloon may be graded for improving a strength by adding resistance to the arm in the form of weights, and endurance may be improved by adding more repetitions of the movement. Passive range of motion, answer A, and Codman's exercises, answer B, are both using passive movements of the upper extremities. A person who pops a balloon, answer C, would be able to increase the resistance needed for upper extremity performance by adding weight to the arms or using a balloon with thicker rubber. However, there would not be an appropriate method to increase the number of repetitions, since the repeated noise would be annoying. See reference: Pedretti (ed): Pedretti, L, and Wade, I: Therapeutic modalities.

74. (B) Remote memory. The ability to recall events from one's distant past is remote memory and is commonly assessed through verbal interviews and informal testing such as this question about an individual's recall of childhood events. Retention is determined by giving the individual information and asking about the same information a few minutes later. Orientation is determined by asking about the current time and date. Recent memory is determined by asking about meals eaten that day. See reference: Christiansen and Baum (eds): Cognitive dimensions of performance.

75. (C) Developing the group. Facilitating discussion based on similarities that are seen on the completion of an activity are aspects of the development phase. The opening phase (answer A) generally includes introducing member names, group goals, and expected length of the group. Answer B, processing, is not a phase of group development. Processing is reflecting on the group with another therapist after the group session. Answer D, group closure, involves restating the purpose as well as giving and receiving feedback. See reference: Borg and Bruce: Through put—The group as a system of change.

76. (B) Photosensitivity. Photosensitivity is a side effect of neuroleptic medications that increases the reactions one has to the sun. Answers A and D are also known to be side effects of neuroleptic but would generally not be problematic for a community outing. Answer C is not a side effect of these medications. See reference: Hopkins and Smith (eds): Gibson, D, and Richert, GZ: The therapeutic process.

77. (B) A therapeutic device in helping. How the occupational therapist uses "the self" is a tool in the therapy process but is not the central focus of the therapy. The therapeutic use of self has a few qualities of a friendship but also requires the therapist to understand and manage some of their reactions. Empathy, not sympathy, is recommended in the therapeutic relationships. See reference: Hopkins and Smith (eds): Schwartzberg, SL: Therapeutic use of self.

78. (C) Major impairment in several areas (e.g., defiant at home and failing at school). Axis V of DSM-IV contains information about overall level of function and can be measured with GAF. GAF is the individual's Global Assessment of Functioning score. GAF is a numerical scale ranging from persistent danger of hurting self (1) to superior functioning (100). Major impairments are scored between 31 and 40. Answer A would be a score between 71 and 80. Answer B would be score between 51 and 60. Answer D would be scored between 21 and 30. See reference: American Psychiatric Association: Multiaxial assessment.

79. (C) Constructional. Constructional play involves building and creating things and it is in this area of play that the child particularly develops a sense of mastery and problem-solving skills. Answer A is not correct because sensorimotor play primarily develops a child's body awareness and sensory experiences. Answer B is not correct because imaginary play involves manipulating people and objects in fantasy as a prelude to dealing with reality. Answer D is not correct because the child is primarily learning rules through games and play. See reference: Kramer and Hinojosa (eds): Olsen, L: Psychosocial frame of reference.

80. (D) Thorazine.   Thorazine is an antipsychotic medication. Lithium, answer A, and Elavil, answer B, are used to treat mood disorders. Xanax, answer C, is an antianxiety medication. See reference: Hopkins and Smith (eds): Gibson, D, and Richert, GZ: The evolution of occupational therapy.

81. (C) Assertiveness training.   Broken record is a specific assertiveness skill concerned with repeating your position without losing control. Music therapy is a creative arts discipline. Psychodrama is a group technique for expressing catharsis. Self-awareness groups tend to focus on feeling identification and expression versus skill building. See reference: Posthuma: Appendix A.

82. (D) Smoking during the group is prohibited.   Norms are guidelines for behavior in groups, whether stated explicitly or implicitly shared by the members. Answer A is an individual's behavior versus the group's guidelines. Answer B is a group activity. Answer C is a general group goal. See reference: Posthuma: Groups and norms.

83. (A) Polyarticular.   Because Janet's condition had a sudden onset, she has several joints involved and has a low grade fever, she demonstrates the signs and symptoms of the polyarticular form of JRA. Answer B is not correct because the systemic type of JRA is characterized by a high grade fever and involvement of the lymph nodes and spleen. Answer C is not correct because there are only a few joints involved with pauciarticular JRA. And, because Still's disease is another name for systemic JRA, this answer is also not correct. See reference: Case-Smith, Allen, and Pratt (eds): Gordon, CY, Schanzenbacher, KE, Case-Smith, J, and Carrasco, RC: Diagnostic problems in pediatrics.

84. (D) 15 percent.   Only 15 percent of children diagnosed with JRA have a remaining permanent disability. See reference: Case-Smith, Allen, and Pratt (eds): Gordon, CY, Schanzenbacher, KE, Case-Smith, J, and Carrasco, RC: Diagnostic problems in pediatrics.

85. (B) Information on JRA.   According to Schanzenbacher, the most essential information for parents and teachers to receive from the occupational therapist is information on JRA. Information on the occupational therapy evaluation and treatment program are of lesser importance. (Answers A, C, and D are less important.) See reference: Case-Smith, Allen, and Pratt (eds): Gordon, CY, Schanzenbacher, KE, Case-Smith, J, and Carrasco, RC: Diagnostic problems in pediatrics.

86. (C) Prevent deformity.   A child with JRA will need splinting to prevent deformity and maintain range of motion. Answer A is not correct because hypertonus is not a characteristic of this condition. Answer B is not correct because, due to the active nature of the child's condition, increasing range of motion may be contraindicated. The correction of deformity may also be contraindicated with this child due to the active nature of her disease. Therefore, answer D is not correct. See reference: Case-Smith, Allen, and Pratt (eds): Gordon, CY, Schanzenbacher, KE, Case-Smith, J, and Carrasco, RC: Diagnostic problems in pediatrics.

87. (C) Pencil gripper.   These are all adaptive devices that can be used with a child who has JRA. However, the correct answer is C, because the pencil gripper will probably make grasping the pencil easier and reduce hand grasp fatigue. This adaptation is needed because of weak hands and because printing and handwriting are common tasks for this child's age. It is important that fatigue be reduced with these children. The reacher, answer A, is not correct because it frequently requires grasp strength even though it does adapt for children who have problems with extended reach. The jar opener, answer B, is not incorrect in terms of its adaptation for hand strength problems, but it is not a frequent task performed by a school-aged child (such as handwriting). The plate guard, answer C, will provide adaptation for coordination, one-handedness, and lack of hand and arm movements, but is not particularly necessary when hand strength is decreased (adapting the utensil handle would be more reasonable). See reference: Case-Smith, Allen, and Pratt (eds): Gordon, CY, Schanzenbacher, KE, Case-Smith, J, and Carrasco, RC: Diagnostic problems in pediatrics.

88. (C) Self concept.   Self concept is defined as the value of one's physical and emotional self. Stating one's strengths and limitations about one's own performance is a reflection of an individual's self concept. Values are more globally stated ideas or beliefs such as being a "perfectionist." Termination of the activity involves knowing who to stop working on the activity. See reference: Bonder: Appendix B—Uniform terminology for reporting occupational therapy services.

89. (D) Each member will remain in the group without disrupting the work of others for 30 minutes.   People who are in parallel groups do not have the ability to interact with the other group members other than some casual greetings. Therefore, appropriate expectations for parallel groups focus on remaining in the group and working alongside others. Taking leadership roles is a goal consistent with egocentric-cooperative groups. Sharing materials with some of the other group members is a project group goal. Expressing feelings within a group is consistent with a cooperative group. See reference: Mosey: Recapitulation of ontogenesis.

90. (D) Encouragement to begin involvement in girl or boy scouts.   Parents of children with severe psychiatric conditions tend to either over or underestimate their child's play and social interaction skills. It is important for occupational therapists to provide education to parents about realistic expectations. Organized activities that are peer focused, for example scouts, are often important to 8-

and 9-year-old children. Competition is more appropriate for 10- to 12-year-olds and would be an "overestimation" of skills. Board games with rule changes and focusing on playing by the rules are examples of underestimating the skills of the eight year old. See reference: Hopkins and Smith (eds): Florey, LL: Psychiatric disorders in childhood and adolescence.

91. (D) Regression. Regression involves a patient's decreased responsibility, increased dependency, and disregard for others. Regression is a risk for patients who remain in treatment settings longer than necessary. Countertransferences are feelings the therapist and patient have about one another that are interfering with the process therapy. Continuity of care is a term that described a range of services differing along treatment structure and intensity. Posttraumatic stress disorder is a psychiatric diagnosis versus a risk factor. See reference: Hopkins and Smith (eds): Richert, GZ, and Gibson, D: Practice setting.

92. (C) Ascertain facts and impressions. Similar to the assessment process for treating a patient is the process for approaching an ethical dilemma. The Savage Model outlines 14 steps of ethical contemplation. The first four steps were the answers to this question. Initially, facts and impressions need to be gathered. Once this is done, information needs to be verified with key players. The third step is to identify problems to be solved and finally to sort the decisions to be made. Answers A, B, and D are incorrect. See reference: Bair and Gray (eds): Opacich, KJ, and Welles, C: Ethical dimensions in occupational therapy.

93. (A) Medicare. Medicare was established in 1965 by an act of Congress as Title XVIII of the Social Security Act. The program consists of two parts. Medicare part "A" pays for inpatient hospitalization, skilled care, and hospice services. Medicare part "B" covers outpatient services along with physician and other professional medical services. Medicaid, answer B, provides health care for the poor and medically indigent. Answer C, third-party payors, represent the largest source of payment in the United States. These providers may be either for profit or not for profit and they adhere to state insurance codes, which require set levels of coverage. Private pay, answer D, is when the patient is responsible for the financial payment of services rendered. See reference: Bair and Gray (eds): Scott, SJ, and Somers, FP: Payment for occupational therapy services.

94. (C) Workers' compensation. Workers' compensation is a state supported program into which employers pay. Beneficiaries will receive coverage for those services which are identified to be covered within their respective state. Medicare, answer A, is a federal program for health coverage for individuals 65 years or older, disabled individuals, or people in the end stages of renal disease. Medicaid, answer B, is a joint state and federal program that provides coverage for the poor and medically indigent. The Education for All Handicapped Children, answer D, is assisted through the provision of state and federal grants. See reference: Bair and Gray (eds): Scott, SJ, and Somers, FP: Payment for occupational therapy services.

95. (A) Standards of Practice. Membership in the American Occupational Therapy Association is voluntary and the AOTA does not have jurisdiction over therapists who are not members. The *Standards of Practice* outlines the values and basic beliefs that are to be exemplified by occupational therapists. The Standards and Ethics Commission (SEC) is responsible for the Code of Ethics and Standards of Practice. The SEC monitors compliance with the ethics and standards from which members practice. However, the SEC does not have any recourse against nonmembers who do not follow these standards. Even though employers may otherwise benefit from employees being members of AOTA, accountability to the professional standards is by far the most beneficial. See reference: Hopkins and Smith (eds): Hopkins, HL: Scope of occupational therapy.

96. (C) Blood, semen, and saliva from dental procedures. OSHA has identified materials that require universal precautions to be blood, semen, vaginal secretions, cerebrospinal fluid, synovial fluid, pleural fluid, any body fluid with visible blood, any unidentifiable body fluid, and saliva from dental procedures. Answers A, B, and D all contain fluids that are not on this list. Items that OSHA identified as not needing universal precautions are feces, nasal secretions, sputum, sweat, tears, urine, and vomitus. See reference: Hopp and Rogers: Elder, HA: Transmission of HIV and prevention of AIDS.

97. (C) Contact with supervisor once a month. The description of general supervision given by the AOTA includes a minimum of monthly direct contact with supervision available as needed by phone or other forms of communication. Answer A describes close supervision with direct contact occurring daily. Answer B refers to routine supervision or direct contact occurring a minimum of every 2 weeks. Answer D is minimal supervision, which occurs on an as-needed basis. See reference: AOTA: The Occupational Therapy Roles Task Force: Occupational Therapy Roles.

98. (A) Efficacy studies. Efficacy studies demonstrate positive results in the ideal circumstances. Answer B, efficiency studies, compare outcomes of service compared to costs. Answer C, effectiveness studies, just look at the outcomes. Answer D, expenditure studies, just look at the cost of services. See reference: Punwar: Overview of occupational therapy.

99. (A) An exposure has occurred and she should use universal precautions. OSHA has identified materials that require universal precautions to be blood, semen, vaginal secretions, cerebrospinal fluid, synovial fluid, pleural fluid, any body fluid with visible blood, any unidentifiable body fluid, and saliva from dental procedures. Since the urine did have blood in it, it would be considered an exposure. Answers B and D are incorrect because they indicate that an exposure has not occurred. Answer C is incorrect because any time an exposure occurs, universal precautions must be followed. In addition, it should be noted that items OSHA has identified as not needing universal precautions are feces, nasal secretions, sputum, sweat, tears, urine, and vomitus. See reference:

Hopp and Rogers: Elder, HA: Transmission of HIV and prevention of AIDS.

100. (B) Manual rocking while in prone on a therapy ball. Answer B employs slow, regular vestibular input in a comfortable and safe position, which is inhibitory. Answers A, C, and D are vestibular activities, but they involve fast or irregular movements, which will increase the level of arousal. See reference: Hopkins and Smith (eds): Kinnealey, M, and Miller, L: Sensory integration and learning disabilities.

101. (C) Lower extremity, trunk, and mild upper extremity. Answer C is correct because diplegia refers to these specific areas of the body. Involvement of both legs, answer B, is called paraplegia and answer D, all extremities, and neck involvement describes quadriplegia. Answer A is also incorrect as there is no specific classification or name for involvement of both upper limbs when describing cerebral palsy. See reference: Case-Smith, Allen, and Pratt (eds): Gordon, CY, Schanzenbacher, KE, Case-Smith, J, and Carrasco, RC: Diagnostic problems in pediatrics.

102. (B) Stage 4. Brunnstrom defined the recovery of muscle function in six stages: (1) flaccidity, (2) development of synergies, (3) voluntary movement within synergy, (4) gross motor movement within synergy, (5) movement outside of synergies, and (6) near normal movement with isolated joint movement. Brunnstrom also defined three movements to represent stage 4: (1) placing the hand behind the back, (2) shoulder flexion at 90 degrees with the elbow fully extended, and (3) pronating and supinating the forearm. See reference: Trombly: Movement therapy of Brunnstrom.

103. (C) Object relations. The psychoanalytic and object relations perspectives view the past as a determining influence on an individual's current functioning. Particularly important to these perspectives is that unconscious factors influence behaviors and are important to address in treatment. Occupational behavior, human occupation, and role acquisition are more concerned with the here-and-now adaptivity of behaviors regardless of the past. See reference: Christiansen and Baum (eds): Borg, B, and Bruce, MA: Assessing psychological performance factors.

104. (B) SOAP notes. The problem-oriented medical record is based on assessing an individual's limitations and listing problem areas. A SOAP note is a structured format of documentation that consists of four sections: subjective, objective, assessment, and plan. This format may be used in initial, progress, and discharge notes as well as consultation documentation. Answer A is incorrect because most checklists are not designed to assess and list problem areas. Answer C is incorrect because the answer is vague and does not indicate whether the format is structured or assess and document problem areas. Answer D is incorrect in that a structured format is not followed. See reference: Hopkins and Smith (eds): Perinchief, JM: Service management.

105. (B) After back extension in prone develops. Back extension developed in prone is a basic requirement for trunk control in sitting. Answer A is incorrect because lifting the head in prone is only the beginning of back extension and the child has little trunk control. Answer C is not correct because primitive reflexes interfere with development of back control. Answer D is incorrect because walking alone requires further development of trunk and leg control than sitting alone. See reference: Case-Smith, Allen, and Pratt (eds): Gordon, CY, Schanzenbacher, KE, Case-Smith, J, and Carrasco, RC: Diagnostic problems in pediatrics.

106. (C) Flexor synergy and voluntary or associated reactions. While in stage 2 of muscle return, the individual's arm will exhibit increased presence of synergy. Some of the characteristics of synergy may be elicited on a voluntary basis or as an associated reaction. Flexor synergy is characterized by shoulder abduction and external rotation, elbow flexion, wrist flexion, and finger flexion or extension. Associated reactions are movements of the affected extremity, which are elicited by forceful movements in other areas of the body. Brunnstrom defined the recovery of muscle function in six stages: (1) flaccidity, (2) development of synergy, (3) voluntary movement within synergies, (4) gross motor movement within synergy, (5) movement outside of synergy, and (6) near normal movement with isolated joint movement. Brunnstrom also defined three movements that are possible in stage 4: (1) placing the hand behind the back, (2) shoulder flexion, at 90 degrees with the elbow fully extended, and (3) pronating and supinating the forearm. See reference: Trombly (ed): Mathiowetz, V, and Bass Haugen, J: Evaluation of motor behaviors, traditional and contemporary views.

107. (D) Rice. There are many serious side effects with MAOI inhibitors. Foods that are known to include aged proteins (smoked meats and aged cheese) should be avoided as well as limiting chocolate and coffee. See reference: Bonder: Fischer, PJ: Psychopharmacotherapy.

108. (B) Any modification to a job that will allow a disabled worker to perform the essential functions. "Reasonable accommodation" refers to the modification of an environment being of realistic and fiscally responsible. An example would be that if the offices for a small company were on the second floor of a building and could only be accessed by stairs, it may be impossible to complete the accommodation due to the expense of putting in an elevator. However, other options such as a stair lift may be considered for an employee in a wheelchair. See reference: Hopkins and Smith (eds): Reed, K: The beginnings of occupational therapy.

109. (A) Observation. The "uncontrived" activity setting allows the therapist to observe the child's natural use of functional abilities and social and play skills without structure or adult influence. In this way the therapist can compare interview and test findings with observation information to formulate recommendations. See reference: Case-Smith, Allen, and Pratt (eds): Richardson, PK: Use of standardized tests in pediatric practice.

110. (D) Prepare the child mentally and physically for visual tasks. Children with poor visual attention will find visual tasks facilitated by being prepared mentally and physically for the task. Answer A is not correct because concentration and task persistence are enhanced by motivation, comprehension, and intrinsic interest in the visual task. Answer B is not correct because stimulation surrounding the task should be minimized. Answer C is not correct because the novelty of the task increases visual attention. See reference: Kramer and Hinojosa: Todd, VR: Visual perceptual frame of reference: An information processing aproach.

111. (B) Good (4). The individual's "available" range is the range that the joint may be moved through passively. Therefore, if an individual is able to move the joint actively through the entire movement that is completed passively and then take maximum resistance, the grade is normal (5). Good (4) is the grade given when a part moves through the available range but against gravity and is able to sustain moderate resistance. Fair (3) is the grade given when an individual is able to move a part through full range against gravity but lacks strength for any resistance. Fair minus (3–) is the grade given when an individual moves a part against gravity through less than full range of motion. Fair minus is the last graded range for movement against gravity. Muscle grades poor and trace are for gravity eliminated movements. See reference: Trombly: Evaluation of biomechanical and physiological aspects of motor performance.

112. (A) Hot is 40 to 45 degrees, cold is 5 to 10 degrees. Temperature levels are set so that there is a difference between the hot and cold, but not extreme enough to be painful or slight enough so as to be indistinguishable. The temperature in degrees Fahrenheit are 105 to 114 for hot and 40 to 50 degrees Fahrenheit for cold. See reference: Trombly (ed): Bentzel, K: Evaluation of sensation.

113. (B) Decreased muscle tone. Decreased muscle tone is usually characterized by joints that are lax and hyperextensible. Low muscle tone and joint hyperextensibility are also frequent characteristics of Down syndrome. Answer A is incorrect as loss of range of motion would be the joint characteristic of increased muscle tone. Answers C and D are incorrect because they are diagnoses that cannot be made on the basis of joint laxness, even though instability at the joint may occur with either of these conditions. The observation of joint hyperextensibility is merely an indication of below normal muscle tone, and is not necessarily the indication of a specific condition or disease process. See reference: Hopkins and Smith (eds): Simon, CJ, and Daub, MM: Human development across the lifespan.

114. (D) Chaining. Chaining is frequently used when teaching a multiple-step task, as it is easier to teach only one step at a time than a complete activity. Repetition and rehearsal involve repeating the whole activity over and over until the activity is learned. Cueing uses an external source to remind a person of the next step or part of that step. See reference: Zoltan, Siev, and Freishtat: Explanations for use of this manual.

115. (B) Temperature and pain. The sensations of pain and temperature are carried along small, unmyelinated nerve fibers, which recover more rapidly than senses carried by larger, myelinated fibers. The sensations of pain and temperature are also part of the "protective" or primary sensory systems, which are the receivers of simple information. More complex information is carried through the "discriminative or epicritic system." The senses carried on this system are vibration, light touch, proprioception, and tactile localization. See reference: Trombly (ed): Bentzel, K: Evaluation of sensation.

116. (A) Using the strongest joint, avoiding positions of deformity, and ensuring correct patterns of movement. These principles of joint protection are beneficial for all individuals. The significance of utilizing these principles for individuals with pre-existing joint deformities or adverse musculoskeletal changes may help to restore function as well as prevent further impairments. Answers B, C, and D involve muscle relaxation and stress management. See reference: Trombly (ed): Bear-Lehman, J: Orthopeadic conditions.

117. (B) Improve ability to grade movement. The "grading of movement" goal best addresses difficulty with control of the midrange of a movement pattern (common with athetosis). Answer A is incorrect because this goal would be appropriate for a child who cannot break up a flexion or extension pattern during a movement. Answer C is not correct because this goal is appropriate for a child who has difficulty with an arm or hand movement being too fast or too slow (graded movements are also too fast). Answer D is incorrect because this goal is appropriate for a child who has difficulty bringing both arms to midline and using them effectively together. See reference: Case-Smith, Allen, and Pratt (eds): Exner, CE: Development of hand skills.

118. (B) A call system for emergency and nonemergency use. A call system is necessary for a person with a high-level spinal cord injury to allow the caretaker to leave the room, but still remain available to answer the person's call for assistance for daily needs or an emergency. This is frequently the first opportunity that a person with a spinal cord injury would have to control some part of his or her life, giving some feeling of independence or choice. An environmental control unit does allow independence in operating appliances, lights, and so on, through the use of switches or voice control, but would not be a necessity for safety. A remote control power door opener, which would allow a caretaker to enter, would be useless if the person is unable to call for assistance. An electric page turner is useless without the ability to call for someone to position or replace reading materials. See reference: Hill, Intagliata, and Allen (eds): Jones, R: Home environment control.

119. (D) A frame of reference. A treatment approach (answer D) is the concept on which a program of treatment is based and directs what methods or techniques are used in treatment by a therapist. A treatment technique, (answer A) is based on the frame of reference or treatment approach and is a specialized activity or method used to improve a person's performance. An exercise (answer B) is an activity to improve the mind or body and is a generic term to describe an activity without referring to the treatment approach. A treatment plan (answer C) includes the specific techniques, methods, or approaches used to reach a goal for a person who is receiving treatment. See reference: Pedretti: Occupational performance: A model for practice in physical dysfunction.

120. (B) Sip and puff switch. A sip-and-puff switch is operated by breath control and would be unaffected by random movements of the extremities. An infrared switch (answer A) sends an infrared beam from the switch to some surface that would reflect the light back to the switch. When the beam is broken, the switch would be activated. The switch may be activated by an eye blink or finger twitch. Random movements of the extremities may misalign the person's head or body causing false activation. A p-switch (answer C) is a piezoelectric sensor that is activated by a muscle tensing and being relayed to the switch. A rocking lever switch activates a device when one side is pushed of the switch and turns the device off when the other side of the switch is pushed. An infrared switch, a p-switch, and a rocking lever switch (answer D) could all be activated by random movements of the extremities moving or pushing the rest of the body out of alignment. See reference: Church and Glennen: Adaptive toys and environmental controls.

121. (D) Scoop dish. This is the most correct answer because the sides of the scoop dish will provide a shape that aides the scooping movement. A high back to the plate provides a surface to push the food against to aide in getting the food onto the spoon. Answer A is not correct because the swivel spoon primarily helps when supination is limited. Answer B is not correct because the nonslip mat helps stabilize the plate itself. Answer D is incorrect because the mobile arm support positions the arm and helps weak shoulder and elbow muscles to position the hand. See reference: Case-Smith, Allen, and Pratt (eds): Case-Smith, J, and Humphry, R: Feeding and oral motor skills.

122. (B) Physician's written consent and medical precautions. No part of the work hardening evaluation or treatment program may begin without a physician's written consent and medical precautions for the patient, as the patient's physical abilities and tolerances are analyzed through the program. Answers A and D are incorrect, since information regarding patient's work history and job site may be obtained after the program has been initiated. Answer C is incorrect because insurance information is obtained by the business office when the referral is made and evaluation is scheduled. This information is passed on to the therapist as necessary. See reference: Pedretti (ed): Burt, C, and Smith, P: Work hardening.

123. (B) 118 degrees to 126 degrees F. At 118 degrees F to 126 degrees F (47.8 degrees C to 52.2 degrees C) the paraffin stays melted without forming a film on the surface, but is not too hot to burn the skin. A temperature of 108 degrees F to 116 degrees F (answer A) would be comfortable to a person's skin, however a film of cooling paraffin would form on the top and interfere with the proper coating of the hand.

Temperatures of 128 degrees F to 136 degrees F (answer C) and 138 degrees to 146 degrees F (answer D) would be too hot for the skin to tolerate comfortably and may cause a burn to sensitive skin. This modality is commonly used in the treatment of arthritis. See reference: Rothstein, Serge, and Wolf: Modalities.

124. (D) The individual's view of the problem and overall goal. The interview is generally the component of the assessment process where the occupational therapist asks about the individual's goals for treatment and gains an understanding of the problems from the person's perspective. Answers A and B are most often found in a review of the chart. Ability, answer C, is determined through performance measures. See reference: Denton: Assessment.

125. (B) Schroeder Block Campbell (SBC). The only evaluation method in the list that assesses adult sensory integrative functions is the SBC. The BaFPE and COTE assesses a variety of basic skills The SCSIT is used only with children. See reference: Hopkins and Smith (eds): Stress management.

126. (A) Prepare a can of soup. Grading activities according to complexity is an important part of the therapist's selection of appropriate activities for an individual's abilities. Complexity increases as the number of steps, number of different ingredients or tools used, and time to complete the task increases. Answers B, C, and D all require more steps and materials and time than preparing a can of soup. See reference: Bruce and Borg: Appendix I.

127. (C) Locate a puncture resistant container that the copper piece could be placed into before disposing of it. Answer C is the only action that is consistent with universal precautions guidelines. Answers A and D do not dispose of blood exposed items in a manner that would protect others from contact. Answer B does not include any blood exposure protection for the person applying the bandage. See reference: Hopkins and Smith (eds): Pizzi, M: HIV infection and AIDS.

128. (C) Conduct disorder. Conduct disorders often involve aggression to people or animals and property destruction. Individuals with Asperger's disorder, answer A, demonstrate restricted or limited social behaviors. Answer B, attention deficit disorders, involve impulsive but not typically violent behaviors. Answer D, oppositional defiant disorders, involve similar but less severe behaviors as conduct disorders. See reference: American Psychiatric Association: Disorders usually first diagnosed in infancy, childhood, or adolescence.

129. (B) Developmental stimulation. Because these children are confined at a very young age and are restricted for repair of the hip dislocation, a primary concern of the therapist should be to evaluate and provide a developmental program. Answers A, C, and D are not correct because although they could be worthy secondary goals as time proceeds, initial goals should be focused on dealing with the child's risk for developmental delay and ability to deal with restriction. See reference: Hopkins and Smith (eds): Atkins, J: Neural tube defect.

130. (C) Assessing and submitting reports determining an individual's ability to manage his or her own funds for a competency hearing. Forensics is a specialty area dealing with problems linking psychiatry and the law. Answer C is the situation that clearly links psychiatry and the law and is a common role for occupational therapists. Answer A does not describe the type of "help" provided so that the occupational therapy role is not addressed. Answer B is typically the role of therapeutic recreation or activity therapy. Answer D does not specify if patients with legal involvement are being treated by the occupational therapist. See reference: Hopkins and Smith (eds): Gibson, D, and Richert, GZ: The therapeutic process.

131. (C) The individual's complaints focus on physical concerns, denies feeling depressed but feels less energy, has lost weight, and complains of some concentration and memory problems. The general presentation of depression varies somewhat with an individual's age group. Answer A is more descriptive of adolescent depression and answer C is descriptive of middle adult depression. Depression and dementia are also important for care givers to distinguish between in working with geriatric patients. Answer D is a description of complaints consistent with dementia. See reference: Hopkins and Smith (eds): Rogers, JC: Geriatric psychiatry.

132. (B) Provide enough chairs around a round table. Circular seating arrangements generally facilitate the most communication among members. Rectangle-shaped tables can lead to unbalanced communications. Difficulties in maintaining comfort and attention are problems related to floor seating arrangements. Using available chairs and couches frequently provide different seating heights and rectangular or square arrangements. See reference: Posthuma: Group dimensions.

133. (B) Improve vestibular processing. Answer B is correct because the vestibular system has "considerable influence on postural tone, ocular pursuits, the coordination of input from the two body sides, the establishment of laterality, language function, and visual perception." Answer A, C, and D are not correct, because ocular pursuits, muscle tone, and postrotary nystagmus can all be affected by vestibular processing, and by emphasizing this sensory system, there may be a positive effect on these functions. In addition, it should be noted that answer D, increasing postrotary nystagmus, is not an appropriate goal of sensory integration therapy, since it is regarded as an expression of only one aspect of intact vestibular functioning in response to rotary stimulation. See reference: Case-Smith, Allen, and Pratt (eds): Parham, LD, and Mailloux, Z: Sensory integration.

134. (C) Rolling in a carpeted barrel. Answer C would appear to be the most appropriate initial activity for this child's treatment program. Because tactile defensiveness is an area of sensory integration treatment that should be approached cautiously, the child-controlled rolling on a textured surface would be less intrusive to her nervous system than answer A, where the therapist provides the sensory stimulation to the most sensitive areas of the

body. In general, sensory integration therapy involves child-directed adaptive responses, and it is recommended that occupational therapists have consultation from a sensory integration therapist when applying direct sensory input. Answers B and D are not correct because balancing and swinging activities generally do not address a problem of tactile defensiveness. See reference: Ayres: Developmental dyspraxia: A motor planning problem.

135. (D) Flushing, blanching, or perspiration. The most correct answer is D because these responses are autonomic nervous system signs of sensory overload. Answers A, B, and C are not correct because they do not describe autonomic responses to the activity. See reference: Case-Smith, Allen, and Pratt (eds): Parham, LD, and Mailloux, Z: Sensory integration.

136. (C) Games of chance. Because winning a game of chance is based essentially on luck, many functional levels have "equal" opportunities at winning. Hobbies are not considered a category of games. Puzzles and strategy games both require specific skills to succeed. See reference: Early: Leisure skills.

137. (A) Punctuality, accepting responsibility for oneself, accepting directions from a supervisor and appropriately interacting with peer coworkers. Psychosocial components include time management, social conduct and self-control. Punctuality, accepting responsibility and accepting feedback are examples of prevocational skills within these psychosocial performance components and are important prevocational skills. Memory, decision making and sequencing are considered to be cognitive components. Standing tolerance, endurance, and eye-hand coordination are categorized as sensory motor components. Grooming and adhering to safety precautions are work performance areas and not psychosocial performance components. See reference: Bonder: Appendix B—Uniform terminology for reporting occupational therapy services.

138. (D) Program evaluation. Program evaluations are various systems that measure the combined outcomes of patients and effectiveness of the program. These systems are designed to report information so that the facility may improve quality, increase organizational ability to plan and allocate resources, and justify to payors the outcomes and services. Qualify improvement, answer A is a systematic approach to monitor patient care. Peer review, answer B, is a component of quality improvement. Cost accounting, answer C, is a method of tracking the costs of specific services or costs incurred by diagnosis specific groups. See reference: Bair and Gray (eds): Scammahorn, G: Program planning.

139. (D) Summarizes the approach of management of an individual. The treatment plan or plan of care is usually a multidisciplinary approach to a patient's treatment. Each member of the treatment team contributes to the plan, which may be documented on a specific form. Specific directions for the therapist in treatment (answer A), measurements of the patient's progress (answer B), and organization of the patient's priorities (answer C) are all pieces of information included in the occupational therapy departmental documentation. See reference: Jacobs and Logigian: Pagonis, J: Documentation.

140. (A) The process of giving an individual sufficient information so that they may make an informed decision about their own care. Answer B is clinical reasoning which is completed by the therapist in planning treatment. Answer C is acceptance of the job offer. Answer D is the result of the Americans with Disabilities Act, which was enacted in 1992. See reference: Jacobs and Logigian: Bloom, G: Ethics.

141. (B) Education for all Handicapped Children Act. This bill was enacted in Congress in 1975. It requires that school systems receiving federal funds provide handicapped children with free appropriate education in the least restrictive manner. The Americans with Disabilities Act, answer A, was passed in 1990 and enacted in 1992 to provide accessibility to individuals with disabilities. Answer C, Children's Protective Services, is an agency that investigates the home environment and removes children from families who neglect or abuse children. Medicare, answer D, was established in 1965 by an act of Congress as Title XVIII of the Social Security Act. The program consists of two parts. Medicare part A pays for inpatient hospitalization, skilled care, and hospice services. Medicare part B covers outpatient services, physician and other professional medical services. See reference: Bair and Gray (eds): Scott, SJ, and Somers, FP: Payment for occupational therapy services.

142. (C) Collaborative. The supervision for a certified occupational therapy assistant is intended to be collaborative. This term takes into account the sharing of information and utilization of each individual's skills in the process of working with patients. Answer A places the COTA in a role of not being able to provide information or have input into the treatment of the patient. Answer B is not appropriate in that it would have the COTA working independently without the supervision of an OTR. Answer D is incorrect in that open communication between the COTA and OTR is vital for a team approach. See reference: AOTA: The Occupational Therapy Roles Task Force: Occupational Therapy Roles.

143. (A) Complete the chart reviews. An identified role of the certified occupational therapy assistant is to complete data collection records such as a record review, general observation checklist, or behavior checklist. Answers B, C, and D indicate that the assistant is independently collecting nonstandardized data and interpreting the data. These roles are not appropriate for an assistant. See reference: Hopkins and Smith (eds): Entry Level Role Delineation Task Force for the Intercommission Council: Appendix F.

144. (B) Protect consumers of occupational therapy. The purpose of licensure was to protect consumers of occupational therapy services to improve the status of occupational therapy and thereby provide for increased coverage of service. Answer A, is the delineation of roles between occupational therapists and certified occupational therapy assistants. Even though licensure guidelines will identify generalities of the roles of OTRs and COTAs, they do not go into depth and provide detail as to their roles. Answer C, ensuring the continued levels of competency of therapists is not the primary purpose of licensure boards. Recently, many state's have initiated requiring evidence of CEUs to maintain licensure. Answer D, justifying occupational therapy services for Medicare and Medicaid reimbursement is also incorrect in that this may occur but primarily from third-party payors. See reference: Hopkins and Smith (eds): Hopkins, HL: Scope of occupational therapy.

145. (A) Provision of information and feedback to coworkers. Functional supervision occurs between peers. This type of supervision is frequently observed as fieldwork educators provide guidance and direction to therapists who are supervising students. This is also the type of feedback that may occur on self-directed work teams who coordinate services without a formal supervisor. Answers B describes formal supervision. Answer C describes minimal supervision and Answer D describes general supervision. See reference: AOTA: The Occupational Therapy Roles Task Force: Occupational Therapy Roles.

146. (C) Program evaluation. Answer C, program evaluation, is the compilation of the intervention results for a population of individuals. One of the most frequently used program evaluation systems is the Functional Independence Measure (FIM). FIM scores may be compiled and compared to regional and national norms. Answer A, a process, is the manner in which services are rendered. Each process has an order in which activities occur. An example of the process of interaction between the consumer and therapist may progress from initial interview to evaluation to treatment to family training to discharge intervention. Answer B, outcome, is the results of service intervention that an individual receives. These measures are taken at the completion of service intervention. Answer D, utilization review, reviews the care that is provided to ensure that services were appropriate and not over or under used. Overall, utilization review analyzes the services to ensure that the interventions were provided in an economical manner. See reference: Hopkins and Smith (eds): Perinchief, JM: Service management.

147. (D) Utilization review. Utilization reviews assess the care that is provided to assure that services were appropriate and not over or under used. Overall, utilization review analyzes the services to assure that the interventions were provided in an economical manner. Answer A, a process, is the manner in which services are rendered. Each process has an order in which activities occur. An example of the process of interaction between the consumer and therapist may progress from initial interview to evaluation to treatment to family training to discharge intervention. Answer B, outcome, is the results of service intervention that an individual receives. These measures are taken at the completion of service intervention. Answer C, program evaluation, is the compilation of the intervention results for a population of individuals. One of the most frequently used program evaluation systems is the FIM. FIM scores may be compiled and compared to regional and national norms. See reference: Hopkins and Smith (eds): Perinchief, JM: Service management.

148. (D) Lightweight wheelchair and hospital bed. Durable medical equipment is defined by Medicare as "that which can withstand repeated use, is primarily and customarily used to serve a medical purpose, and generally is not useful to a person in the absence of illness or injury." Answers A, B, and C are incorrect because they included items that are not considered as "durable medical equipment" (i.e., reachers, a shower chair, or a hand held shower). Depending on the patient's medical condition, a bedside commode may be covered. See reference: Bair and Gray (eds): Scott, SJ, and Somers, FP: Payment for occupational therapy services.

149. (A) Capital equipment. Equipment pieces that cost in excess of $500 are considered capital equipment and will generally last for more than 2 years (i.e., filing cabinets). Items that cost less than $500 are considered expendable, answer B, and may last up to approximately 2 years (i.e., pinch meter). Adaptive equipment, answer C, such as reachers may be used during therapy or sold to a patient. Supplies, answer D, are items such as forms, pens, which may be used by staff. See reference: Bair and Gray (eds): Scammahorn, G: Program planning.

150. (B) Expendable equipment. Items that cost less than $500 are considered expendable and may last up to approximately 2 years (i.e., pinch meter). Equipment pieces that cost in excess of $500 are considered capital equipment, answer A, and will generally last for more than 2 years (i.e., filing cabinet). Adaptive equipment, answer C, such as reachers may be used during therapy or sold to a patient. Supplies, Answer D, are items such as forms, pens that may be used by staff. See reference: Bair and Gray (eds): Scammahorn, G: Program planning.

151. (D) Consider and treat underlying sensory integration problems as a possible cause. Very often children's sensory integration problems interfere with the development of hand dominance. The cause could be decreased ability to cross body, poor sensory perception in the arms and hands, delayed integration of reflex patterns, and so on. Answers A, B, and C are incorrect because they do not address possible underlying causes for poorly established hand dominance. See reference: Case-Smith, Allen, and Pratt (eds): Parham, LD, and Mailloux, Z: Sensory integration.

152. (D) The individual asks for more beverages during meals, but appears surprised when beverages in closed containers are indicated on the meal tray. The subjective portion of the SOAP note should contain information that is gained through a chart review, or communication with patient, their family or staff. This information is not measurable and is therefore considered subjective. Answer A would be in the program plan. Answers B and C would be in the objective portion because they are either

measurable or based on specific observations. See reference: Trombly (ed): Bentzel, K: Remediating sensory impairment.

153. (A) Counted cross stitch needlework projects. Blurred vision is a common side effect of tricyclic antidepressants and small detailed activities can be quite difficult to work on. Food precautions are important with monomamine oxidase inhibitors (MAOIs). Sun precautions are important with antipsychotics. Although blood pressure may change during gross motor activities, METS is a cardiac endurance-based grading method. See reference: Bonder: Fischer, PJ: Psychopharmacotherapy.

154. (A) The goals have been met and the individual can no longer benefit from occupational therapy services. Discontinuation of occupational therapy should occur when an individual has met the goals and further progress is not anticipated within the therapeutic environment. Answer C is incorrect because sometimes, individuals may achieve their goals and new goals are established since it is anticipated that further progress may be made. Answer B is incorrect because if the therapist does not anticipate progress and the goals have not been met, it is necessary for the therapist to discharge the individual. Depending on an individual's status at discharge, recommendations may be made for community services, outpatient care, day care, or home health services. A vital role of the occupational therapist is to provide appropriate linkages to the community for those individuals served. The preparation for discharge planning should include the patient's support system, discharge environment, and possible need for continued health care services. Answer D is incorrect because discharge of an individual should be made on objective information. If an individual does not "feel" that they are making progress, the therapist should be able to clarify with the individual the status based on objective measurements and observations. See reference: Reed and Sanderson: Service functions.

155. (C) 9 and 12 months. Children usually begin to "cruise" (walk sideways holding on to a rail) between 9 and 12 months. See reference: Case-Smith, Allen, and Pratt (eds): Gordon, CY, Schanzenbacher, KE, Case-Smith, J, and Carrasco, RC: Diagnostic problems in pediatrics.

156. (A) Successful for hypersensitivity. Hyposensitivity retraining cannot be done secondary to sensory system damage. Hypersensitivity retraining may be successfully done on an intact sensory system and is most beneficial when the individual controls the stimuli. See reference: Trombly (ed): Bentzel, K: Remediating sensory impairment.

157. (C) The precipitating conditions and events that elicit stress reactions. The conditions and events that elicit stress reactions are known as stressors. Stressors can be both short term or long term. Answer A describes coping, answer B describes stress, and answer D describes adaptation. See reference: Christiansen and Baum (eds): Christiansen, C: Performance deficits as sources of stress—Coping theory and occupational therapy.

158. (B) Writing qualitative and quantitative facts in the results section. The results section should only contain measurable results. Conclusions and interpretive and analytical information appear in the summary or conclusion of the research. Subjective information is not typically included into research. See reference: Hopkins and Smith (eds): Dietz, J: Research: A systematic process for answering questions.

159. (C) Body righting. The body righting reaction replaces the neonatal neck righting reflex (log rolling) and provides the infant with the ability to rotate the trunk on the vertebral axis. The asymmetrical tonic neck reflex interferes with development of rotation because of arm extension on the face side and shoulder retraction on the skull side. The tonic labyrinthine reflex interferes with development of rotation also because it acts on the body in flexion and extension patterns only. See reference: Hopkins and Smith (eds): Simon, CJ, and Daub, MM: Human development across the lifespan.

160. (C) Combine task with additional sensory input (i.e., tactile, proprioceptive, auditory). Additional sensory input, when combined with a visual memory task, will facilitate memory. Answer A is not correct because interest in the task should be high in order to enhance visual memory. Answer B is not correct because visual attention is a prerequisite to visual memory. Answer D is not correct because serial or varied repetition enhances visual memory. See reference: Kramer and Hinojosa: Todd, VR: Visual perceptual frame of reference: An information processing aproach.

161. (A) An electric razor. An electric razor is safer shaving since a rotary head or foil would be in contact with the skin instead of a blade. Any shaving over the incision area or near it would not be recommended until the incision area is healed. The other razors have blades that could nick or cut the skin, which would need to be avoided until the patient is off blood thinners and normal blood coagulation can occur. See reference: Trombly (ed): Feinberg, JR, and Trombly, CA: Arthritis.

162. (D) At the midrange of the joint. Proprioception (or position sense) is demonstrated when the therapist passively positions the joint being tested and the individual is able to imitate the position with the opposite extremity. The joint should not be moved through range to an extent that would elicit a stretch or pain response, which would be at the end ranges of the joint. Movement should be at a rate of approximately 10 degrees per second to prevent the stretch reflex from being elicited. The end points of the range are used as the starting positions from which proprioception testing is started, for it is in these positions that the stretch or pain response would occur. See reference: Trombly (ed): Bentzel, K: Evaluation of sensation.

163. (A) Poor modulation of tactile input. This is the only answer that describes both his hypersensitive and hyposensitive responses to tactile input. The child with autism, as with many children who have sensory processing problems, may be unpredictable in terms of response to sensory stimuli, and many avoid stimulation at various times. Answers B and C are incorrect because they describe only one part of the problem. Answer D is wrong because he appears to be craving deep pressure or proprioceptive input in order to modulate the tactile system. See reference: Hopkins and Smith (eds): Kinnealey, M, and Miller, L: Sensory integration/Learning disabilities.

164. (D) A long handled bath sponge. A person with a total hip arthroplasty needs to avoid hip flexion of 80 degrees or more, hip adduction with internal rotation at the knee or ankle, or to lift the knee higher than the hip during self care or home management activities. A wire basket attached to the walker would not allow the person to come close to a counter without having to step sideways, which causes hip adduction to either move toward or away from the counter. A padded toilet seat of 1 inch height or a short handle sponge would cause the person to flex the hip past 80 degrees during the performance of self care activities. See reference: Trombly (ed): Bear-Lehman, J: Orthopedic conditions.

165. (C) Manual Muscle Test. The Manual Muscle Test is an example of a nonstandardized test. It has instructions for the administration and scoring of the test, however, it lacks validity and reliability. The results or interpretation of a nonstandardized test often depend on the skill, judgment, and bias of the evaluator. A standardized test has instructions for the administration and scoring as well as information regarding the validity and reliability, which have established norms from a specific population. The Motor Free Visual Perception Test (answer A), the Minnesota Rate of Manipulation Test (answer B), and the Purdue Pegboard Evaluation (answer D) all have information available regarding the reliability and validity based on the established norms. See reference: Pedretti: Occupational therapy evaluation of physical dysfunction.

166. (D) The therapist has the man trace letters through a pan of rice with his fingers. This method involves a larger input of sensory information to the brain by performing a gross movement in a more stimulating environment. A verbal description of how to make a letter (answer A), watching his grip (answer B), or performing strengthening exercises (answer C) would not give the man proprioceptive feedback on his letter formation through tactile input. See reference: Fisher, Murray, and Bundy: Cermak, S: Somatodyspraxia.

167. (C) Weight bearing on hands. This is the only activity that will facilitate hand function in the preparation phase. Weight bearing on the hands gives deep pressure to the surface of the hand and facilitates wrist and arm extension, as well as shoulder cocontraction, to prepare the arm for reach and stabilization of the hand for grasping. The other answers all provide different types of grasp activities which could be used as therapy. See reference: Case-Smith, Allen, and Pratt (eds): Exner, CE: Development of hand skills.

168. (A) Terminal behavior. The terminal behavior is the behavior or performance that is expected to be demonstrated by the patient. Answer B, the condition, is the circumstances under which performance of the patient will be evaluated. Answer C, the criteria, is the degree of competence of a patient's performance, which is stated in specific, measurable terms. Answer D, the plan, is the method or approach used to achieve a treatment objective as a proposal of treatment. See reference: Pedretti (ed): Foti, D, and Pedretti, L: Activities of daily living.

169. (A) Isometric exercises. Isometric exercises involve contracting the muscles without joint movement or a change in muscle length (answer A). Isotonic exercises (answer B) shorten the muscle length with joint movement occurring. The progressive resistive exercises in answer C are a type of isotonic exercise that use an increase in weight during consecutive exercise repetitions. A person who has a cast obstructing movement would be unable to perform isotonic exercises. Passive exercises (answer D) are performed by an outside force to the arm with no muscle contraction, with joint motion occurring. Passive exercises could not be performed to a casted joint. See reference: Pedretti (ed): Pedretti, L, and Wade, I: Therapeutic modalities.

170. (D) 82 cm. A minimum accessible width would be 82 cm or 32 inches to allow a wheelchair to pass through easily. All the other widths, answers A, B, and C, respectively, would be too narrow to allow a wheelchair to pass through a door into the next room. Answer A, 46 cm, would be too narrow to allow a standard walker entry easily even if the person side stepped. See reference: Rothstein, Serge, and Wolf: Wheelchairs and standards for access.

171. (C) The mother on the first floor, the grandmother in the basement. A master bedroom should be placed on the first floor to allow easy access for the woman with as few steps as possible. The grandmother also would want to use as few steps as possible, but there would not be room for a grandmother's suite on the first floor since the kitchen, dining area, living room, and master bedroom with bath would be located on that floor. The most available area with the least steps would be in the basement for the grandmother's suite, allowing her access to the basement from the exterior basement door (no steps) or the interior door (one flight of steps). This would also place her living quarters close to the recreation area where her grandsons would be able to play after school. Placing the mother and grandmother on the second floor, answer A, would cause too many trips for them to reach the main living areas on the first floor. Placing the mother on the first floor and the grandmother on the second, answer B, eliminates steps for the mother, but not the grandmother. The mother and grandmother in the basement, answer D, would place them close to the boys' play area, but would involve steps for the mother. See reference: O'Sullivan and Schmitz: Schmitz, T: Environmental assessment.

172. (D) 5 feet by 5 feet. An outward-opening door needs a space of 5 feet by 5 feet to allow for the wheelchair to be maneuvered around the door. A standard wheelchair requires 5 feet of turning space for a 180 or 360 degree turn. An area that is 3 feet by 5 feet, answer A,

4 feet by 4 feet, answer B, or 4.5 feet by 3 feet, answer C, would not provide enough space to allow the wheelchair to be turned. See reference: Rothstein, Serge, and Wolf: Wheelchairs and standards for access.

173. (B) 33 to 36 inches. This is the proper height for grab bars to allow for the upper extremities to lift the body with enough clearance to transfer onto the toilet seat. A height of 28 to 31 inches (answer A) would be too low to allow the body to clear the toilet seat when the arms are straightened. A height of 38 to 41 inches or 43 to 46 inches, answers C and D, respectively, would be too high to effectively push down with the arms to lift the body onto the toilet seat. See reference: O'Sullivan and Schmitz: Schmitz, T: Environmental assessment.

174. (C) Changes necessary for furniture arrangement. It is necessary to document how furniture should be arranged, in order to give the individual greatest accessibility. A report will supply the necessary information to other team members, the family, or therapists who will treat the woman as an outpatient or in the home. The outpatient therapy recommendations, answer A, and the status of the woman at the time of discharge, answer B, would be information needed in the discharge summary. The appropriate method of transportation, answer D, would be determined by the woman's physical abilities and by what is available to the family, not by the home visit. See reference: O'Sullivan and Schmitz: Schmitz, T: Environmental assessment.

175. (B) Tranxene. Tranxene is considered to be an antianxiety medication. Tegretol is an anticonvulsant medication and Trilafon is an antipsychotic medication. Tofranil is classified as an antidepressant. See reference: Hopkins and Smith (eds): Gibson, D, and Richert, GZ: The therapeutic process.

176. (C) Acute care hospitalization. The emphases of acute care hospitalization are symptom reduction, medications, and discharge planning. The club house treatment format emphasizes belonging and security. Community mental health centers focus on medication management, crisis intervention, and outpatient therapy. Quarterway houses emphasize increasing autonomy and decreasing supervision. See reference: Hopkins and Smith (eds): Richert, GZ and Gibson, D: Practice settings.

177. (C) Alcoholics Anonymous (AA). Self-help groups focus on personal growth in which leadership comes from the membership. AA is an example of such a group. MADD is an example of an advocacy group focusing on changing the legal system. Group therapy involves leadership and expertise from outside of the membership itself. Al-Anon is a combination of support group and self-help group for the family members of the alcoholic. See reference: Hopkins and Smith (eds): Richert, GZ: Program planning, development, and implementation.

178. (B) To evaluate the individual's occupational performance. Discharge planning in short-term hospitalizations should begin at admission. The therapist's evaluation of occupational performance is the first step in the occupational therapy discharge planning. Answers A, C, and D all would occur later in the treatment process. See reference: Sederer: Schwartzberg, SL, and Abeles, J: Occupational therapy.

179. (C) Slow and predictable movement. According to Kennealey and Miller, sensory integration treatment is a highly complex and individualized form of treatment. Within this consideration, they describe the use of sensory input with the therapy ball for children with vestibular hypersensitivity as providing "slow predictable rhythmic movement tolerance, heavy bounce tactile input simultaneously all pressure." Answer A is not correct because movement in any position or direction is used with children who have vestibular hyposensitivity. Answer B is not correct because adaptation to movement will be an important goal for comfort in the child's life activities. Answer D is not correct because it describes the type of movement most likely to be used in therapy when children are hyposensitive to movement. See reference: Hopkins and Smith (eds): Kinnealey, M, and Miller, L: Sensory integration/Learning disabilities.

180. (B) Activity adaptation. Modifying the directions that are provided is one way to adapt activities. Activity adaptations enable the individuals to become functional in task performance. Activity analysis is the process of identifying aspects, steps, and materials used in performing an activity. Activity sequencing is one method of grading activities. Early: Analyzing, adapting, and grading activities.

181. (D) Recovery. Tangential (topic jumping) speech, elated mood and some hyperactivity are known as prodromal of first stages of manic depressive illness. People in recovery are moving back through the stages to the first stages of the disease. Regression and decompensation both are processes of decline. Progression is a general term of improvement but is not specific enough to describe this client's changes. See reference: Bonder: Mood disorders.

182. (B) Ventricular septal defect. Eisenmenger's complex is the pooling of blood in the right ventricle as a result of the heart's inability to pump against a pulmonary vascular obstruction. The latter occurs because of prolonged exposure to the increased blood flow and high pressure associated with the presence of a ventricular septal defect. Children with a severe defect need to be monitored when in therapy for the possibility of the occurrence of this life-threatening situation. None of the other conditions listed (rheumatic fever, sickle-cell anemia, or asthma) include a heart defect that can create an Eisenmenger's complex. See reference: Case-Smith, Allen, and Pratt (eds): Gordon, CY, Schanzenbacher, KE, Case-Smith, J, and Carrasco, RC: Diagnostic problems in pediatrics.

183. (D) Support reactions. The term "support reaction" refers to the ability to coactivate muscle groups of the appropriate extremity or about the midline in order to support the body weight or posture in a certain position. Answer A is incorrect because protective reactions follow the development of support reactions in the arms, which protect the child when falling, and require that the body is free from support. Answer B is not correct because equilibrium reactions are compensatory movements used to regain stability, not to maintain stability. Answer C is not correct because rotational righting reactions involve turning of the head or trunk in order to maintain body alignment. See reference: Gilfoyle, Grady, and Moore: Strategies for developmental and purposeful sequences.

184. (B) Raise the handle bars. Raising the handle bars demands that the arms are raised, thus bringing the child to the upright posture. Answers A and D are not correct because the hips and lower extremities are already positioned correctly and this positioning would be disrupted. Answer C is not correct because the arms would be lowered and trunk forward flexion would be increased. See reference: Kramer and Hinojosa (eds): Colangelo, CA: Biomechanical frame of reference.

185. (D) 5 to 6 years. Nighttime bowel and bladder control may not be accomplished until the child is 5 or 6 years of age. Other developmental trends in toilet training are that daytime control is usually attained by 30 months, and that girls may precede boys by 2.5 months. See reference: Case-Smith, Allen, and Pratt (eds): Shepherd, J, Procter, SA, and Coley, IL: Self-care and adaptations for independent living.

186. (A) Specific measurable statements with time frames. Goals can be either short term (meaning in the immediate future) or long term (meaning over an extended period of time). The purpose of a goal is to provide a specific statement that is measurable and indicates what is to be accomplished. Patients and significant others play a vital role in working with the therapist to establish goals that are meaningful and realistic. Time frames, answer B, may only be a part of a measurable goal or objective. Specific measurements of the patient's skill and performance, answer C, is a part of the assessment information which assists the therapist in establishing appropriate goals and objectives for treatment. Activities to be completed that correspond with the goals. Answer D is part of the objective and treatment plan. See reference: Jacobs and Logigian: Pagonis, J: Documentation.

187. (D) Statements of how the goals will be achieved. An objective is a statement of the plan for how a goal will be achieved. This is the vital link that connects a patient's status on admission to how he or she will make progress so as to meet the goals for discharge. Statements of what will be accomplished with time frames, answer A, are referred to as goals. Time frames of what will be accomplished, answer B, are the component that make goals and objectives measurable. Specific measurements of an individual's skill and performance, answer C, are part of the assessment portion of an evaluation or SOAP note that indicate his or her status. See reference: Jacobs and Logigian: Pagonis, J: Documentation.

188. (C) Completing a literature review. Review of the written material is necessary in the preparation for the design of the research project. The literature review will help the researcher to clearly state the purpose and establish boundaries. Stating the purpose and the hypothesis follows the identification of the research question, therefore, answer A is incorrect. The design of the research and establishing the boundaries are affected by information from the literature review and therefore answers C and D are incorrect. See reference: Bailey: Reviewing the literature.

189. (C) PROs. PROs are state organizations that were established to ensure appropriate and cost effective patient care. These organizations numerically assess unnecessary procedures, patient deaths, and substandard care. Answer A is incorrect in that JCAHO (Joint Commission on Accreditation of Hospital Organizations) is an agency that reviews medical care provided by hospitals, psychiatric facilities, hospice, long-term care agencies, and MR/DD programs. CARF stands for the Commission of Accreditation of Rehabilitation Facilities. CARF reviews free-standing rehabilitation facilities as well as those within hospital systems. ARA stands for the American Rehabilitation Association. This organization was formerly known as NARF (National Association of Rehabilitation Facilities). A majority of rehabilitation facilities belong to the ARA, which provides professional support services and information to its members. See reference: Bair and Gray (eds): Joe, B: Quality assurance.

190. (D) An increase in the amount of services available on an outpatient basis. Current trends in health care are reducing inpatient hospital stays and increasing the types and amounts of services which are available on an outpatient basis. Answers A and C are incorrect because it is projected that with the population getting older and patients moving out of hospitals faster, utilization of nursing homes and home health will increase. Answer B is incorrect because hospitalizations are anticipated to decrease as only individuals with more serious illnesses and higher acuities of illness will be admitted. See reference: Punwar: Current trends and future outlook.

191. (A) Refine the question and develop the background. Once the question has been identified, a review of the literature is to occur. The next step in research is to refine the question and develop the background. Answer B, is the next step of the process which is deciding on the methodology. Answers C and D come later in the research as the researcher establishes the boundaries and then collects and analyzes qualitative data. See reference: Bailey: Introduction.

192. (B) A mobile arm support. A C5 quadriplegic with fair shoulder flexors and abductors and at least poor minus biceps, upper trapezius, and external rotators will be able to operate a mobile arm support for self feeding and facial hygiene activities. A wrist-driven flexor hinge splint would be used for a lower level spinal cord injury (C6-C8) in which the individual had functional use of the shoulder and arm muscles and has fair plus or better wrist

extension strength. This splint is indicated for individuals who lack prehension power. An electric feeder is indicated for individuals with a higher level of involvement (C4) and demonstrate poor plus or weaker shoulder strength. Built-up silverware may be indicated for individuals with C8 or T1 injuries in that they may lack the strength to tightly grasp regular utensils. See reference: Trombly (ed): Hollar, L: Spinal cord injury.

193. (D) Have him place his feet through loops of a therapeutic band. A prefunctional activity is when an individual is unable to perform a specific task, so an activity is used that practices the same movement as placing his feet into his pants legs. Activities that teach him to pull his pants up do not practice the same skill, and doffing socks is an activity that practices the opposite skill-removing feet from something. The other choices are also functional tasks that practice a specific skill. A prefunctional activity provides a base to improve a functional activity and may be practiced before or at the same time as a functional task. See reference: Kovich and Bermann (eds): Van Dam-Burke, A, and Kovich, K: Self-care and homemaking.

194. (B) The Holmes-Rahe Life Change Index. Answers A, C, and D are all designed to identify an individual's responses or reactions to stressors. Stressors are the triggers to the reactions, not the reactions. The Holmes-Rahe lists major social and environmental stressors. See reference: Hopkins and Smith (eds): Stress management.

195. (B) Begin the assessment process when patients are admitted on the weekends. The OTR will finish the assessment on Monday. The primary role of the COTA is to implement treatment such as that described in answers A, C, and D. 1990 AOTA guidelines about supervising COTAs state that a COTA may not independently evaluate patients. Working on weekends, the COTA would be independently initiating evaluations. See reference: Hopkins and Smith (eds): Appendix F: Entry-level role delineation for registered occupational therapists (OTRs) and certified occupational therapy assistants (COTAs).

196. (D) Block out all areas of the page except important words. Answer D is correct because this compensatory technique represents methods for dealing with visual figure-ground or visual discrimination problems. The child needs to learn how to rule out extraneous stimuli and focus on the important area of a task, such as reading. Answer A is not correct because this is a technique used to orient the child with left-right visual tracking problems. Answer B is not correct because it is a technique used to deal with visual attention problems. Answer C is not correct because it is a technique used to help children deal with visual memory problems. See reference: Kramer and Hinojosa: Todd, VR: Visual perceptual frame of reference: An information processing aproach.

197. (A) Provide the student with the opportunity to apply theory to practice. The main purpose of fieldwork education is to compliment the student's academic preparation with practical experience. See reference: Commission on Education: Guide to Fieldwork Education.

198. (B) Form constancy perception. Form constancy perception refers to the ability to match similar shapes regardless of change in their orientation in space. Answer A is not correct because figure-ground perception refers to the ability to distinguish a form or shape against a distracting background. Answer C is not correct because visual sequencing requires the ability to copy the same sequence of shapes or objects presented to the child. Although the latter is required when stringing the geometric beads, the error described refers to a form constancy error. See reference: Kramer and Hinojosa: Todd, VR: Visual perceptual frame of reference: An information processing approach.

199. (B) Have at least 1 year of experience as a registered occupational therapist. Based on the Essentials for level II fieldwork, an occupational therapist supervising a Level II OTR student is required to have a minimum of 1 year of experience. OTRs with 6 months of experi-

ence may supervise level I or II COTA student's. See reference: AOTA: Commission on Education: Guide to Fieldwork Education.

200. (A) Managed care. Managed care companies act as intermediaries between insurance companies and health care providers with the intent to reduce overall health care costs by requiring the individual to use providers who have pre-negotiated rates. In addition, the managed care entities work to reduce hospital lengths of stay by limiting hospital days or therapeutic visits. Managed competition is the concept of utilizing outcome data and charge efficiencies of health care providers to award health business to the systems with the best ratings. It is anticipated that the concept of managed competition will drive the cost of health care down and potentially put some facilities out of business. Medicare and Medicaid are governmental systems that are not currently under managed care systems. However, within the next decade, it is anticipated that the enrollees of these systems will be in some form of managed care system. See reference: Hopkins and Smith (eds): Hansen, RA: Ethics in occupational therapy.

BIBLIOGRAPHY

Allen, CK, Earhart, CA, and Blue, T: Occupational Therapy Treatment Goals for the Physically and Cognitively Disabled. The American Occupational Therapy Association, Rockville, MD, 1992.

American Occupational Therapy Association Inc: Terminology Task Force (1994): Uniform terminology for occupational therapy, ed 3. Am J Occup Ther 48:1047–1054.

American Occupational Therapy Association Inc: Commission on Standards and Ethics: Occupational Therapy Code of Ethics. Am J Occup Ther 48:1037–1038, 1994.

American Occupational Therapy Association Inc: Commission on Practice: Standards of Practice for Occupational Therapy. Am J Occup Ther 48:1039–1043, 1994.

American Occupational Therapy Association Inc: Intercommission Council: Occupational Therapy Roles. Am J Occup Ther 47:1087–1099, 1993.

American Occupational Therapy Association Inc: Commission on Education: Guide to Fieldwork Education. American Occupational Therapy Association, Rockville, MD, 1991.

American Psychiatric Association: Diagnostic and Statistical Manual IV. American Psychiatric Association, Washington, DC, 1994.

American Psychological Association: Publication Manual of the American Psychological Association, ed 3. American Psychological Association, Washington, DC, 1992.

Ayres, AJ: Sensory Integration and the Child. Western Psychological Services, Los Angeles, 1983.

Bailey, DM: Research for the Health Professional: A Practical Guide. FA Davis, Philadelphia, 1991.

Bair, J, and Gray, M (eds): The Occupational Therapy Manager. The American Occupational Therapy Association, Rockville, MD, 1992.

Bonder, BR: Psychopathology and Function, ed 2. Slack, Thorofare, NJ, 1995.

Bonder, BR, and Wagner, MB (eds): Functional Performance in Older Adults. FA Davis, Philadelphia, 1994.

Borg, B, and Bruce, MA: The Group System—The Therapeutic Activity Group in Occupational Therapy. Slack, Thorofare, NJ, 1991.

Bruce, MA, and Borg, B: Frames of Reference in Psychosocial Occupational Therapy, ed 2. Slack, Thorofare, NJ, 1993.

Butler, RN, and Lewis, MI: Aging and Mental Health—Positive Psychosocial and Biomedical Approaches, ed 3. Mosby, St. Louis, 1982.

Cailliet, R: Hand Pain and Impairment, ed 4. FA Davis, Philadelphia, 1994.

Cailliet, R: Shoulder Pain, ed 3. FA Davis, Philadelphia, 1991.

Case-Smith, J, Allen, AS, and Pratt, PN (eds): Occupational Therapy for Children, ed 3. CV Mosby, St. Louis, 1996.

Christiansen, C, and Baum, C: Occupational Therapy: Overcoming Human Performance Deficits. Slack, Thorofare, NJ, 1991.

Church, G, and Glennen, S: The Handbook of Assistive Technology. Singular Publishing Group, San Diego, 1992.

Conners, G, and Hilling, L: Guidelines for Pulmonary Rehabilitation Programs. Human Kinetics, Champaign, IL, 1993.

Crist, PH: Community Living Skills: A psychoeducational community-based program. Occup Ther Mental Health 6:51–64, 1986.

Cromwell, FS (Ed): Computer Applications in Occupational Therapy. The Haworth Press, New York, 1986.

Davies, PM: Steps to Follow: A Guide to the Treatment of Adult Hemiplegia. Springer-Verlag, Tokyo, 1985.

Denton, PL: Psychiatric Occupational Therapy: A Workbook of Practical Skills. Little, Brown, Boston, 1987.

Drake, RE, and Sederer, L: Inpatient psychosocial treatment of chronic schizophrenia: Negative effects and current guidelines. Hosp Community Psychiatry, 37:897–901.

Drake, M: Crafts in Therapy and Rehabilitation. Slack, Thorofare, NJ, 1992.

Duncombe, LW, Howe, MC, and Schwartzberg, SL: Case Simulations in Psychosocial Occupational Therapy, ed 2. FA Davis, Philadelphia, 1988.

Dunn, W: Pediatric Occupational Therapy. Slack, Thorofare, NJ, 1991.

Early, MB: Mental Health Concepts and Techniques for the Occupational Therapy Assistant, ed 2. Raven Press, New York, 1993.

Eichmann, MA, Griffin, BP, Lyons, JS, Larson, DB, and Finkel, S: An estimation of the impact of OBRA-87 on nursing home care in the United States. Hosp Community Psychiatry, 43:781–788, 1992.

Erhardt, RP: Developmental Hand Dysfunction; Theory Assessment Treatment. Tucson Therapy Builders, Tucson, 1989.

Fess, EE, and Philips, CA: Hand Splinting, ed 2. CV Mosby, St. Louis, 1987.

Fidler, GS: Design of Rehabilitation Services in Psychiatric Hospital Settings. American Occupational Therapy Association, Rockville, MD, 1991.

Finnie, NR: Handling the Young Cerebral Palsied Child at Home. JB Lippincott, New York, 1993.

Fisher, AG, Murray EA, and Bundy AC: Sensory Integration: Theory and Practice. FA Davis, Philadelphia, 1991.

Gilfoyle, EM, Grady, AP, and Moore, JC: Children Adapt. Slack, Thorofare, NJ, 1990.

Glickstein, JK: Therapeutic Interventions in Alzheimer's Disease: A Program of Functional Communication Skills for Daily Living. Aspen Publishers, Rockville, MD, 1988.

Green, JH: Frequent rehospitalization and noncompliance with treatment. Hosp Community Psychiatry 39:963–966, 1988.

Green, MA, and Florey, L: Child psychiatry and middle childhood: A guide to play for parents, Mental Health Special Interest Section Newsletter, 15 3:1–2, 1992.

Griffith, ER, and Lemberg, S: Sexuality and the Person with Traumatic Brain Injury. FA Davis, Philadelphia, 1993.

Hemphill, BJ: Mental Health Assessment in Occupational Therapy. Slack, Thorofare, NJ, 1988.

Hemphill, BJ: The Evaluative Process in Psychiatric Occupational Therapy. Slack, Thorofare, NJ, 1982.

Hill, JP: Spinal Cord Injury: A Guide to Functional Outcomes in Occupational Therapy. A Rehabilitation Institute of Chicago procedure manual. Aspen Publishers, Rockville, MD, 1988.

Hopp, JW, and Rogers, EA: AIDS and the Health Professions. FA Davis, Philadelphia, 1989.

Howe, MC, and Schwartzberg, SL: A Functional Approach to Group Work in Occupational Therapy, ed 2. JB Lippincott, Philadelphia, 1995.

Hughes, PL, and Mullins, L: Acute Psychiatric Care: An Occupational Therapy Guide to exercises in Daily Living Skills. Slack, Thorofare, NJ, 1982.

Hunter, J, Schneider, M, Mackin, E, and Bell J (eds): Rehabilitation of the Hand: Surgery and Treatment, ed 3. CV Mosby, Philadelphia, 1990.

Hopkins, HL, and Smith, HD: Willard and Spackman's Occupational Therapy, ed 8, JB Lippincott, Philadelphia, 1993.

Jacobs, K, and Logigian, M: Functions of a Manager In Occupational Therapy. Slack, Thorofare, NJ, 1989.

Jaffe, EG, and Epstein, CF: Occupational Therapy Consultation: Theory Principles and Practice. Mosby Year Book, St. Louis, 1992.

Joint Commission on Accreditation of Healthcare Organizations: How to Prepare for a Survey: Physical Rehabilitation Services. Checklist Publication, Oakbrook, IL, 1992.

Kesselman-Turkel, J, and Peterson, F: Test Taking Strategies. Contemporary Books, Chicago, 1981.

Kielhofner, G: Conceptual Foundations of Occupational Therapy. FA Davis, Philadelphia, 1992.

Kisner, C, and Colby, LA: Therapeutic Exercise Foundations and Techniques, ed 2. FA Davis, Philadelphia, 1985.

Kovich, KM, and Bermann, DE (eds): Head Injury: A Guide to Functional Outcomes in Occupational Therapy. A Rehabilitation Institute of Chicago procedure manual. Aspen Publishers, Rockville, MD, 1988.

Kramer, P, and Hinojosa, J: Frames of Reference for Pediatric Occupational Therapy. Williams & Wilkins, Baltimore, 1993.

Lavine, E, and the American Occupational Therapy Association: Manual On Administration. Kendall/Hunt, Dubuque, IA, 1982.

Lewis, SC: Elder Care in Occupational Therapy. Slack, Thorofare, NJ, 1989.

Lorig, K, and Fries, JF: The Arthritis Helpbook: A Tested Self-Management Program for Coping with Arthritis and Fibromyalgia, ed 4. Addison-Wesley, Reading, MA, 1995.

Mattingly, C, and Fleming, MH: Clinical Reasoning: Forms of Inquiry in a Therapeutic Practice. FA Davis, Philadelphia, 1994.

McFadden, S, and Woolridge, E: Certification. OT Week: Today's Student. The American Occupational Therapy Association, Rockville, MD, 1994.

Mosey, AC: Psychosocial Components of Occupational Therapy. Raven Press, New York, 1986.

National Safety Council: Bloodborn Pathogens. Jones and Bartlett, London, 1993.

Norkin, CC, and Levangie, PK: Joint Structure and Function: A Comprehensive Analysis, ed 2. FA Davis, Philadelphia, 1992.

Norkin, CC, and White, DJ: Measurement of Motion: A Guide to Goniometry, ed 2. FA Davis, Philadelphia, 1995.

Novak, ES: Improving payment for occupational therapists in mental health through effective documentation strategies. Proceedings–Acute care psychiatry: Practical strategies and collaborative approaches. American Occupational Therapy Association, Rockville, MD, 1988.

O'Sullivan, SB, and Schmitz, TJ: Physical Rehabilitation: Assessment and Treatment, ed 3. FA Davis, Philadelphia, 1994.

Palmer, ML, and Toms, JE: Manual for Functional Training, ed 3. FA Davis, Philadelphia, 1992.

Pedretti, L: Occupational Therapy; Practice Skills for Physical Dysfunction, ed 4, Mosby-Yearbook, St. Louis, 1996.

Polimeni-Walker, I, Wilson, KG, and Jewers, R: Reasons for participating in occupational therapy groups: Perceptions of adult psychiatric inpatients and occupational therapists. Canadian Journal of Occupational Therapy, 59:241–247, 1992.

Posthuma, BW: Small Groups in Counseling Therapy: Process and Leadership, ed 2. Allyn and Bacon, Needham Heights, MA, 1996.

Punwar, AJ: Occupational Therapy Principles and Practice, ed 2. Williams and Wilkins, Baltimore, 1994.

Schneinberg, LC (ed): Multiple Sclerosis: A Guide for Patients and Their Families. Raven Press, New York, 1983.

Reed, KL: Quick Reference to Occupational Therapy. Aspen Publications, Rockville, MD 1991.

Reed, KL, and Sanderson, SN: Concepts of Occupational Therapy, ed 3. Williams & Wilkins, Baltimore, 1992.

Rose, SM, Peabody, CG, and Stratigeas, B: Undetected abuse among intensive case management clients. Hosp Community Psychiatry, 42:499–503, 1991.

Rothstein, JM, Roy, SH, and Wolf, SL: The Rehabilitation Specialist's Handbook. FA Davis, Philadelphia, 1991.

Roy, S, and Irvin, R: Sports Medicine—Prevention Evaluation, Management and Rehabilitation. Prentice-Hall, Englewood Cliffs, NJ, 1983.

Rules and Regulations. Federal Register. August 24, 1987; 52: 163.

Sederer, LI (ed): Inpatient Psychiatry: Diagnosis and Treatment, ed 2. Williams & Wilkins, Baltimore, 1986.

Taylor, E: Anger Intervention. Am J Occup Ther, 42:147–155, 1989.

Thomas, CL (ed): Taber's Cyclopedic Medical Dictionary, ed 17. FA Davis, Philadelphia, 1993.

Trace, A, and Howell, T: Occupational therapy in geriatric mental health. Am J Occup Ther, 45:833–938, 1991.

Trombly, CA (ed): Occupational Therapy for Physical Dysfunction, ed 4. Williams & Wilkins, Baltimore, 1995.

Wilson, DJ, McKenzie, M, and Barber, LM: Spinal Cord Injury. Slack, Thorofare, NJ, 1974.

Zoltan, B, Siev, E, and Freishtat, B: The Adult Stroke Patient, ed 2 rev. Slack, Thorofare, NJ, 1986.